Frontiers in Cardiovascular Drug Discovery

(Volume 4)

Edited by

Atta-ur-Rahman, *FRS*

Honorary Life Fellow,
Kings College, University of Cambridge, Cambridge, UK

&

M. Iqbal Choudhary

H.E.J. Research Institute of Chemistry, International Center for Chemical
and Biological Sciences, University of Karachi, Karachi, Pakistan

Frontiers in Cardiovascular Drug Discovery

Volume # 4

Editors: Prof. Atta-ur-Rahman and Prof. M. Iqbal Choudhary

ISSN (Online): 1879-6648

ISSN (Print): 2452-3267

ISBN (Online): 978-1-68108-399-5

ISBN (Print): 978-1-68108-400-8

need for a court order if at any point you breach any terms of this License Agreement. In no event will any delay or failure by Bentham Science Publishers in enforcing your compliance with this License Agreement constitute a waiver of any of its rights.

3. You acknowledge that you have read this License Agreement, and agree to be bound by its terms and conditions. To the extent that any other terms and conditions presented on any website of Bentham Science Publishers conflict with, or are inconsistent with, the terms and conditions set out in this License Agreement, you acknowledge that the terms and conditions set out in this License Agreement shall prevail.

Bentham Science Publishers Ltd.
Executive Suite Y - 2
PO Box 7917, Saif Zone
Sharjah, U.A.E.
Email: subscriptions@benthamscience.net

BENTHAM SCIENCE

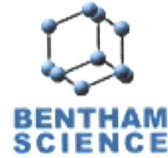

CONTENTS

Amparo Hernándiz, José Luis Díez, Antonio Moscardó, Ana Latorre, Maria Dolores Domenech, Maria Teresa Santos and Juana Vallés

Sule Apikoglu-Rabus, Murat B. Rabus and Rashida Muhammad Umar

PREFACE

Cardiovascular diseases (CVDs) are among the leading causes of mortality and morbidity. In several regions of the world, CVDs have reached to epidemic proportions. Despite high prevalence, the some of the causes and risks of CVDs are still far from clear. The 4th volume of book series, "*Frontiers in Cardiovascular Drug Discovery*", is an excellent compilation of five reviews contributed by the leading authorities in the selected fields.

Norgard *et al*. present a comprehensive review on the pattern and optimum doses of the wonder drug "aspirin" for CVDs prevention. With an excellent background of mechanism of action of aspirin, the authors have concluded that with the accelerated platelet turnover, the frequency of consumption of aspirin is more important than its dose. Nayeem *et al*. have contributed a comprehensive review on the physiological and pathological role of adenosine, particularly in the cardiovascular system. As a result , various adenosine receptors were identified as targets in the development of drugs against cardiovascular diseases. They have reviewed the clinical potential of various adenosine receptor ligands, and their potential as CVD drugs. Merits and demerits of dual anti-platelet therapy (DAPT) with aspirin (ASA) and clopidogrel in patients after cardiovascular interventions (bioactive stenting or everolimus-coated stenting) are reviewed by Hernandiz *et al*. The review by Apikoglu-Rabus *et al*. focuses on the role of immunosuppressant drugs after heart transplant to prevent hyperacute and acute rejections. They have also discussed the complications associated with the induction and maintenance of common immunosuppressive regimens. Morales-Villegas and Rays have contributed an excellent review on the inhibition of PCSK9 by MAb-PCSK9 (Evolocumab) antibody, as an approach to reduce atherosclerotic burden, and cardiovascular diseases. PCSK9 is a protease enzyme which catalyzes LDLR proteolysis, and plays an important role in increasing the intracellular concentration of cholesterol. The results of clinical studies on evolocumab and its derivatives in the treatment of hypercholesterolemia are presented.

We are graceful to Mr. Mahmood Alam (Director Publications), Ms. Mariam Mehdi (Assistant Manager Publications), and other members of Bentham Science Publishers for excellent coordination with the authors, and timely compilation of the 4th volume of this book series.

Prof. Dr. Atta-ur-Rahman, FRS
Honorary Life Fellow,
Kings College,
University of Cambridge,
Cambridge
UK

&

Prof. Dr. M. Iqbal Choudhary
H.E.J. Research Institute of Chemistry,
International Center for Chemical and Biological Sciences,
University of Karachi,
Pakistan

List of Contributors

Antonio Moscardó	Hemostasis, Thrombosis, Atherosclerosis, and Vascular Biology Unit, Health Research Institute La Fe, Valencia, Spain
Ana Latorre	Hemostasis, Thrombosis, Atherosclerosis, and Vascular Biology Unit, Health Research Institute La Fe, Valencia, Spain
Amparo Hernándiz	Cardiology Research Unit, Health Research Institute La fe, Torre A lab 5.04 Avda. Fernando Abril Martorell nº 106, 46026 Valencia, Spain
Ahmad Hanif	Department of Pharmaceutical Sciences, West Virginia University, School of Pharmacy, São Bernardo do Campo, Morgantown, USA
Enrique C. Morales-Villegas	Cardiometabolic Research Center, Aguascalientes, Mexico
José Luis Díez	Department of Cardiology, University and Polytechnic Hospital La Fe, Valencia, Spain
Juana Vallés	Hemostasis, Thrombosis, Atherosclerosis, and Vascular Biology Unit, Health Research Institute La Fe, Valencia, Spain
Jonathon R. Enriquez	School of Medicine, University of Missouri, Kansas City, USA
Kausik K. Ray	Department of Biophysics, Imperial Centre for Cardiovascular Disease Prevention, London, UK
Maan T. Khayat	Department of Pharmaceutical Sciences, West Virginia University, School of Pharmacy, São Bernardo do Campo, Morgantown, USA Department of Pharmaceutical Chemistry, King Abdulaziz University, School of Pharmacy, São Bernardo do Campo, Jeddah, Saudi Arabia
Maria Dolores Domenech	Cardiology Department Dr Peset Aleixandre Hospital, Valencia, Spain
Maria Teresa Santos	Hemostasis, Thrombosis, Atherosclerosis, and Vascular Biology Unit, Health Research Institute La Fe, Valencia, Spain
Mohammed A. Nayeem	Department of Pharmaceutical Sciences, West Virginia University, School of Pharmacy, São Bernardo do Campo, Morgantown, USA
Murat B. Rabus	Cardiovascular Surgery Department, Kartal Kosuyolu Higher Specialization Training and Research Hospital, Istanbul, Turkey
Nicholas B. Norgard	Kansas City School of Medicine, University of Missouri, M4-325, 2411 Holmes St, Kansas City, USA
Priya Jain	School of Medicine, University of Missouri, Kansas City, USA
Rashida Muhammad Umar	Clinical Pharmacy Department, Marmara University Faculty of Pharmacy, Istanbul, Turkey
Sule Apikoglu-Rabus	Clinical Pharmacy Department, Marmara University Faculty of Pharmacy, Istanbul, Turkey
Werner J. Geldenhuys	Department of Pharmaceutical Sciences, West Virginia University, School of Pharmacy, São Bernardo do Campo, Morgantown, USA

CHAPTER 1

Should the Argument About Aspirin Dosing be About Frequency Rather the Dose?

Nicholas B. Norgard[1,*], **Priya Jain**[2] and **Jonathon R. Enriquez**[2]

[1] *Kansas City School of Medicine, University of Missouri, M4-325, 2411 Holmes St, Kansas City, MO, USA*

[2] *School of Medicine, University of Missouri-Kansas City, USA*

Abstract: Aspirin is known to have inter-individual variability in its pharmacodynamic response. Clinical investigators continue their empirical search for the optimum aspirin dose to safely prevent athero-thrombosis. Several patient populations have an accompanied accelerated platelet turnover that is associated with a time-dependent loss of aspirin efficacy. Increasing the dosing frequency has been shown to elicit better and more sustained platelet inhibition compared to a dose increase in these patient populations. This review explores the role of accelerated platelet turnover in aspirin pharmacodynamics and the benefits of multiple daily aspirin dosing.

Keywords: Antiplatelet, Aspirin, Essential Thrombocythemia, High On-Aspirin Platelet Reactivity, Platelet Turnover.

INTRODUCTION

Daily low-dose aspirin therapy is strongly recommended for all patients with established cardiovascular (CV) disease and for primary prevention of atherothrombotic disease in high-risk patients. Notwithstanding, clinical investigators continue their empirical search for the optimum aspirin dose to safely prevent thrombogenesis [1]. Aspirin doses ranging from 75 to 325 mg have become standard of care. There are differences of opinion on whether daily doses from 75-100 mg or 300-325 mg are more appropriate [1]. Thus, wide variations in aspirin-dosing have been seen in national registries analyzing practice patterns for treatment of patients with cardiovascular disease [2].

Numerous studies have shown inter-individual variability in the pharmacodynamic response to aspirin therapy [3 - 13]. It has been estimated that up to

* **Corresponding author Nicholas B. Norgard:** the Kansas City School of Medicine, University of Missouri, M4-325, 2411 Holmes St, Kansas City, MO, USA; Tel: 816-235-1911; E-mail: norgardn@umkc.edu, ORCID ID: 0000-000--4612-0107

Atta-ur-Rahman & M. Iqbal Choudhary (Eds.)

45% of patients do not derive adequate platelet inhibition from aspirin, putting them at increased risk of myocardial infarction, stroke, and CV death [3 - 13]. Estimates of high on-aspirin platelet reactivity (HAPR) prevalence differ widely due to distinct drug doses, definitions, platelet function tests and time interval between aspirin dosing and measurements of platelet inhibition [8].

Higher aspirin doses (~325 mg/day) are often used in situations of observed HAPR or in patient populations (*e.g.* diabetes mellitus) known to be at greater risk of a poor aspirin pharmacodynamic effect [14]. Another aspirin dosing strategy that may be better suited to provide a more sustained antiplatelet effect is to increase dosing frequency rather than dose. This review explores the role of accelerated platelet turnover in aspirin pharmacodynamics and the benefits of multiple daily aspirin dosing.

ACCELERATED PLATELET TURNOVER

The key mechanism by which aspirin protects against atherothrombosis is the inhibition of thromboxane (TX) production *via* permanent inactivation of platelet cyclooxygenase (COX)-1 activity. This platelet inactivation occurs pre-systemically, in the portal blood, and is cumulative with repeated daily dosing [15]. Nearly complete suppression of platelet COX-1 activity is ensured by presystemic acetylation of the enzyme, however cumulative acetylation and the long-lasting duration of the aspirin effect is determined by the rate of platelet turnover [16]. After aspirin administration, recovery of platelet TX synthesis requires new platelets with functional COX-1 to be released from the bone marrow. Aspirin that does not bind to COX-1 remains in circulation for only a short time (~20 min). Following the elimination of unbound aspirin, new platelets released into circulation will not be exposed to aspirin and will have fully functional COX-1 activity and the capacity to convert arachidonic acid into TX. While it can take up to 10 days to restore the platelet population to full COX-1 activity, it only takes a very small portion of newly formed platelets with intact COX-1 activity to sustain a substantial platelet response [16]. Full suppression of TX-dependent platelet function requires >95% inhibition of COX-1 activity and even a modest recovery of this activity can normalize hemostasis [17]. Normal hemostasis can be achieved in the presence of as few as 20% unacetylated platelets with normal COX activity [18].

With the daily generation of 10-12% new platelets, near normal hemostasis can be recovered within 2-3 days after the last aspirin dose in patients with a typical rate of platelet turnover [19]. COX expression is positively correlated with platelet turnover, therefore the accelerated platelet turnover also restores COX levels at an accelerated rate [20, 21]. At a normal rate of thrombopoiesis, negligible amounts of unacetylated COX enzymes are resynthesized following an aspirin dose and a daily dose of aspirin is able to maintain 24-hour inhibition of COX-1–dependent TX production. When the platelet turnover rate is higher than normal, a more rapid renewal of COX-1 can limit the duration of the aspirin effect, leading to a partial recovery of TX-dependent platelet function during the 24-hour dosing interval [22 - 25]. This leads to an important question surrounding increased incidence of both myocardial infarction and stroke in the early morning hours, usually around 24 hours after most patients have taken their once-daily dose of aspirin [26, 27].

Quantification of the number and fraction of reticulated platelets can be used as a proxy for platelet turnover [28 - 30]. The number of circulating reticulated platelets reflects the rate of thrombopoiesis, increasing with increased synthesis and decreasing with decreased production [29]. Reticulated platelets are large, immature platelets that are both metabolically and enzymatically more active than mature platelets and have a greater prothrombotic potential [31]. These mRNA-containing platelets, in contrast to more mature, anucleate platelets, are capable of producing membrane and secretory proteins. This includes COX-2, a contributor to TX production that is not inhibited by low-dose aspirin [32, 33]. High levels of reticulated platelets are associated with increased markers of platelet reactivity, increased TX production, and have been shown to be a powerful independent predictor of impaired platelet responses to several antiplatelet drugs including aspirin [34 - 37].

ASPIRIN PHARMACODYNAMICS IN ESSENTIAL THROMBO-CYTHEMIA

The time-dependent loss of aspirin efficacy seen in essential thrombocythemia (ET) provides a practical link between accelerated platelet turnover and aspirin pharmacodynamics. Aspirin is a recommended treatment for ET, a myeloproliferative neoplasm characterized by enhanced platelet generation and high arterial thrombotic complications [38]. This patient population has a high prevalence of HAPR (~80%) while on daily aspirin therapy [39 - 41]. The altered megakaryopoiesis associated with ET leads to a faster release of immature platelets from the bone marrow, an augmented renewal of COX, and the recovery of TX-dependent platelet function [39, 41]. It also leads to an incomplete response to a conventional regimen of once-daily aspirin administration, in particular between 12 and 24 hours after dosing [39 - 41].

Larger doses of aspirin extend the duration of the antiplatelet response in ET patients but are unable to cause complete TXA2 suppression throughout the 24-hour dosing interval [41, 42]. An elevated dose increases aspirin bioavailability and the amount of aspirin that makes it to the systemic circulation [43]. This causes more acetylation of megakaryocyte COX-1, thereby inhibiting TXA2 production in some of the newly released platelets as well as those already in the circulation [44, 45]. However, this strategy does not overcome the high rate of COX renewal, given the short half-life of aspirin. In contrast, shortening the dosing interval to 12 hours addresses the time-dependent loss of aspirin efficacy. After an initial dose, a second aspirin dose 12 hours later acetylates the newly formed COX from rapidly proliferating megakaryocytes and produces a more sustained inhibition of TX production over a 24-hour period [39, 41, 42].

HIGH PLATELET TURNOVER STATES

Like ET, other disease states associated with accelerated platelet turnover experience a similar time-dependent recovery of TX-dependent platelet function during the 24-hour dosing interval. Diabetes mellitus (DM), obesity, hemodialysis, ischemic stroke, coronary artery disease (CAD), and coronary bypass surgery are marked by a high risk of atherothrombotic complications and have been associated with a higher than normal rate of entry of platelets into the circulation, likely as a consequence of higher than normal platelet consumption [34, 46 - 50]. In these patient populations, an elevated rate of platelet turnover is a predictor of poor thrombotic outcome and has been linked with residual platelet reactivity while taking a conventional regimen of daily low-dose aspirin [34, 46 - 54].

Diabetes Mellitus

Patients with DM have a higher prevalence of HAPR compared to nondiabetics [14, 55]. The rate of platelet turnover has also been found to be higher is diabetics compared to nondiabetics, related to DM-associated oxidative stress and inflammation, and can generate pharmacodynamic variability in aspirin response [56, 57]. Among patients with DM, the recovery rate of platelet COX-1 twelve to 24 hours after aspirin administration was found to be the main mechanism contributing to the interindividual variability in aspirin response [22]. Accelerated renewal of platelet COX-1 also altered aspirin pharmacodynamics in patients without DM. In this population, elevated body weight was the major determinant of more rapid recovery of the drug target and provides a mechanistic explanation for the high rate of HAPR seen in obesity [22].

To counter HAPR, higher doses of aspirin may augment the antiplatelet effect but only a twice daily aspirin regimen is able to demonstrate complete reversal of the accelerated recovery of platelet COX-1 [14, 22, 58]. Several different studies have consistently reported a greater and more sustained inhibition of platelet function and/or platelet TX production by twice daily *vs.* once daily dosing in DM

(Table **1**) [22, 59 - 63].

Coronary Artery Disease

Patients with CAD have a higher rate of platelet turnover compared to healthy subjects [36, 64]. The platelet turnover rate is highest during acute coronary syndromes and is a predictor of poor thrombotic outcome after coronary intervention [50, 54, 65 - 67]. CAD patients with a high platelet turnover have a reduced antiplatelet effect of once-daily aspirin [34, 68, 69]. These patients exhibit a time-dependent loss of aspirin efficacy over a 24 hour period similar to ET and DM [69 - 72]. Twice-daily aspirin regimens, not higher aspirin doses, were more effective at providing sustained TX and platelet function suppression (Table **1**) [22, 59 - 63]. These studies were done in CAD patients who also had DM. The pharmacodynamic benefit of twice-daily aspirin dosing would be expected in CAD patients without DM given the time-dependent loss of aspirin efficacy shown in this population. However, confirmatory studies are needed.

Table 1. Prior Studies of Multiple Day Aspirin Dosing.

Authors	Patient Population	Dose Comparisons	Study Conclusion
Bethel MA, *et al.* 2016 [62];	DM n = 24	100 mg once daily *vs.* 200 mg once daily *vs.* 100 mg twice daily	Aspirin 100 mg twice daily, but not 200 mg daily, was more effective than aspirin 100 mg daily
Rocca B, *et al.* 2012 [22];	DM n = 100	100 mg once daily *vs.* 200 mg once daily *vs.* 100 mg twice daily	Aspirin 100 mg twice daily was only regimen to completely reverse abnormal TX recovery
Spectre G, *et al.* 2011 [59];	DM n = 25	75 mg once daily *vs.* 75 mg twice daily *vs.* 320 mg once daily	Twice-daily aspirin dosing improved laboratory responses to aspirin compared to once daily dosing
Addad F, *et al.* 2010 [60];	DM, Coronary artery disease n = 25	100 mg daily *vs.* 100 mg twice daily	100 mg aspirin twice-daily dosing rather than a once-daily dose significantly improved the aspirin effect
Capodanno D, *et al.* 2011 [61];	DM, Coronary artery disease n = 20	81 mg daily *vs.* 81 mg twice daily *vs.* 162 mg daily *vs.* 162 mg twice daily *vs.* 325 mg daily	Twice-daily low-dose aspirin administration was associated with greater platelet inhibition than a once-daily administration
Dillinger JG, *et al.* 2010 [63];	DM, Coronary artery disease n = 92	150 mg daily *vs.* 75 mg twice daily	Twice daily aspirin was more effective at suppressing platelet reactivity at 24 hours

(Table 1) cont.....

Authors	Patient Population	Dose Comparisons	Study Conclusion
Cavlaca V, *et al.* 2017 [74];	Coronary artery bypass grafting surgery n = 37	100 mg once-daily *vs.* 100 mg twice-daily *vs.* 200 mg once-daily	Twice daily aspirin, but not a double once-daily dose, rescued the impaired antiplatelet effect of low-dose aspirin
Paikin JS, *et al.* 2015 [76];	Coronary artery bypass grafting surgery n = 68	81 mg once-daily *vs.* 325 mg once-daily *vs.* 162 mg twice-daily	Multiple daily dosing of ASA was more effective than ASA 81 mg once-daily or 325 mg once-daily at suppressing serum TXB2 formation after CABG surgery
Paikin JS, *et al.* 2017 [77];	Coronary artery bypass grafting surgery n = 110	81 mg once-daily *vs.* 325 mg once-daily *vs.* 81 mg four-times daily	Aspirin given four times daily was more effective than once-daily dosing at suppressing serum TX formation and platelet aggregation

Coronary Artery Bypass Surgery

Coronary artery bypass graft (CABG) surgery is associated with an increase in platelet turnover rate corresponding with systemic inflammation in the early post-operative period [73, 74]. The accelerated rate of platelet turnover is thought to lead to a transient impairment of aspirin pharmacodynamic response and is a proposed mechanism for early graft failure [73, 75]. A once-daily aspirin dose has been found to incompletely inhibit serum TX production during the first week after CABG surgery [76]. Only multiple daily aspirin doses were able to overcome HAPR and completely suppresses TX formation over 24 hours [74, 76, 77]. While low-dose aspirin has become the standard for long-term therapy in patients with CAD, clinical practice guidelines from the American Heart Association and American College of Cardiology for treatment of patients after CABG recommend treatment with higher dose aspirin (162-325mg daily) for graft patency, which further underpins potential benefit of exploration of variation in aspirin frequency as a mechanism for accomplishing the same goal [78].

End Stage Renal Disease

Patients on chronic hemodialysis or peritoneal dialysis were found to have an accelerated platelet turnover compared to healthy subjects and may contribute to the platelet dysfunction and HAPR in these patients [79]. An increase in platelet turnover was associated with a reduced pharmacodynamic effect of aspirin [80]. The rate of platelet turnover is increased in renal transplant patients and is a proposed mechanism for associated CV risk [81, 82]. Multiple daily aspirin dosing studies have not been performed in this population.

Ischemic Stroke

Platelet turnover is elevated in patients with ischemic stroke as a consequence of platelet consumption during thrombogenesis [48]. HAPR is prevalent in patients presenting with acute ischemic stroke [83, 84]. A signal that platelet turnover plays a role in aspirin pharmacodynamics is that the platelet response to aspirin is reduced in the early phase of ischemic stroke when inflammation and platelet turnover are highest, but aspirin begins to have a greater effect on platelet function as healing begins and inflammation decreases [85]. Multiple daily aspirin dosing studies have not been performed in this population.

DISCUSSION

The optimal dose of aspirin is still not fully defined from large, randomized, controlled trials (1). Clinical evidence has failed to show a dose-response relationship for the efficacy of aspirin as high dose (300 to 325 mg daily) showed no differences in CV end points at 30 days versus low dose (75 to 100 mg daily) in patients with a recent acute coronary syndrome [86]. As the dose of aspirin increases there is greater inhibition of COX-2 with resultant decreases in prostaglandin I2 production, which may offset aspirin's ischemic benefit [87]. The risk of adverse effects, specifically gastrointestinal bleeding, also escalates and as the dose of aspirin increases [88 - 90]. Evidence supports the use of aspirin doses that maximize efficacy and minimize toxicity.

It is conceivable that in clinical settings of accelerated platelet turnover, the rapid renewal rate of COX-1 during the 24-hour aspirin dosing interval accounts for a partial recovery of TXA2-dependent platelet function and represents a major mechanism contributing to the interindividual variability in aspirin's pharmacodynamic response. This provides an explanation for the significantly improved and sustained aspirin effect consistently observed with twice daily dosing compared to once-daily dosing. Another dosing strategy that may improve the pharmacodynamic profile is moving the timing of administration a daily dose from morning to bedtime rather than adding an additional dose [91]. A bedtime dose may be more appropriate for the body's circadian rhythm and can more effectively attenuate morning platelet reactivity. The presence of a bedtime dose in a twice-daily dosing strategy may also be an explanation for improved the pharmacodynamics.

While twice daily aspirin dosing provides a more optimal pharmacodynamic profile, it is difficult to fully assess the effectiveness of this strategy based on pharmacodynamic studies alone. Pharmacodynamic testing of aspirin response is fraught with limitations. A multitude of tests are currently available to assess inhibition of platelet function induced by aspirin and their methodologies are diverse. Many studies test platelet function during a single time point during the day and may not accurately portray the diurnal changes that may be seen from new platelet development after aspirin administration [70]. Conclusions drawn in these studies are highly dependent on the test used and results from various assays are not interchangeable [92]. The true value of increasing aspirin dosing frequency needs to be established in large randomized clinical studies in CV patients, both with and without DM.

Limitations

While benefits may vary with aspirin dosing, potential risks, specifically bleeding risk may also vary across dosing frequency of aspirin therapy. Prior analyses have demonstrated a dose-dependent relationship between aspirin dose and bleeding risk [93]. Further studies are needed to determine the net clinical benefit of aspirin dosing frequency balanced against potential bleeding risk.

Medication adherence also remains a continual challenge in clinical practice. As dosing frequency increases, an inverse relationship is seen resulting in worse compliance [94]. Thus, even if benefits of increased frequency of aspirin dosing would be noted, real world data would need to be assessed to see if this would translate into better outcomes when balanced against potentially lower adherence rates.

CONCLUSION

Heterogeneity in treatment benefits, risks, and outcomes often exists such that the same treatment may not affect every patient the same. It is possible that there may not be an ideal one-size fits all dose for aspirin across patients and disease states, and it is also possible that there may not be an ideal one-size fits all dosing frequency. Recognition of high platelet reactivity and its association with adverse events has received considerable attention in cardiovascular pharmacology; however, current trends in dealing with this problem have been primarily to develop newer and more expensive anti-platelet agents, including prasugrel, ticagrelor, cangrelor, leading to trends in higher healthcare costs and disparities in care between those who can afford versus not afford these treatments. One of the newest antiplatelet agents, cangrelor, has an estimated cost of over $700 per dose. Aspirin is one of the most widely available and most affordable medications in modern medicine. It is incredible that simpler and exceedingly more cost-effective strategies like variations in aspirin dosing have not been explored further as potential strategies to improve outcomes across many disease states.

CONSENT FOR PUBLICATION

Not applicable.

CONFLICT OF INTEREST

The author declares no conflict of interest, financial or otherwise.

ACKNOWLEDGEMENTS

Declared none.

REFERENCES

[1]   DiNicolantonio JJ, Norgard NB, Meier P, *et al.* Optimal aspirin dose in acute coronary syndromes: an emerging consensus. Future Cardiol 2014; 10(2): 291-300.
        [http://dx.doi.org/10.2217/fca.14.7] [PMID: 24762255]

[2]   Hall HM, de Lemos JA, Enriquez JR, *et al.* Contemporary patterns of discharge aspirin dosing after acute myocardial infarction in the United States: results from the National Cardiovascular Data Registry (NCDR). Circ Cardiovasc Qual Outcomes 2014; 7(5): 701-7.
        [http://dx.doi.org/10.1161/CIRCOUTCOMES.113.000822] [PMID: 25116897]

[3]   Gum PA, Kottke-Marchant K, Poggio ED, *et al.* Profile and prevalence of aspirin resistance in patients with cardiovascular disease. Am J Cardiol 2001; 88(3): 230-5.
        [http://dx.doi.org/10.1016/S0002-9149(01)01631-9] [PMID: 11472699]

[4]   Eikelboom JW, Hirsh J, Weitz JI, Johnston M, Yi Q, Yusuf S. Aspirin-resistant thromboxane biosynthesis and the risk of myocardial infarction, stroke, or cardiovascular death in patients at high risk for cardiovascular events. Circulation 2002; 105(14): 1650-5.
        [http://dx.doi.org/10.1161/01.CIR.0000013777.21160.07] [PMID: 11940542]

[5]   Maree AO, Curtin RJ, Dooley M, *et al.* Platelet response to low-dose enteric-coated aspirin in patients with stable cardiovascular disease. J Am Coll Cardiol 2005; 46(7): 1258-63.
        [http://dx.doi.org/10.1016/j.jacc.2005.06.058] [PMID: 16198840]

[6]   Ohmori T, Yatomi Y, Nonaka T, *et al.* Aspirin resistance detected with aggregometry cannot be explained by cyclooxygenase activity: involvement of other signaling pathway(s) in cardiovascular events of aspirin-treated patients. J Thromb Haemost 2006; 4(6): 1271-8.
        [http://dx.doi.org/10.1111/j.1538-7836.2006.01958.x] [PMID: 16706971]

[7]   Chen W-H, Cheng X, Lee P-Y, *et al.* Aspirin resistance and adverse clinical events in patients with coronary artery disease. Am J Med 2007; 120(7): 631-5.
        [http://dx.doi.org/10.1016/j.amjmed.2006.10.021] [PMID: 17602938]

[8]   Hovens MMC, Snoep JD, Eikenboom JCJ, van der Bom JG, Mertens BJA, Huisman MV. Prevalence of persistent platelet reactivity despite use of aspirin: a systematic review. Am Heart J 2007; 153(2): 175-81.
        [http://dx.doi.org/10.1016/j.ahj.2006.10.040] [PMID: 17239674]

[9]   Snoep JD, Hovens MM, Eikenboom JC, van der Bom JG, Huisman MV. Association of laboratory-defined aspirin resistance with a higher risk of recurrent cardiovascular events: a systematic review and meta-analysis. Arch Intern Med 2007; 167(15): 1593-9.
        [http://dx.doi.org/10.1001/archinte.167.15.1593] [PMID: 17698681]

[10]   Krasopoulos G, Brister SJ, Beattie WS, Buchanan MR. Aspirin "resistance" and risk of cardiovascular morbidity: systematic review and meta-analysis. BMJ 2008; 336(7637): 195-8.
        [http://dx.doi.org/10.1136/bmj.39430.529549.BE] [PMID: 18202034]

[11]   Sofi F, Marcucci R, Gori AM, Abbate R, Gensini GF. Residual platelet reactivity on aspirin therapy and recurrent cardiovascular events--a meta-analysis. Int J Cardiol 2008; 128(2): 166-71.
[http://dx.doi.org/10.1016/j.ijcard.2007.12.010] [PMID: 18242733]

[12]   Frelinger AL III, Li Y, Linden MD, *et al.* Association of cyclooxygenase-1-dependent and -independent platelet function assays with adverse clinical outcomes in aspirin-treated patients presenting for cardiac catheterization. Circulation 2009; 120(25): 2586-96.
[http://dx.doi.org/10.1161/CIRCULATIONAHA.109.900589] [PMID: 19996015]

[13]   Pettersen A-ÅR, Seljeflot I, Abdelnoor M, Arnesen H. High On-Aspirin Platelet Reactivity and Clinical Outcome in Patients With Stable Coronary Artery Disease: Results From ASCET (Aspirin Nonresponsiveness and Clopidogrel Endpoint Trial). J Am Heart Assoc 2012; 1(3): e000703.
[http://dx.doi.org/10.1161/JAHA.112.000703] [PMID: 23130135]

[14]   DiChiara J, Bliden KP, Tantry US, *et al.* The effect of aspirin dosing on platelet function in diabetic and nondiabetic patients: an analysis from the aspirin-induced platelet effect (ASPECT) study. Diabetes 2007; 56(12): 3014-9.
[http://dx.doi.org/10.2337/db07-0707] [PMID: 17848625]

[15]   Patrignani P, Filabozzi P, Patrono C. Selective cumulative inhibition of platelet thromboxane production by low-dose aspirin in healthy subjects. J Clin Invest 1982; 69(6): 1366-72.
[http://dx.doi.org/10.1172/JCI110576] [PMID: 7045161]

[16]   Patrono C, Ciabattoni G, Patrignani P, *et al.* Clinical pharmacology of platelet cyclooxygenase inhibition. Circulation 1985; 72(6): 1177-84.
[http://dx.doi.org/10.1161/01.CIR.72.6.1177] [PMID: 3933848]

[17]   Santilli F, Rocca B, De Cristofaro R, *et al.* Platelet cyclooxygenase inhibition by low-dose aspirin is not reflected consistently by platelet function assays: implications for aspirin "resistance". J Am Coll Cardiol 2009; 53(8): 667-77.
[http://dx.doi.org/10.1016/j.jacc.2008.10.047] [PMID: 19232899]

[18]   Altman R, Luciardi HL, Muntaner J, Herrera RN. The antithrombotic profile of aspirin. Aspirin resistance, or simply failure? Thromb J 2004; 2(1): 1.
[http://dx.doi.org/10.1186/1477-9560-2-1] [PMID: 14723795]

[19]   Awtry EH, Loscalzo J. Aspirin. Circulation 2000; 101(10): 1206-18.
[http://dx.doi.org/10.1161/01.CIR.101.10.1206] [PMID: 10715270]

[20]   Rubak P, Kristensen SD, Hvas AM. Flow cytometric analysis of platelet cyclooxygenase-1 and -2 and surface glycoproteins in patients with immune thrombocytopenia and healthy individuals. Platelets 2017; 28(4): 387-93.
[http://dx.doi.org/10.1080/09537104.2016.1224829] [PMID: 27715371]

[21]   Dragani A, Pascale S, Recchiuti A, *et al.* The contribution of cyclooxygenase-1 and -2 to persistent thromboxane biosynthesis in aspirin-treated essential thrombocythemia: implications for antiplatelet therapy. Blood 2010; 115(5): 1054-61.
[http://dx.doi.org/10.1182/blood-2009-08-236679] [PMID: 19887674]

[22]   Rocca B, Santilli F, Pitocco D, *et al.* The recovery of platelet cyclooxygenase activity explains interindividual variability in responsiveness to low-dose aspirin in patients with and without diabetes. J Thromb Haemost 2012; 10(7): 1220-30.
[http://dx.doi.org/10.1111/j.1538-7836.2012.04723.x] [PMID: 22471290]

[23]   Rocca B, Dragani A, Pagliaccia F. Identifying determinants of variability to tailor aspirin therapy. Expert Rev Cardiovasc Ther 2013; 11(3): 365-79.
[http://dx.doi.org/10.1586/erc.12.144] [PMID: 23469916]

[24]   Armstrong PC, Hoefer T, Knowles RB, *et al.* Newly Formed Reticulated Platelets Undermine Pharmacokinetically Short-Lived Antiplatelet Therapies. Arterioscler Thromb Vasc Biol 2017; 37(5): 949-56.

[http://dx.doi.org/10.1161/ATVBAHA.116.308763] [PMID: 28279968]

[25]   Freynhofer MK, Gruber SC, Grove EL, Weiss TW, Wojta J, Huber K. Antiplatelet drugs in patients with enhanced platelet turnover: biomarkers versus platelet function testing. Thromb Haemost 2015; 114(3): 459-68.
[PMID: 26272640]

[26]   Willich SN, Linderer T, Wegscheider K, Leizorovicz A, Alamercery I, Schröder R. ISAM Study Group. Increased morning incidence of myocardial infarction in the ISAM Study: absence with prior beta-adrenergic blockade. Circulation 1989; 80(4): 853-8.
[http://dx.doi.org/10.1161/01.CIR.80.4.853] [PMID: 2571430]

[27]   Marler JR, Price TR, Clark GL, *et al.* Morning increase in onset of ischemic stroke. Stroke 1989; 20(4): 473-6.
[http://dx.doi.org/10.1161/01.STR.20.4.473] [PMID: 2648651]

[28]   Harrison P, Robinson MS, Mackie IJ, Machin SJ. Reticulated platelets. Platelets 1997; 8(6): 379-83.
[http://dx.doi.org/10.1080/09537109777050] [PMID: 16793671]

[29]   Freitas LG, Carvalho Md, Dusse LM. Reticulated platelets: how to assess them? Clin Chim Acta 2013; 422: 40-1.
[http://dx.doi.org/10.1016/j.cca.2013.04.008] [PMID: 23588062]

[30]   Ault KA, Knowles C. *In vivo* biotinylation demonstrates that reticulated platelets are the youngest platelets in circulation. Exp Hematol 1995; 23(9): 996-1001.
[PMID: 7635185]

[31]   Dusse LM, Freitas LG. Clinical applicability of reticulated platelets. Clin Chim Acta 2015; 439: 143-7.
[http://dx.doi.org/10.1016/j.cca.2014.10.024] [PMID: 25451948]

[32]   Weber AA, Zimmermann KC, Meyer-Kirchrath J, Schrör K. Cyclooxygenase-2 in human platelets as a possible factor in aspirin resistance. Lancet 1999; 353(9156): 900.
[http://dx.doi.org/10.1016/S0140-6736(99)00498-5] [PMID: 10093990]

[33]   Rocca B, Secchiero P, Ciabattoni G, *et al.* Cyclooxygenase-2 expression is induced during human megakaryopoiesis and characterizes newly formed platelets. Proc Natl Acad Sci USA 2002; 99(11): 7634-9.
[http://dx.doi.org/10.1073/pnas.112202999] [PMID: 12032335]

[34]   Grove EL, Hvas AM, Mortensen SB, Larsen SB, Kristensen SD. Effect of platelet turnover on whole blood platelet aggregation in patients with coronary artery disease. J Thromb Haemost 2011; 9(1): 185-91.
[http://dx.doi.org/10.1111/j.1538-7836.2010.04115.x] [PMID: 20955349]

[35]   Perl L, Lerman-Shivek H, Rechavia E, *et al.* Response to prasugrel and levels of circulating reticulated platelets in patients with ST-segment elevation myocardial infarction. J Am Coll Cardiol 2014; 63(6): 513-7.
[http://dx.doi.org/10.1016/j.jacc.2013.07.110] [PMID: 24148715]

[36]   Cesari F, Marcucci R, Caporale R, *et al.* Relationship between high platelet turnover and platelet function in high-risk patients with coronary artery disease on dual antiplatelet therapy. Thromb Haemost 2008; 99(5): 930-5.
[PMID: 18449424]

[37]   Stratz C, Bömicke T, Younas I, *et al.* Comparison of Immature Platelet Count to Established Predictors of Platelet Reactivity During Thienopyridine Therapy. J Am Coll Cardiol 2016; 68(3): 286-93.
[http://dx.doi.org/10.1016/j.jacc.2016.04.056] [PMID: 27417007]

[38]   Tefferi A, Vainchenker W. Myeloproliferative neoplasms: molecular pathophysiology, essential clinical understanding, and treatment strategies. J Clin Oncol 2011; 29(5): 573-82.
[http://dx.doi.org/10.1200/JCO.2010.29.8711] [PMID: 21220604]

[39]   Dragani A, Pascale S, Recchiuti A, *et al.* The contribution of cyclooxygenase-1 and -2 to persistent thromboxane biosynthesis in aspirin-treated essential thrombocythemia: implications for antiplatelet therapy. Blood 2010; 115(5): 1054-61.
[http://dx.doi.org/10.1182/blood-2009-08-236679] [PMID: 19887674]

[40]   Dillinger JG, Sideris G, Henry P, Bal dit Sollier C, Ronez E, Drouet L. Twice daily aspirin to improve biological aspirin efficacy in patients with essential thrombocythemia. Thromb Res 2012; 129(1): 91-4.
[http://dx.doi.org/10.1016/j.thromres.2011.09.017] [PMID: 22014557]

[41]   Pascale S, Petrucci G, Dragani A, *et al.* Aspirin-insensitive thromboxane biosynthesis in essential thrombocythemia is explained by accelerated renewal of the drug target. Blood 2012; 119(15): 3595-603.
[http://dx.doi.org/10.1182/blood-2011-06-359224] [PMID: 22234683]

[42]   Cavalca V, Rocca B, Squellerio I, *et al. In vivo* prostacyclin biosynthesis and effects of different aspirin regimens in patients with essential thrombocythaemia. Thromb Haemost 2014; 112(1): 118-27.
[PMID: 24671522]

[43]   Pedersen AK, FitzGerald GA. Dose-related kinetics of aspirin. Presystemic acetylation of platelet cyclooxygenase. N Engl J Med 1984; 311(19): 1206-11.
[http://dx.doi.org/10.1056/NEJM198411083111902] [PMID: 6436696]

[44]   Patrono C, Ciabattoni G, Pinca E, *et al.* Low dose aspirin and inhibition of thromboxane B2 production in healthy subjects. Thromb Res 1980; 17(3-4): 317-27.
[http://dx.doi.org/10.1016/0049-3848(80)90066-3] [PMID: 7368167]

[45]   Burch JW, Stanford N, Majerus PW. Inhibition of platelet prostaglandin synthetase by oral aspirin. J Clin Invest 1978; 61(2): 314-9.
[http://dx.doi.org/10.1172/JCI108941] [PMID: 413839]

[46]   Aksu HU, Oner E, Celik O, *et al.* Aspirin resistance in patients undergoing hemodialysis and effect of hemodialysis on aspirin resistance. Clin Appl Thromb Hemost 2015; 21(1): 82-6.
[http://dx.doi.org/10.1177/1076029613489597] [PMID: 23698727]

[47]   Larsen SB, Grove EL, Hvas AM, Kristensen SD. Platelet turnover in stable coronary artery disease - influence of thrombopoietin and low-grade inflammation. PLoS One 2014; 9(1): e85566.
[http://dx.doi.org/10.1371/journal.pone.0085566] [PMID: 24465602]

[48]   Nakamura T, Uchiyama S, Yamazaki M, Okubo K, Takakuwa Y, Iwata M. Flow cytometric analysis of reticulated platelets in patients with ischemic stroke. Thromb Res 2002; 106(4-5): 171-7.
[http://dx.doi.org/10.1016/S0049-3848(02)00131-7] [PMID: 12297121]

[49]   Santilli F, Vazzana N, Liani R, Guagnano MT, Davì G. Platelet activation in obesity and metabolic syndrome. Obes Rev 2012; 13(1): 27-42.
[http://dx.doi.org/10.1111/j.1467-789X.2011.00930.x]

[50]   Funck-Jensen KL, Dalsgaard J, Grove EL, Hvas AM, Kristensen SD. Increased platelet aggregation and turnover in the acute phase of ST-elevation myocardial infarction. Platelets 2013; 24(7): 528-37.
[http://dx.doi.org/10.3109/09537104.2012.738838] [PMID: 23216571]

[51]   Würtz M, Grove EL, Wulff LN, *et al.* Patients with previous definite stent thrombosis have a reduced antiplatelet effect of aspirin and a larger fraction of immature platelets. JACC Cardiovasc Interv 2010; 3(8): 828-35.
[http://dx.doi.org/10.1016/j.jcin.2010.05.014] [PMID: 20723855]

[52]   Guthikonda S, Lev EI, Patel R, *et al.* Reticulated platelets and uninhibited COX-1 and COX-2 decrease the antiplatelet effects of aspirin. Journal of Thrombosis and Haemostasis 2007; 5(3): 490-6.
[http://dx.doi.org/10.1111/j.1538-7836.2007.02387.x] [PMID: 17319904]

[53]   Grove EL, Würtz M, Hvas AM, Kristensen SD. Increased platelet turnover in patients with previous definite stent thrombosis. J Thromb Haemost 2011; 9(7): 1418-9.

[http://dx.doi.org/10.1111/j.1538-7836.2011.04304.x] [PMID: 21501377]

[54]   Eisen A, Lerman-Shivek H, Perl L, *et al.* Circulating reticulated platelets over time in patients with myocardial infarction treated with prasugrel or ticagrelor. J Thromb Thrombolysis 2015; 40(1): 70-5.
        [http://dx.doi.org/10.1007/s11239-014-1156-4] [PMID: 25481810]

[55]   Simpson SH, Abdelmoneim AS, Omran D, Featherstone TR. Prevalence of high on-treatment platelet reactivity in diabetic patients treated with aspirin. Am J Med 2014; 127(1): 95.e1-9.
        [http://dx.doi.org/10.1016/j.amjmed.2013.09.019] [PMID: 24384107]

[56]   Tschoepe D, Roesen P, Esser J, *et al.* Large platelets circulate in an activated state in diabetes mellitus. Semin Thromb Hemost 1991; 17(4): 433-8.
        [http://dx.doi.org/10.1055/s-2007-1002650] [PMID: 1803514]

[57]   Winocour PD. Platelet turnover in advanced diabetes. Eur J Clin Invest 1994; 24 (Suppl. 1): 34-7.
        [http://dx.doi.org/10.1111/j.1365-2362.1994.tb02424.x] [PMID: 8013530]

[58]   Schwartz K, Chivu S, Davis J. Amount of Platelet Inhibition Produced When Initiating Aspirin Therapy: Comparison of Two Doses 81 *Vs.* 325. Blood 2011; 118(21): 1250.

[59]   Spectre G, Arnetz L, Östenson C-G, Brismar K, Li N, Hjemdahl P. Twice daily dosing of aspirin improves platelet inhibition in whole blood in patients with type 2 diabetes mellitus and micro- or macrovascular complications. Thromb Haemost 2011; 106(3): 491-9.
        [http://dx.doi.org/10.1160/TH11-04-0216] [PMID: 21800009]

[60]   Addad F, Chakroun T, Elalamy I, *et al.* Antiplatelet effect of once- or twice-daily aspirin dosage in stable coronary artery disease patients with diabetes. Int J Hematol 2010; 92(2): 296-301.
        [http://dx.doi.org/10.1007/s12185-010-0652-3] [PMID: 20725815]

[61]   Capodanno D, Patel A, Dharmashankar K, *et al.* Pharmacodynamic effects of different aspirin dosing regimens in type 2 diabetes mellitus patients with coronary artery disease. Circ Cardiovasc Interv 2011; 4(2): 180-7.
        [http://dx.doi.org/10.1161/CIRCINTERVENTIONS.110.960187] [PMID: 21386092]

[62]   Bethel MA, Harrison P, Sourij H, *et al.* Randomized controlled trial comparing impact on platelet reactivity of twice-daily with once-daily aspirin in people with Type 2 diabetes. Diabet Med 2016; 33(2): 224-30.
        [http://dx.doi.org/10.1111/dme.12828] [PMID: 26043186]

[63]   Dillinger J-G, Drissa A, Sideris G, *et al.* Biological efficacy of twice daily aspirin in type 2 diabetic patients with coronary artery disease. Am Heart J 2012; 164(4): 600-606.e1.
        [http://dx.doi.org/10.1016/j.ahj.2012.06.008] [PMID: 23067920]

[64]   Guthikonda S, Alviar CL, Vaduganathan M, *et al.* Role of reticulated platelets and platelet size heterogeneity on platelet activity after dual antiplatelet therapy with aspirin and clopidogrel in patients with stable coronary artery disease. J Am Coll Cardiol 2008; 52(9): 743-9.
        [http://dx.doi.org/10.1016/j.jacc.2008.05.031] [PMID: 18718422]

[65]   Freynhofer MK, Iliev L, Bruno V, *et al.* Platelet turnover predicts outcome after coronary intervention. Thromb Haemost 2017; 117(5): 923-33.
        [http://dx.doi.org/10.1160/TH16-10-0785] [PMID: 28229159]

[66]   Lakkis N, Dokainish H, Abuzahra M, *et al.* Reticulated platelets in acute coronary syndrome: a marker of platelet activity. J Am Coll Cardiol 2004; 44(10): 2091-3.
        [http://dx.doi.org/10.1016/j.jacc.2004.05.033] [PMID: 15542299]

[67]   Grove EL, Hvas AM, Kristensen SD. Immature platelets in patients with acute coronary syndromes. Thromb Haemost 2009; 101(1): 151-6.
        [http://dx.doi.org/10.1160/TH08-03-0186] [PMID: 19132202]

[68]   Guthikonda S, Alviar CL, Vaduganathan M, *et al.* Role of Reticulated Platelets and Platelet Size Heterogeneity on Platelet Activity After Dual Antiplatelet Therapy With Aspirin and Clopidogrel in Patients With Stable Coronary Artery Disease 2008; 52(9): 743-9.

[69]   Christensen KH, Grove EL, Würtz M, Kristensen SD, Hvas AM. Reduced antiplatelet effect of aspirin during 24 hours in patients with coronary artery disease and type 2 diabetes. Platelets 2015; 26(3): 230-5.
[http://dx.doi.org/10.3109/09537104.2014.901497] [PMID: 24750015]

[70]   Henry P, Vermillet A, Boval B, *et al.* 24-hour time-dependent aspirin efficacy in patients with stable coronary artery disease. Thromb Haemost 2011; 105(2): 336-44.
[http://dx.doi.org/10.1160/TH10-02-0082] [PMID: 21136023]

[71]   Lordkipanidzé M, Pharand C, Schampaert E, Palisaitis DA, Diodati JG. Heterogeneity in platelet cyclooxygenase inhibition by aspirin in coronary artery disease. Int J Cardiol 2011; 150(1): 39-44.
[http://dx.doi.org/10.1016/j.ijcard.2010.02.025] [PMID: 20207433]

[72]   Würtz M, Hvas AM, Jensen LO, *et al.* 24-hour antiplatelet effect of aspirin in patients with previous definite stent thrombosis. Int J Cardiol 2014; 175(2): 274-9.
[http://dx.doi.org/10.1016/j.ijcard.2014.05.013] [PMID: 24861258]

[73]   Arazi HC, Doiny DG, Torcivia RS, *et al.* Impaired anti-platelet effect of aspirin, inflammation and platelet turnover in cardiac surgery. Interact Cardiovasc Thorac Surg 2010; 10(6): 863-7.
[http://dx.doi.org/10.1510/icvts.2009.229542] [PMID: 20233808]

[74]   Cavalca V, Rocca B, Veglia F, *et al.* On-pump Cardiac Surgery Enhances Platelet Renewal and Impairs Aspirin Pharmacodynamics: Effects of Improved Dosing Regimens. Clin Pharmacol Ther 2017; 102(5): 849-58.
[http://dx.doi.org/10.1002/cpt.702] [PMID: 28379623]

[75]   Gluckman TJ, McLean RC, Schulman SP, *et al.* Effects of aspirin responsiveness and platelet reactivity on early vein graft thrombosis after coronary artery bypass graft surgery. J Am Coll Cardiol 2011; 57(9): 1069-77.
[http://dx.doi.org/10.1016/j.jacc.2010.08.650] [PMID: 21349398]

[76]   Paikin JS, Hirsh J, Ginsberg JS, *et al.* Multiple daily doses of acetyl-salicylic acid (ASA) overcome reduced platelet response to once-daily ASA after coronary artery bypass graft surgery: a pilot randomized controlled trial. J Thromb Haemost 2015; 13(3): 448-56.
[http://dx.doi.org/10.1111/jth.12832] [PMID: 25546465]

[77]   Paikin JS, Hirsh J, Ginsberg JS, *et al.* Once versus twice daily aspirin after coronary bypass surgery: a randomized trial. J Thromb Haemost 2017; 15(5): 889-96.
[http://dx.doi.org/10.1111/jth.13667] [PMID: 28267249]

[78]   Hillis LD, Smith PK, Anderson JL, *et al.* 2011 ACCF/AHA Guideline for Coronary Artery Bypass Graft Surgery: a report of the American College of Cardiology Foundation/American Heart Association Task Force on Practice Guidelines. Circulation 2011; 124(23): e652-735.
[PMID: 22064599]

[79]   Himmelfarb J, Holbrook D, McMonagle E, Ault K. Increased reticulated platelets in dialysis patients. Kidney Int 1997; 51(3): 834-9.
[http://dx.doi.org/10.1038/ki.1997.117] [PMID: 9067918]

[80]   Würtz M, Wulff LN, Grove EL, Kristensen SD, Hvas A-M. Influence of renal function and platelet turnover on the antiplatelet effect of aspirin. Thromb Res 2012; 129(4): 434-40.
[http://dx.doi.org/10.1016/j.thromres.2011.07.019] [PMID: 21839494]

[81]   Zanazzi M, Cesari F, Rosso G, *et al.* Reticulated platelets and platelet reactivity in renal transplant recipients receiving antiplatelet therapy. Transplant Proc 2010; 42(4): 1156-7.
[http://dx.doi.org/10.1016/j.transproceed.2010.03.042] [PMID: 20534248]

[82]   Cesari F, Marcucci R, Gori AM, *et al.* High platelet turnover and reactivity in renal transplant recipients patients. Thromb Haemost 2010; 104(4): 804-10.
[PMID: 20694276]

[83]   Ozben S, Ozben B, Tanrikulu AM, Ozer F, Ozben T. Aspirin resistance in patients with acute ischemic

stroke. J Neurol 2011; 258(11): 1979-86.
[http://dx.doi.org/10.1007/s00415-011-6052-7] [PMID: 21509427]

[84]   Fiolaki A, Katsanos AH, Kyritsis AP, *et al.* High on treatment platelet reactivity to aspirin and clopidogrel in ischemic stroke: A systematic review and meta-analysis. J Neurol Sci 2017; 376: 112-6.
[http://dx.doi.org/10.1016/j.jns.2017.03.010] [PMID: 28431593]

[85]   Kim JT, Heo SH, Choi KH, *et al.* Clinical Implications of Changes in Individual Platelet Reactivity to Aspirin Over Time in Acute Ischemic Stroke. Stroke 2015; 46(9): 2534-40.
[http://dx.doi.org/10.1161/STROKEAHA.115.009428] [PMID: 26219647]

[86]   Mehta SR, Tanguay J-F, Eikelboom JW, *et al.* CURRENT-OASIS 7 trial investigators. Double-dose versus standard-dose clopidogrel and high-dose versus low-dose aspirin in individuals undergoing percutaneous coronary intervention for acute coronary syndromes (CURRENT-OASIS 7): a randomised factorial trial. Lancet 2010; 376(9748): 1233-43.
[http://dx.doi.org/10.1016/S0140-6736(10)61088-4] [PMID: 20817281]

[87]   FitzGerald GA, Oates JA, Hawiger J, *et al.* Endogenous biosynthesis of prostacyclin and thromboxane and platelet function during chronic administration of aspirin in man. J Clin Invest 1983; 71(3): 676-88.
[http://dx.doi.org/10.1172/JCI110814] [PMID: 6338043]

[88]   van Gijn J, Algra A, Kappelle J, Koudstaal PJ, van Latum A. Dutch TIA Trial Study Group. A comparison of two doses of aspirin (30 mg vs. 283 mg a day) in patients after a transient ischemic attack or minor ischemic stroke. N Engl J Med 1991; 325(18): 1261-6.
[http://dx.doi.org/10.1056/NEJM199110313251801] [PMID: 1922220]

[89]   Peters RJG, Mehta SR, Fox KAA, *et al.* Clopidogrel in Unstable angina to prevent Recurrent Events (CURE) Trial Investigators. Effects of aspirin dose when used alone or in combination with clopidogrel in patients with acute coronary syndromes: observations from the Clopidogrel in Unstable angina to prevent Recurrent Events (CURE) study. Circulation 2003; 108(14): 1682-7.
[http://dx.doi.org/10.1161/01.CIR.0000091201.39590.CB] [PMID: 14504182]

[90]   Berger JS, Sallum RH, Katona B, *et al.* Is there an association between aspirin dosing and cardiac and bleeding events after treatment of acute coronary syndrome? A systematic review of the literature. Am Heart J 2012; 164(2): 153-162.e5.
[http://dx.doi.org/10.1016/j.ahj.2012.04.001] [PMID: 22877800]

[91]   Bonten TN, Saris A, van Oostrom MJ, *et al.* Effect of aspirin intake at bedtime versus on awakening on circadian rhythm of platelet reactivity. A randomised cross-over trial. Thromb Haemost 2014; 112(6): 1209-18.
[http://dx.doi.org/10.1160/th14-05-0453] [PMID: 25208590]

[92]   Lordkipanidzé M, Pharand C, Schampaert E, Turgeon J, Palisaitis DA, Diodati JG. A comparison of six major platelet function tests to determine the prevalence of aspirin resistance in patients with stable coronary artery disease. Eur Heart J 2007; 28(14): 1702-8.
[http://dx.doi.org/10.1093/eurheartj/ehm226] [PMID: 17569678]

[93]   Serebruany VL, Steinhubl SR, Berger PB, *et al.* Analysis of risk of bleeding complications after different doses of aspirin in 192,036 patients enrolled in 31 randomized controlled trials. Am J Cardiol 2005; 95(10): 1218-22.
[http://dx.doi.org/10.1016/j.amjcard.2005.01.049] [PMID: 15877994]

[94]   Claxton AJ, Cramer J, Pierce C. A systematic review of the associations between dose regimens and medication compliance. Clin Ther 2001; 23(8): 1296-310.
[http://dx.doi.org/10.1016/S0149-2918(01)80109-0] [PMID: 11558866]

CHAPTER 2

Adenosine Receptors and Drug Discovery in the Cardiovascular System

Maan T. Khayat[1,2,a], Ahmad Hanif[1,a], Werner J. Geldenhuys[1] and Mohammed A. Nayeem[1,*]

[1] *Department of Pharmaceutical Sciences, West Virginia University, School of Pharmacy, Morgantown, WV, USA*

[2] *Department of Pharmaceutical Chemistry, King Abdulaziz University, School of Pharmacy, Jeddah, Saudi Arabia*

[a] *equally share first authorship in this book chapter*

Abstract: The signaling nucleoside adenosine is produced intra- and extracellularly under physiologic and, more importantly, under pathologic conditions. Adenosine modulates cellular functions involved in injury, metabolic derangement, energy perturbations, and inflammation. The biologic effects of adenosine are mediated by four adenosine receptor (AR) subtypes of the G-protein coupled receptors (GPCRs) family: A_1AR, $A_{2A}AR$, $A_{2B}AR$ and A_3AR. In the cardiovascular (CV) system, adenosine and its receptors are intricately involved in the regulation of myocardial contraction, heart rate, sympathetic control, conductivity, vascular tone, cardiac and vascular growth, inflammation, injury and apoptosis. As such, the modulation of the adenosinergic system has therapeutic potential for cardiovascular diseases (CVDs) such as metabolic disorders, atherosclerosis, hypertrophy, ischemic heart diseases, and heart failure. Nevertheless, despite the many years of investigation and experimentation only a few drugs targeting the adenosinergic system were developed and actually have reached clinical application. This chapter outlines the unique role adenosine plays in the CV system in physiology, pathology, and potentially therapeutic pharmacology. It also presents an updated review of the different adenosine receptors ligands, and their clinical potential in different CVDs.

Keywords: 4′-oxonucleosides, 4′-selenonucleoside, Adenosine, Adenosine receptors, Allosteric modulator, Atherosclerosis, Binding affinity, Capadenoson, Cardiac hypertrophy, Cardiovascular system, CGS 21680, Heart failure, Ischemic heart disease, Istradefylline, Metabolic disorders, Receptor desensitization, Receptor dimerization, Regadenoson, Rolofylline, Tecadenoson, Xanthine.

* **Corresponding author Mohammed A. Nayeem:** Department of Pharmaceutical Sciences, School of Pharmacy, West Virginia University, Biomedical Research Building, 2ⁿᵈ floor, Room # 220, Health Science Center – North, 1 Medical Center Drive, PO Box 9530, Morgantown, WV 26506-9530, USA; Tel: 304-293-4484; Fax: 304-293-2576; E-mail: mnayeem@hsc.wvu.edu

Atta-ur-Rahman & M. Iqbal Choudhary (Eds.)

ADENOSINE IN PHYSIOLOGY AND PATHOPHYSIOLOGY

Introduction

Adenosine is a signaling purine nucleoside generated primarily from the breakdown of adenosine triphosphate (ATP) [1] in response to cell damage or stress [2]. It is produced both intra- and extracellularly by physiologic and pathologic stimuli and mediates a plethora of actions throughout the body [3]. Among adenosine's actions in the central nervous system (CNS) are the control of synaptic plasticity [4], neuroprotection during ischemia [5], and modulation of neurotransmitter release [6]. In the cardiovascular (CV) system, adenosine impacts major functions, such as cardiac contractility, conductivity, heart rate, autonomic regulation of the heart, and coronary blood flow [3]. Also, adenosine enhances the cellular energy balance, and protects the heart against ischemia [7] through its actions on its receptors to deliver more blood to an oxygen-poor cell or tissue. Additionally, regulates vascular tone [8 - 12]. In fact, the importance of adenosine to the CV system begins in utero; it is essential for the development of healthy hearts and for protecting the embryo against intrauterine stress [13]. The ubiquitous nature of adenosinergic system in the body in general, and in the CV system in particular, makes it an attractive target to investigate its potential in the management of CV diseases.

Production and Metabolism

Under physiologic conditions, adenosine is constitutively generated intracellularly and extracellularly [14] (Fig. **1**). Intracellularly, adenosine is produced by dephosphorylation of AMP by 5′-nucleotidase [15], or by the transmethylation pathway, in which S-adenosylhomocysteine (SAH) hydrolase hydrolyzes SAH to adenosine and homocysteine [16]. Under normoxic, or physiologic, conditions, the latter pathway is the main contributor to adenosine generation intracellularly [17], whereas the former gains more significance during hypoxia [15] (Fig. **1**). Similarly, extracellular adenosine is produced by a chain of enzymatic dephosphorylation of adenine nucleotides, such as ATP, ADP, and AMP by ectonucleotidases [14]. These dephosphorylation reactions take a few hundred milliseconds, where dephosphorylation of AMP to adenosine by ecto-5′-nucleotidase (also known as CD73) is the rate-limiting step [18]. Adenosine receptors are surface receptors and adenosine will eventually have to be available in the extracellular space to activate its receptors. Under such physiologic conditions, the extracellular concentration of adenosine ranges from 40 to 600 nM [2], most of which is produced intracellularly and then transferred passively through equilibrative transport proteins (ENT) [19].

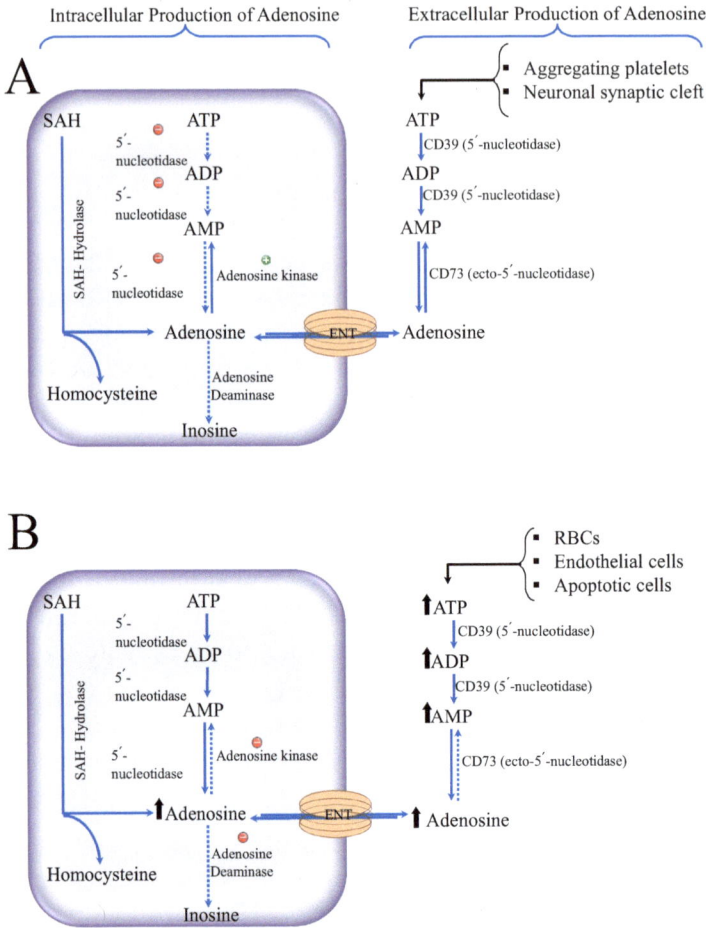

Fig. (1). Adenosine production and metabolism during normoxia and hypoxia:
(**A**) Under physiologic conditions, where normoxia prevails, adenosine signaling is not very pronounced. Here, the transmethylation pathway, in which S-adenosylhomocysteine (SAH) hydrolase hydrolyzes SAH to adenosine and homocysteine, is the main contributor to adenosine generation intracellularly [17]. Cytosolic 5′-nucleotidases, which generate adenosine from nucleotides (ATP, ADP, and AMP), are constitutively inhibited by ATP during normoxia [237]. Adenosine rephosphorylation to AMP, by adenosine kinase, dominates over adenosine deamination into inosine by adenosine deaminase [238].
(**B**) Under pathologic conditions, such as ischaemia, hypoxia, inflammation, or tissue damage, adenosine production increases significantly both extracellularly, through increased ATP production by different cell types, and intracellularly, through enhanced dephosphorylation of ATP, ADP by removing the constitutive inhibition of cytosolic 5′-nucleotidases.

Under physiologic conditions, equal intracellular and extracellular concentrations of adenosine exist thanks to the equilibrative transport proteins (ENT) which facilitate adenosine's movement across the plasma membrane down its concentration gradient [14]. Both intracellular and extracellular sources of adenosine are important [20]. Depletion of cellular fuel (ATP) in response to excessive consumption, ischemia [14] or hypoxia [21] are associated with increased adenosine levels by up to a 100-fold [22], which is primarily produced from the breakdown of adenine nucleotides, ADP and ATP [2]. When the extracellular production of adenosine is high, it is transported into cells, where it is either phosphorylated by adenosine kinase to AMP and subsequently to ADP and ATP [23] or broken down by adenosine deaminase to inosine [24] (Fig. **1**).

Adenosine Receptors and Signaling Pathways

The biological effects of adenosine are mediated by four adenosine receptor (AR) subtypes: A_1AR, $A_{2A}AR$, $A_{2B}AR$ and A_3AR. Although adenosine is the main agonist at adenosine receptors, its metabolite inosine can activate these receptors [14]. A_1AR and $A_{2A}AR$ have high affinity to adenosine with Kd values of 0.3–3 nM and 1–20 nM, respectively. In contrast, $A_{2B}AR$ and A_3AR have lower affinities (Kd >1 μM) [14, 25]. Adenosine's effects depend on the level of adenosine (which changes dramatically depending on consumption, ischemia, or hypoxia), the affinity of its receptor subtypes to adenosine, and the level of expression of these receptors on cellular membranes [26]. Adenosine receptors are members of the G-protein coupled receptors (GPCRs) family, which have similar general structure of seven-transmembrane α-helical structure with an intracellular carboxy-terminus and an extracellular amino-terminus [14].

Adenosine receptors are distributed widely in the body and, hence, can affect almost all physiologic functions [27]. Experimental tools, such as radioligands and antibodies, allowed decent mapping of where adenosine receptors are distributed in the body [28]. The distribution of adenosine receptors, A_1AR and $A_{2A}AR$, was more extensively studied using these tools. However, the distribution of the other two adenosine receptors, $A_{2B}AR$ and A_3AR, is less well-investigated [14]. The presence and distribution of A_1AR and $A_{2A}AR$ was confirmed using multiple tools, such as receptor localization and mRNA distribution. The evidence for receptor distribution is more solid when either techniques supports the same findings as the other does [14]. All adenosine receptors are expressed on cardiomyocytes, including $A_{2A}AR$ [29]. A_1AR, is found in intermediate-high levels in the central nervous system on neurons of the cortex, cerebellum, hippocampus [14], oligodendrocytes [30], microglia [31], and astrocytes [32]. A_1AR is also detected in adipose tissue, heart, skeletal muscle, liver, and kidneys [33]. In the vascular system, the vasoconstrictive effects of adenosine in some vascular beds, such as renal afferent arterioles and hepatic veins, is mediated by A_1AR [34]. $A_{2A}AR$ is highly distributed, like A_1AR, in the CNS; it is found in the hippocampus [35], on astrocytes, oligodendrocytes, microglia and neurons [36,

37]. In the periphery, $A_{2A}AR$ is highly expressed in spleen, thymus, leukocytes, blood platelets, heart, lung, and blood vessels [14]. mRNA distribution studies indicated that $A_{2B}AR$ is expressed in colon, bladder, lung, blood vessels, eye, and mast cells, whereas A_3AR is found in high levels in heart atria and testis, and in low levels in most of the brain, adrenal gland, spleen, thyroid, liver, kidney, intestine, and testis [14].

The signaling pathways of adenosine receptor subtypes have both common and unique elements. Initial classification of adenosine receptors was based on their effect on adenylyl cyclase and, therefore, cyclic AMP (cAMP) level [38]. $A_{2A}AR$ and $A_{2B}AR$ bind to $G_{s/olf}$ proteins and result in stimulation of cAMP production and increase in protein kinase A (PKA) [1]. These two receptor subtypes mediate adenosine's vasodilatory effect *via* CYP-epoxygenase pathway [11, 39 - 44], epoxyeicosatrienoic acids (EETs) production [45], ATP-sensitive K^+ channels (K_{ATP}) channels [10, 46 - 48], and voltage-dependent K_v channels [49]. Also, adenosine-induced vasodilation could be nitric oxide- (NO-) dependent [46, 50] or NO-independent [49]. CYP-epoxygenases, such as CYP2C and CYP2J families, and ω-hydroxylases, such as CYP4A and CYP4F families, are cytochrome P450s (CYP450) enzymes [51, 52], and are involved in vascular tone regulation [51 - 53]. CYP-epoxygenases metabolize arachidonic acid (AA) to generate EETs, which have vasodilatory and cardioprotective effects [54]. On the other hand, ω-hydroxylases produce the vasoconstrictor metabolites hydroxyeicosatetraenoic acids (HETEs) [55]. In contrast, A_1AR and A_3AR bind to $G_{i/o}$ proteins causing inhibition of cAMP production and decrease in PKA [38]. Also, signaling through the A_1AR, $A_{2B}AR$, and A_3AR involves activation of phospholipase C (PLC)-β-III pathway, which leads to the activation of inositol 1,4,5-trisphosphate (IP3)/diacylglycerol (DAG) [14].

Signal transduction through adenosine receptors is associated with changes in mitogen-activated protein kinases (MAPK), which encompass the stress-activated protein kinases (SAPK), such as p38 and jun-N-terminal kinase (JNK), and the extracellular regulated kinases (ERK), such as ERK1/2 [56]. A_1AR activates ERK1/2 *via* β,γ-subunits released from pertussis toxin-sensitive G proteins $G_{i/o}$ [57], which may involve protein kinase A (PKA), protein kinase C (PKC), Ras, or Src tyrosine kinase [58]. $A_{2A}AR$ activates ERK1/2 using the cAMP-ras-MEK1 pathway [59], whereas $A_{2B}AR$ activates ERK1/2 as well as JNK and p38, which is unique to this receptor subtype [14]. Similarly, ERK1/2 activation ensues A_3AR stimulation [60].

Effects of Adenosine on the Physiology of the Cardiovascular System

Adenosine modulates many aspects of the cardiovascular system's physiology, such as growth and remodeling, and its response and resistance to pathologic conditions, such as ischemia. Adenosine slows heart rate through its A_1AR, which is highly expressed in the atria, by inhibiting impulse generation in the main components of the cardiac conduction system, including the supraventricular tissue (SA and AV nodes), bundle of His, and Purkinje fibers [61]. Adenosine's negative chronotropic effect involves the inactivation of the inward Ca^{2+} current (I_{Ca}), the inwardly rectifying K^+ current, and the funny hyperpolarization-activated current (I_f) [62]. Multiple adenosine receptors seem to be involved in mediating adenosine's effect on myocardial contractility, including A_1AR, $A_{2A}AR$ and $A_{2B}AR$ [3]. The net effect of adenosine on cardiac contractility is negative inotropic effect mediated by A_1AR, which does not directly regulate myocardial contractility [63]. Rather, adenosine decreases contractility, *via* A_1AR, by attenuating the effects of catecholamines on β-adrenoceptors through inhibiting cAMP and PKA activation [63], and inhibiting norepinephrine release from cardiac nerves [64]. These effects of adenosine counter the overstimulation of the heart in cases of reduced energy availability, such as ischemia or hypoxia, and contribute to the cardioprotective properties of adenosine [3]. On the other hand, $A_{2A}AR$ and $A_{2B}AR$ exert positive inotropic effects [65]. In isolated human right atrial myocytes, the expression of $A_{2A}AR$ was confirmed and was shown to increase spontaneous calcium release from the sarcoplasmic reticulum [66]. The interplay and significance of these opposing effects on myocardial contractility among adenosine receptors is yet to be disclosed.

Adenosine induces vasodilation in most vascular beds directly through activating its receptors on vascular smooth muscle cells (VSMCs), or indirectly through activating its receptors on vascular endothelial cells, which in turn release endothelium-derived relaxing factors [27, 67]. In the coronary arteries, all adenosine receptor subtypes are expressed [68], through which adenosine impacts vascular regulation, angiogenesis, and vascular protection and remodeling [69] [70]. $A_{2A}AR$ and $A_{2B}AR$ mediate endothelium-dependent and independent coronary vasodilation by adenosine [3]. They also compensate for each other's reduced level of expression; when either receptor is genetically deleted, the other receptor is upregulated [71]. Although the available data have been conflicting in regards to when adenosine's effects on coronary arteries are more prevalent: during physiologic or pathologic conditions [72], it seems that although adenosine has important roles during both, its role is more pronounced during ischemic episodes [72, 73] as seen in coronary reactive hyperemia studies [74, 75]. A_1AR mediates coronary vasoconstriction through inhibiting $A_{2A}AR$-mediated relaxation [67]. Similarly, A_3AR has inhibitory role on vascular relaxation, possibly indirectly, through mast cell involvement, where A_3AR is expressed [76].

The reported metabolic effects of adenosine on the heart are not consistent; studies indicated mixed effects of enhanced and suppressed glucose utilization as a source of energy [3]. Overall, most studies under physiological conditions suggest enhanced glucose utilization by adenosine [3]. Adenosine also exerts systemic metabolic effects, which may improve insulin resistance by inducing hepatic glucose production through its A_3AR [77], and reducing myocardial fatty acid utilization *via* its A_1AR-mediated anti-lipolytic effects [78].

Remodeling and hypertrophy are both modulated by adenosine in the myocardial and vascular tissues. In the heart, $A_{2A}AR$ and $A_{2B}AR$ mediate the suppression of cardiac fibroblast proliferation and collagen synthesis [79, 80], which may limit harmful fibrosis and remodeling [3]. Adenosine also restricts the production of inflammatory mediators associated with cardiac remodeling, such as cardiac TNFα expression [81], and matrix metalloproteinases (MMPs) secretion by macrophage through $A_{2A}ARs$ and $A_{2B}ARs$ [82]. In the vasculature, adenosine contributes significantly to the angiogenic response to ischemia [83] through effects involving all adenosine receptors [84], and actions on endothelial, vascular smooth muscle, and immune cells [85]. Moreover, adenosine induces vasculogenesis by stimulating vascular endothelial cell proliferation, migration and tube formation [83], promoting pro-angiogenic molecules, such as endothelial IL-8, basic fibroblast growth factor (bFGF), and vascular endothelial growth factor (VEGF) release through $A_{2B}AR$ [86], and inhibiting anti-angiogenic molecules, such as thrombospondin-1 release through $A_{2A}AR$ [87].

Protective Potential of Adenosine in Cardiovascular Pathology

Atherosclerosis

Adenosine positively modulates some important aspects of atherosclerosis, such as vascular injury modulation, anti-inflammatory effects, hepatic lipid metabolism, macrophage cholesterol transport, and foam cell formation [88, 89]. $A_{2A}AR$ stimulates reverse cholesterol transport and, hence, inhibits foam cell formation in macrophages, which reduces vascular cholesterol accumulation and counters the development of atherosclerosis [89]. Arterial injury is associated with upregulation of interferon (IFN)-γ and $A_{2B}AR$, which inhibits the release of inflammatory cytokines and deactivates macrophages [90]. Similarly, through inhibiting IFN-γ, A_3AR inhibits macrophage activation [91]. Hepatic lipogenesis, which affects plasma fatty acid level and atherogenesis, is decreased by $A_{2B}AR$-mediated effects [92].

Ischemic Heart Disease

Compelling evidence of adenosine's cardioprotective role, particularly in response to ischemia, is irrefutable [93 - 95]. The progression and outcome of ischemic heart disease are modulated by adenosine through its effects on atherosclerosis [88, 89], dyslipidemia [92] (see previous section), and post-myocardial infarction remodeling and heart failure [96]. Neuronal stunning, which is the post-ischemic neuronal dysfunction caused by impaired sympathetic neurotransmission, contributes to ischemic damage, and is suppressed by A_1AR [97].

Adenosine's range of actions target many of the inflammatory processes accompanying the ischemia–reperfusion injury, including inflammatory mediators' production, local and systemic inflammatory cells, such as neutrophils, macrophages, lymphocytes and dendritic cells [3]. Also, all adenosine receptors are believed to be involved in curbing the inflammatory processes ensuing reperfusion. For example, $A_{2A}AR$, $A_{2B}AR$, and A_3AR suppress the inflammatory cytokines release by cardiomyocytes, such as TNF-α and IL-6 [98, 99], and A_1AR positively modulates autophagy by removing damaged intracellular organelles such as dysfunctional mitochondria and providing alternative energy source from the broken-down protein when nutrients are deficient [100]. Understandably, aging and comorbidities, such as diabetes, hypertension, ventricular hypertrophy, and obesity, were shown to limit the efficacy of adenosine to counteract the ischemia–reperfusion damage [95, 101].

Cardiac Hypertrophy and Heart Failure

Myocardial adenosine level and function are altered in hypertrophied and failing hearts; it is unclear if these reported changes are part of the mechanistic changes of these disease conditions or adaptive and compensatory to limit their progression [3]. Heart failure is reportedly associated with irregular calcium release from the sarcoplasmic reticulum [66]. $A_{2A}AR$ modulates spontaneous calcium release from the sarcoplasmic reticulum in isolated human right atrial myocytes [66]. Moreover, up-regulation of adenosine $A_{2A}AR$ is linked to abnormal calcium handling in atrial fibrillation [102]. Therefore, $A_{2A}AR$–antagonism could be a viable strategy for investigating the potential benefit of decreasing the spontaneous calcium release from the sarcoplasmic reticulum in patients with atrial fibrillation [102]. There is evidence that changes in adenosine handling and function beneficially modulate cardiac hypertrophy and heart failure [96]. $A_{2A}AR$, A_1AR, and A_3AR are upregulated in response to phenylephrine-induced cardiomyocyte hypertrophy [96], activation of A_1AR attenuates cardiac hypertrophy and prevents heart failure [103], post-MI stimulation of $A_{2B}AR$ prevents cardiac remodeling [104], blocks apoptosis, and inhibits contractile dysfunction [105]. However, overexpression of A_1AR causes adverse, but reversible, changes in cardiac morphology and function, such as dilatation, hypertrophy and dysfunction [106]. In failing hearts, endogenous adenosine levels are enhanced in compensation for the decreased expression of $A_{2A}AR$, $A_{2B}AR$, and A_3AR by reduced adenosine deaminase activity; an adaptation that attenuates the severity of heart failure [3]. Therefore, the described effects of adenosine on fibroblast proliferation, apoptosis, fibrosis, cytokine release, and oxidative stress are relevant to cardiac hypertrophy and heart failure. The many roles $A_{2A}AR$ can potentially play in protecting against or modulating a number of cardiac pathologies, including cardiac hypertrophy, inflammatory cytokines release by cardiomyocytes, failing hearts, and calcium handling, indicate that this receptor subtype could be an important target to investigate in our search of therapeutic options for these conditions.

Metabolic Disorders

Since adenosine impacts the levels of fatty acids, glucose, and insulin, it has the potential to modulate the negative cardiovascular effects of metabolic disorders, such as metabolic syndrome, diabetes, and obesity as well as being part of the pathogenesis of these diseases [3]. In cardiac fibroblasts, glucose upregulates, whereas insulin downregulates, A_1AR and $A_{2B}AR$; at the same time, glucose represses A_3AR [107]. These effects are augmented by the observed upregulation of A_1AR and $A_{2B}AR$ in streptozotocin-induced diabetes [108]. Additionally, $A_{2B}AR$ has an important role in inhibiting dyslipidemia and atherosclerosis due to its effects on hepatic lipid metabolism [92], and A_1AR and is important in glucose disposal, and insulin sensitivity [109].

ADENOSINE AND DRUG DISCOVERY: A MEDICINAL CHEMISTRY PERSPECTIVE

Introduction

The versatility of adenosine's effects in different body systems and their role in a number of pathologies have sparked research interest the modulation of adenosine receptors as a therapeutic strategy against numerous diseases, such as sleep disorder, immune and inflammatory disorders, cerebral and cardiac ischemic disease, and finally cancer [110]. There are some useful, diverse applications of targeting adenosine receptors. For example, adenosine is clinically available under two generic drugs, Adenocard® and Adenoscan® to treat supraventricular tachycardia [110, 111]. Another example is caffeine, a methylxanthine, which is highly consumed by adults globally on a daily basis, blocks adenosine receptors at the regular doses available in different beverages [112] (see Fig. **2A**). Caffeine is utilized in clinical preparation to treat premature apnoea [112]. Moreover, other available medications, such as dipyridamole and methotrexate, interfere and alter the signaling pathway that results in a change of adenosine concentration [112]. Dipyridamole is an adenosine uptake inhibitor; it enhances adenosine's effects by reducing adenosine's uptake by endothelial cells, which increases its endogenous levels [113]. Methotrexate activates 5′-nucleotidase, which catalyzes AMP dephosphorylation to produce adenosine [114]. Many trials are ongoing to investigate the effects and properties of selective adenosine receptors ligands (both agonists and antagonists) [110] in different promising applications [112].

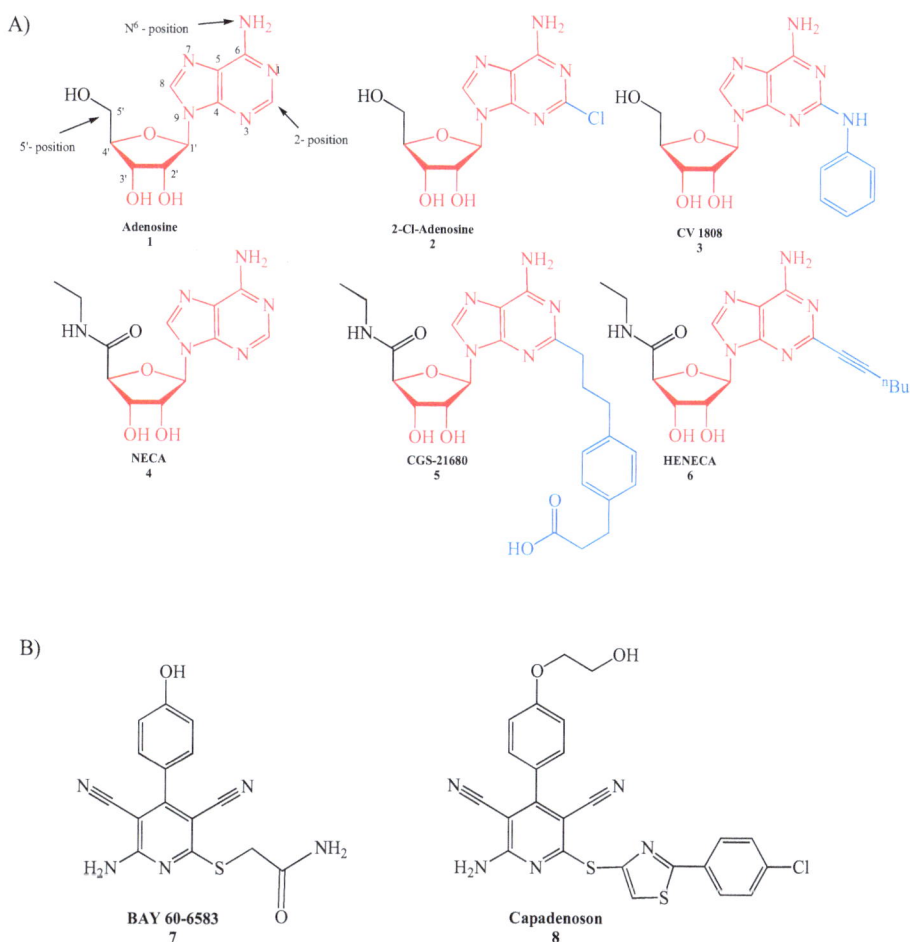

Fig. (2). Different Adenosine Receptors Agonists Structures. **A)** Nucleoside-based structure agonists class. **B)** Non-nucleoside agonists class.

The medicinal chemistry research has provided a huge number of selective agonists and antagonists. Those agents are characterized by potent activity and selectivity (binding affinity within a nanomolar level and selectivity of >100- to 200-fold higher than other adenosine receptor subtypes) for these receptors for several decades [110, 112]. Based on the known many roles of adenosine and its receptors in physiology and pathology, still, drug discovery based on the adenosinergic system is very slow and challenging [110]. The slow progress could be explained by many factors, which will be discussed later in the chapter. Despite the intensive research work and development which continuously provide many selective ARs- agonists and antagonists, only two drugs have approached the clinical application; these are istradefylline and regadenoson [112]. In this section, we will highlight the latest advancement and developments of ligands targeting AR in the cardiovascular system.

Adenosine Receptors' Ligands: A Historical Review

In 1929, Drury and Szent-Gyorgy uncovered that adenosine was involved in many physiological functions, including many cardiovascular effects [115]. Since then, adenosine has become a valuable point of interest for research [115] and new analogs were synthesized and tested [116]. Adenosine has high affinity toward $A_{2A}AR$, A_1AR, and A_3AR, but low affinity toward $A_{2B}AR$ [117] (Fig. **2A**, Table **1**). Since the discovery of adenosine, almost all adenosine agonists have been adenosine structure-based [118]. Adenosine structure is composed of a purine nucleoside moiety, which is made of a purine base and ribose (five-carbon sugar) (Fig. **2A**). Only one class of adenosine agonists, known as pyridine-3,--dicarbonitrile derivatives, was not adenosine structure-based, and was discovered by Beukers *et al.* in 2004 [119]. This group of non-adenosine agonists are very potent and selective to different adenosines receptors subtypes, such as $A_{2B}AR$ and A_1AR [119]. For instance, BAY 60-6583 is a selective $A_{2B}AR$-agonist; it was protective in renal ischemia [120]. Another example is the selective A_1AR agonist capadenoson (BAY 68-4986), which is in clinical trials for stable angina pectoris [121] (Fig. **2B**).

Table 1. Binding Affinities of Historical ARs Agonists.

	Compound name	K_i (nM)			
		A_1	A_{2A}	A_{2B}	A_3
1	Adenosine [a]	~100 (h)[b] 73 (r)[b]	310(h) [b] 150 (r)[b]	15,000 (h) [b] 5100 (r)[b]	290 nM(h) [b] 6500 (r)[b]
2	2-chloro Adenosine	6.7 (r)[c]	76 (r)[c]	24,000 (h)[d]	1890 (r)[e]
3	CV 1808*	400 (r)	100 (r)	ND	ND
4	NECA	14 (h)[b] 5.1 (r)[f]	20 (h)[b] 9.7 (r)[f]	140 (h)[b] 1890 (h)[g] 1900 (m)[f]	25 (h)[b] 113 (r)[f]

(Table 1) cont.....

Compound name		K_i (nM)			
		A_1	A_{2A}	A_{2B}	A_3
5	CGS 21680	289 (h)[l] 1800 (r)[m] 120 (rb)[m]	27 (h)[l] 19 (r)[m]	>10,000 (h)[l] >10,000 (r)[m]	67 (h)[l] 584 (r)[m] 673(rb)[m]
6	HENECA[§]	60 (h)	6.4 (h)	6100b	2.4 (h)
7	BAY 60-6583	>10,000 (h)[a,r]	>10,000 (h)[a,r]	3-10 (h)[r] 330 (m)[s] 750 (d)[s] 340 (rb)[s]	>10,000 (h)[a,r]
8	Capadenoson	N.D	N.D	N.D	N.D

h, human; d, dog; r, rat; rb, rabbit; m, mouse; N.D., no data available;
[a] Data are from functional studies.
[b] Yan *et al.*, 2003 [30].
[c] Daly *et al.*, 1993 [122].
[d] Bruns, 1980 [123].
[e] van Galen *et al.*, 1994 [124].
[f] Müller and Stein, 1996 [125].
[g] Fredholm *et al.*, 2011 [14].
[m] Liang *et al.*, 2010 [126].
[r] Kuno *et al.*, 2007 [127].
[s] Auchampach *et al.,* 2009 [128].
[l] Jacobson and Gao, 2006 [110].

Despite the uniqueness of this non-adenosine class, the core structure of adenosine, the purine nucleoside, remains conserved as the primary scaffold for developing new AR agonists [115].

In addition, most of the structural modification take place on one of three positions: N6 and 2-position of the purine moiety, and 5′-position of the ribose moiety [115]. Modification at these positions have consistently resulted in modulation of the selectivity and stability of the structure [115]. For example, 2-chloroadenosine, which has a chlorine atom in 2-position, was found to have enhanced potency on A_{2A}AR. Moreover, replacing the chlorine atom by an aniline group, as in CV 1808, led to discovering the first adenosine derivative with more selectivity to A_{2A}AR than A_1AR [115]. However, the substitution at the 5′-position, such as small alkylamide group, increased the potency 20-fold compared to 2-chloroadensoine. Substitution at the 2-position and 5'-position provided two agonists, HENECA and CGS 21680, which have a potential application as treatment for a cardiovascular disease [115] (see Fig. **2A**, Table **1**).

As mentioned previously, nearly all ARs-agonists are based on adenosine's purine-sugar structure. On the other hand, all ARs-antagonists lack the ribose part [115]. Moreover, the purine moiety is replaced with other cyclic structure to fit and mimic adenosine binding to its receptors [115]. These cyclic structures can be monocyclic (*e.g.* pyrimidine, 1,2,4-triazoles, and 1,3,5-triazine) [129, 130], bicyclic (*e.g.* purines, triazolopyridazines, and xanthines) [131 - 133], and tricyclic core structures such as indenopyrimidinones, triazoloquinoxalinones, and pyrazolotriazolopyrimidines [134 - 136] (Fig. **3**).

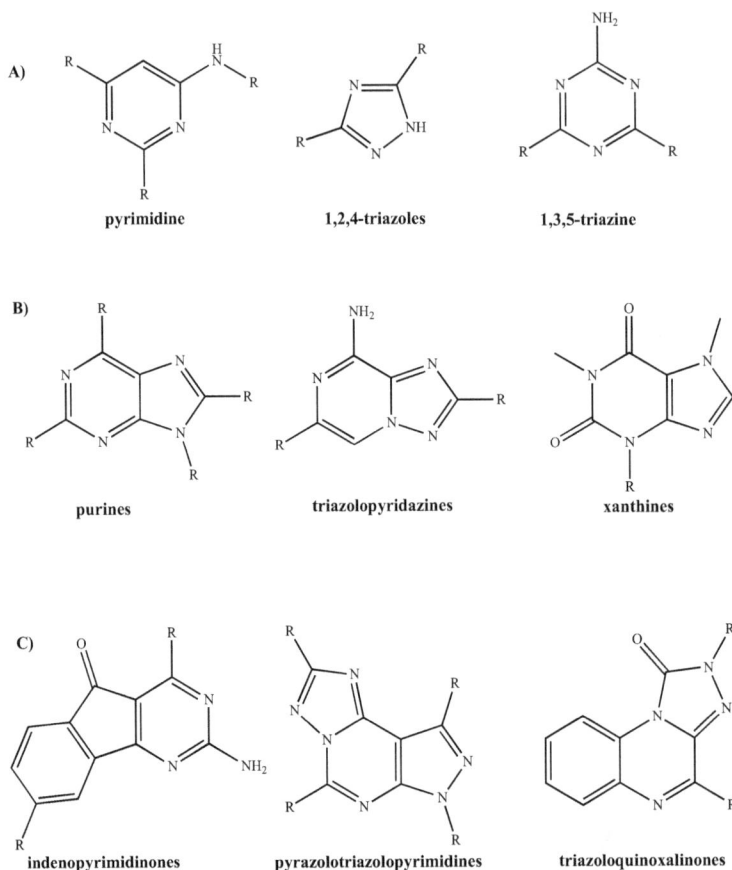

Fig. (3). Different Adenosine Receptors Antagonists Cyclic Structures Classes. **A)** monocyclic core structures, **B)** bicyclic core structures and **C)** tricyclic structures.

There are two classes of AR-antagonist: 1) xanthine-based and 2) nonxanthine derivatives [115, 137, 138]. The best examples of the xanthine derivatives are caffeine and theophylline which were discovered as the first AR-antagonists [115, 118, 139]. Both compounds have comparatively low binding affinity and selectivity toward ARs [139]. The xanthine structure has been used as a major scaffold to design and develop more potent and more selective A_{2A}AR-antagonists [115, 139]. In addition, all xanthine derivatives were mainly focused on the substitution at the positions 1-, 3-, 7-, and 8- of the xanthine scaffold. Since then, numerous screening on these substitutions have been successful, and led to the discovery CSC or 3-chlorostyrylcaffeine, MSX-2, MSX-3, and later istradefylline (Fig. **4**, Table **2**).

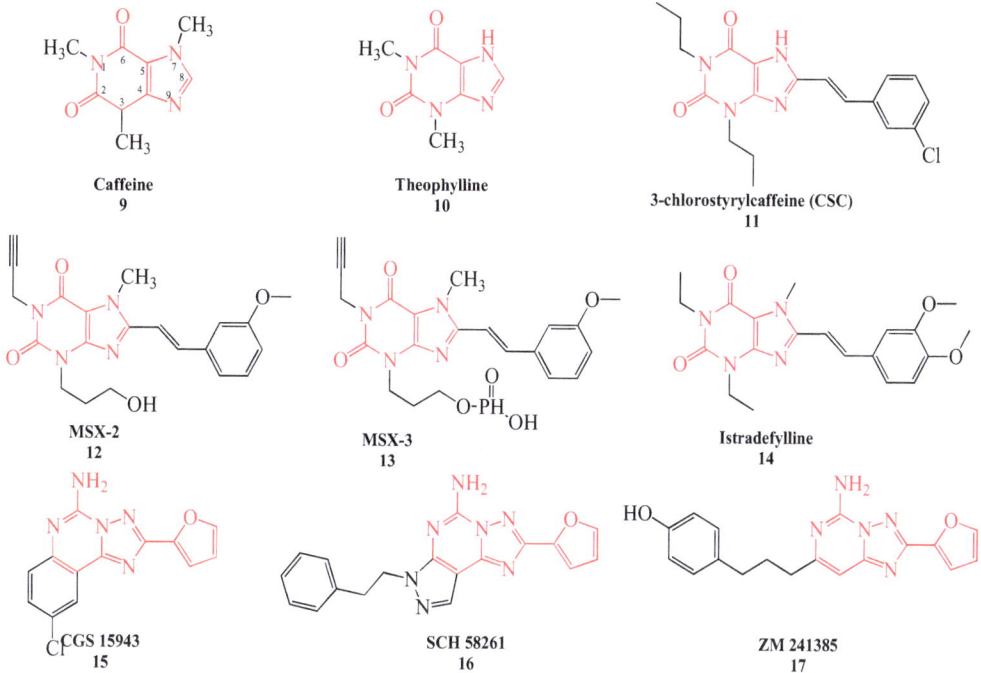

Fig. (4). Different Structures of Adenosine Receptors Antagonists. These antagonists are historical and known for a long time. Some of them have reached clinical trials while others are being used as standard reference *in vitro* experiments.

Table 2. Binding Affinities of Historical ARs Antagonists.

	Compound name	K_i (nM)			
		A_1	A_{2A}	A_{2B}	A_3
9	Caffeine	10,700 (h)[a] 41,000 (r)[f]	23,400 (h)[b] 45,000 (r)[g]	33,800 (h)[c] 20,500 (r)[h]	13,300 (h)[a]
10	Theophylline	6770 (h)[l] 8740 (r)[a]	1710 (h)[l] 22,000 (r)[m]	9070 (h)[d] 5630 (m)[n]	22,300 (h)[a] >100,000 (r)[e]
11	3-chlorostyrylcaffeine (CSC)	28,000 (r)[hh]	54 (r)[hh]	8200[ii]	>10,000 (r)[e]
12	MSX-2	900 (r)[jj]	8.04 (r)[i,jj]	>10,000 (h)[jj]	>10,000 (h)[jj]
14	Istradefylline	841 (h)[dd] 230 (r)[dd]	12 (h)[ee] 91.2 (h)[dd] 2.2 (r)[ff] 4.46 (r)[gg]	>10,000 (h)[dd]	4470 (h)[dd]

(Table 2) cont.....

Compound name		K_i (nM)			
		A_1	A_{2A}	A_{2B}	A_3
15	CGS 15943	3.5 (h)[s]	1.2 (h)[s]	32.4 (h)[n]	35 (h)[s]
16	SCH 58261	725 (h)[aa]	5.0 (h)[aa]	1110 (h)[aa]	1200 (h)[aa]
17	*ZM 241385	255 nM	0.8 nM	50	>10,000

h, human; d, dog; r, rat; rb, rabbit; m, mouse; N.D., no data available;
[a] Jacobson *et al.*, 1999 [140].
[b] Abo-Salem *et al.*, 2004 [141].
[c] Borrmann *et al.*, 2009 [142].
[d] Kim *et al.*, 2002 [143].
[e] van Galen *et al.*, 1994 [124].
[f] Grahner *et al.*, 1994 [144].
[g] Daly *et al.*, 1991 [145].
[h] Bertarelli *et al.*, 2006 [146].
[i] Müller *et al.*, 2000 [147].
[l] Klotz *et al.*, 1998 [148].
[m] Müller *et al.*, 1993b [149].
[n] Auchampach *et al.*, 2009 [128].
[s] Müller, 2000a [147].
[aa] Jacobson and Gao, 2006 [110].
[dd] Fredholm *et al.*, 2011 [14].
[ee] Kase *et al.*, 2003 [150].
[ff] Shimada *et al.*, 1997 [151].
[gg] Pretorius *et al.*, 2008 [152].
[hh] Jacobson *et al.*, 1993a [153].
[ii] Daly and Jacobson, 1995 [154].
[jj] Sauer *et al.*, 2000 [155].

These analogs are known by 8-styrylxanthines derivative (subclass) which was discovered in 1992 as potent and selective A_{2A}AR-antagonists at Kyowa Hakko (a pharmaceutical company), Tokyo, Japan (Fig. **4**). The activity behind the selectivity is due to the trans-styryl substituent at the 8-position [115]. Thereafter, istradefylline (KW-6002) was approved in Japan to treat Parkinson disease (PD), whereas, in the USA, the FDA did not approve it and requested more clinical trial data for safety purposes [151, 156 - 158]. Istradefylline is a selective A_{2A}AR-antagonist. As mentioned earlier, A_{2A}ARs are highly concentrated in the striatum and substantially involved in motor control. Istradefylline was found to reverse the motor disability in rodents and primate of Parkinson's disease without causing dyskinesia [159]. Moreover, when combined with L-DOPA in clinical trials, istradefylline reduced the off time without causing dyskinesia [159] [156]. The development of istradefylline was based on the substitution of a styryl group at the 8-position of xanthine base [139] (Fig. **5**). Moreover, istradefylline is the only 8-styrylxanthines subclass as an A_{2A}AR-antagonist that approached clinical trials and licensed [160]. However, the instability issue of istradefylline analogs was a major drawback that limited their development and led to identify a large number of nonxanthine derivatives [161].

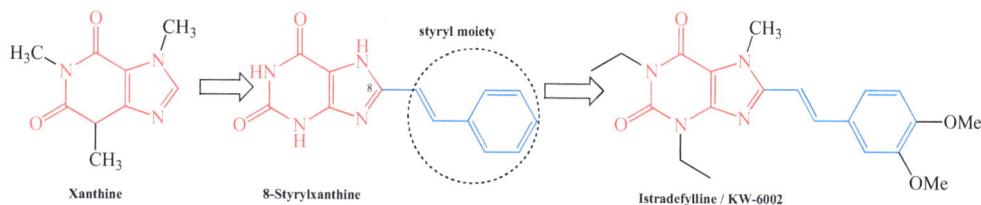

Fig. (5). Rationale of Istradefylline Synthesis that Requires Few Synthesis Steps.

In 1987, Williams *et al.* [162] discovered CGS 15943 as potent, selective $A_{2A}AR$ antagonist among other ARs. In 1993, the phenyl ring of CGS 15943 was substituted with different heterocycles such as imidazole and pyrazole. Unfortunately, the selectivity toward $A_{2A}AR$ did not improve [163]. Later, Baraldi *et al.* [164] introduced SCH 58261, a pyrazolotriazolopyrimidines system, which made a significant discovery by maintaining the antagonist selectivity only to $A_{2A}AR$ and losing the activity on other ARs. With the strong antagonist selectivity, SCH 58261 became very common and popular since it can cross the blood brain barrier (BBB). Therefore, it has many applications on $A_{2A}AR$ such as a tool to characterize $A_{2A}AR$, as a reference for the $A_{2A}AR$ antagonist, and as an exploration tool for the intracellular signaling pathway of $A_{2A}AR$ [164]. Zeneca group [165] discovered a bicyclic nonxanthine $A_{2A}AR$ antagonist ZM 241385 which was developed to overcome the stability and solubility issues discussed for previous analogs (Fig. **4**).

The Allosteric Modulators of AR Function

It is reported that ARs were regulated allosterically and since then, for the past decade, numerous allosteric modulators have been synthesized and evaluated [112, 166 - 170]. An allosteric site is a binding site that is distinct from the active (orthosteric) binding site on the protein [112, 115, 170]. Although allosteric modulators do not interfere with the binding site of orthosteric ligands and endogenous adenosine, for their effects to be elicited, the orthosteric ligands must be in their binding site [112, 115, 170]. Unfortunately, the localization of the allosteric binding pocket is not clear [170]. There are four types of allosteric modulators 1) Positive allosteric modulators (PAM), which enhance the effects of the active ligand [171]; 2) Negative allosteric modulators (NAM), which reduce or inhibit the ligands' effects [115, 172]; 3) Silent allosteric modulators (SAM), also known as a neutral allosteric ligand (NAL), which binds to the allosteric site without affecting the action of the active ligand [173 - 175]; 4) Allosteric / orthosteric ("Dualsteric" or "bitopic") hybrid ligands that bind to both allosteric and orthosteric sites [171, 176, 177] (Fig. **6**).

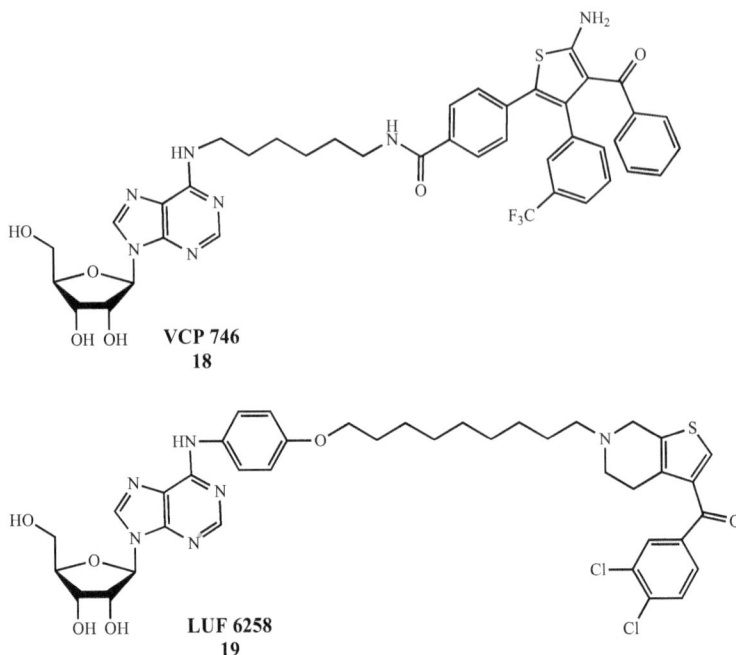

Fig. (6). Examples of Hybrid Allosteric Orthosteric Ligands. the allosteric modulator is connected to AR ligand by variant hydrocarbon bridge.

The first A_1AR allosteric modulators, such as 2-amino-3-benzoylthiophenes, (Fig. 7) were discovered by serendipity as PAM by Bruns *et al.* [178]. The inception of these compounds was initially prepared as intermediates for the synthesis of benzodiazepine-like compounds [179]. Then, some of these compounds, such as PD 81723, were extensively investigated to conclude that they enhanced the endogenous adenosine preconditioning effect on the heart [180]. Therefore, in most of the structure activity relationship studies (SAR), PD 81723 is the reference PAM allosteric modulator for A_1AR [181]. Chordia *et al* presented 2-aminothiazole such as compound **26**, which is the other A_1AR allosteric modulators class with potent PAM activity [182]. In 2001, Fawzi *et al* reported SCH 202676, a thiadiazole class, as an allosteric modulator for both agonist and antagonist coupling to GPCRs [183]. Particularly in A_1AR, both allosteric modulators SCH 202676 and LUF 5794 have PAM activity for the antagonist [³H]-DPCPX [184]. Interestingly, these thiadiazoles were thought to be allosteric modulator, but they were found to be sulfhydryl-modifying agents [181]. The previous classes of A_1AR allosteric modulators were summarized in detail by Göblyös and Guo [170, 172] and more examples are provided in Fig. (7).

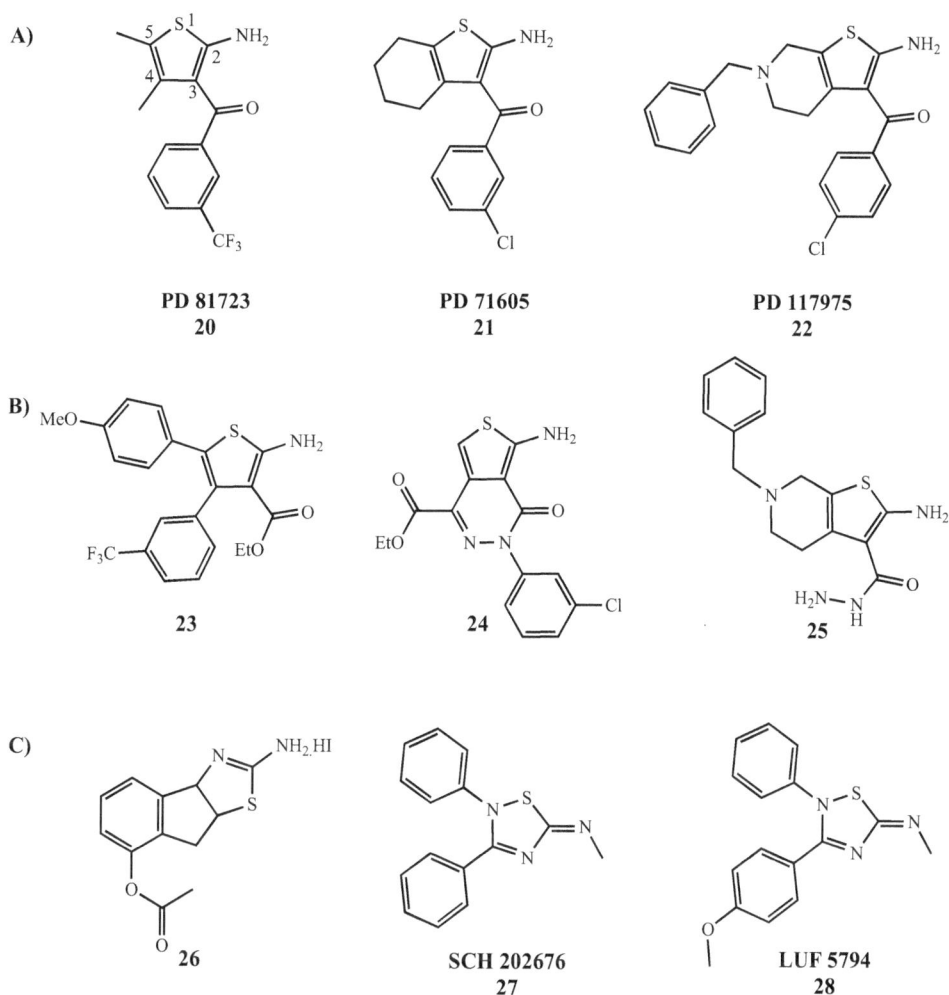

Fig. (7). Examples of A1AR Allosteric Modulators. **A)** The first generation of allosteric modulators A1AR, **B)** Recent A1AR allosteric modulators, and **C)** new allosteric modulaotrs class such as 2-aminothiazoles and [1, 2, 4] thiadiazole analogues.

On the other hand, the allosteric modulators of $A_{2A}AR$ include sodium ions, amiloride (potassium sparing diuretics), and amiloride analogs (DMA and HMA) (Fig. **8**). Sodium ions were found to decrease the dissociation rate of [^{3}H]ZM24185 antagonist, whereas amiloride analogs increased the dissociation rate of the antagonist [^{3}H]ZM24185, and no effect was observed on the agonist [^{3}H]CGS21680 [185]. Giorgi *et al*. studied new derivatives, such as 1-[4- (9-benzyl-2-phenyl-9H-purin-6-ylamino)-phenyl]-3-phenyl-urea derivatives and 1-

[4-(9-benzyl-2-phenyl-9H-8-azapurin-6-ylamino)-phenyl]-3-phenyl-urea, then in the functional studies, they found that compound **31** has PAM with CGS 21680 on rat aortic rings [186]. Thus, modulator **31** has a potential as a lead to develop new allosteric modulators toward $A_{2A}AR$ [186] (Fig. **8**).

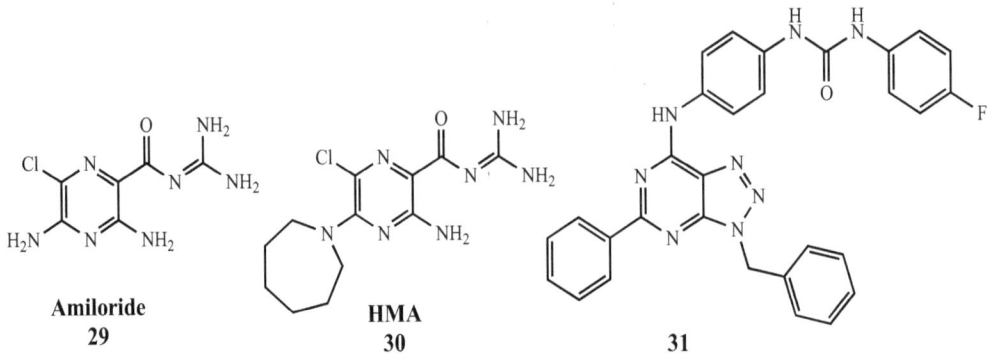

Fig. (8). $A_{2A}AR$ Allosteric Modulators.

The allosteric modulators play an important role in AR functions, especially PAMs. They are important in drug targeting as they may enhance selectivity, prolong functional activity, and reduce side effects [112].

Dimerization of Adenosine Receptors

The GPCRs, as well as adenosine receptors, can from homo-, multi-, and heterodimers of complex structures [139, 187]. A heterodimer as a macromolecular complex composed of two or more functional receptors and displays different biochemical characteristics of each receptor [187]. If the same GPCRs are coupled together, they form a homodimer [1, 139, 187]. Once a portion of the heterodimer complex structure is activated, it can potentially alter the receptor properties of the same heterodimer. Likewise, as reported by Sheth *et al.*, adenosine receptors can couple with each other to form homodimers and heterodimers with other different receptors [1]. An example of A_1AR-A_1AR homodimers as reported in Purkinje cells of the cerebellum and hippocampal pyramidal neurons [188], and in the intact tissue of the cortex [189]. However, the homodimers of $A_{2A}AR$-$A_{2A}AR$ were reported by Canals *et al.* in HeLa and HEK-293T cells, in which $A_{2A}AR$ homodimers co-transfected with different $A_{2A}AR$ receptor structures [190]. On the other hand, Ciruela *et al.* uncovered the heterodimers on the cell surface of HEK-293T co-transfected with their cDNAs in A_1AR-$A_{2A}AR$ [191]. They demonstrated heterodimerization through activating $A_{2A}AR$ on these cells by CGS 21680, which decreased the binding affinity to a selective radioligand and A_1AR [191]. Another example of heterodimers is A_1AR-$A_{2A}AR$ which was found in rat astrocyte cultures [192]. Although adenosine receptors can form homo- and heterodimers among each other, these receptors can also form a heterodimer with different receptors such as dopamine receptor $A_{2A}AR$-D_2R [193]. It is also worthy to mention the importance of heterodimers and homodimers receptors since these dimers mediate the cell surface function [190]. As reported by Sheth *et al*. [1] in CNS, the presence of the heterodimers, A_1AR-$A_{2A}AR$, is necessary to manage the neuronal excitability. Another example by Cristovao is the GABA uptake which was regulated by the heterodimers A_1AR-$A_{2A}AR$ [192]. These data demonstrated that the activation of A_1AR blocked, while the activation of $A_{2A}AR$ enhanced GABA transport [192]. Moreover, the homodimers $A_{2A}AR$-$A_{2A}AR$ coupling is the functional form of receptor found in the plasma membrane [190]. An excellent example that validates the oligomerization as bivalent drug target approach was done by Paulo A *et al*. [194] in the management of tardive dyskinesia (TD) that is characterized by reserpine-induced vacuous chewing movement (VCM) in a mouse model. First, they demonstrated a heteromer interaction between angiotensin receptor type 1 (AT_1R) and $A_{2A}AR$ in cultured cells that led to AT_1R-$A_{2A}AR$ formation. Then in TD mouse model, they co-treated with minimum effective doses of losartan (angiotensin II receptor antagonist) and istradefylline ($A_{2A}AR$ antagonist). Interestingly, the bivalent treatment was able to manage and reduce VCM [194]. Thus, the concept of receptor dimerization since its discovery three decade ago [195, 196] has become significant and it is an indication to search for possible valid target (illustration of adenosine homo-, and heterodimers is provided in Fig. (**9**).

Overall, most of the published adenosine receptor dimerization is focused on the CNS. However, other functional dimerization is still complex and challenging to reveal in other organs [1]. Once these dimers are revealed and fully understood, they can be a potential target as illustrated by Paulo A *et al*. However, the investigation of adenosine receptors dimerization and oligomerization in the vascular system is unclear.

Adenosine Receptors Crystal Structure

The adenosine receptor family protein structure has been studied for the development of novel therapeutic compounds. Fig. (**10**) shows the sequence alignment of the adenosine receptor drug targets, showing the sequence similarity between the different protein sequences. As mentioned, the adenosine receptor family are GPCRs, which were notoriously difficult to crystalize until the group of Jaakola *et al*. published the first crystal structure complex of $A_{2A}AR$ with the ligand ZM241385 [197]. This paved the way for structure-based drug discovery since until this point, the only available method available for development of novel drugs were the use of homology modeling. After this x-ray crystal structure, soon followed by several others, including structures that shed light on agonist, antagonist, and allosteric binding of small molecules [197 - 200]. Fig. (**11**) shows the $A_{2A}AR$ with the endogenous ligand adenosine [198]. Binding of ligands cause the induction of structural changes of the receptor protein structure, which is an evidenced of signaling downstream. For instance, an agonist binds in the active conformation of the receptor, allows the structural changes of the GPCR, which facilitate the secondary signaling events. This illustration is found in the structure of 3QAK where the amino acids ARG102 and GLU228 are "unlocked" and open, whereas the inactive receptor has these amino acids "locked" or in a closed state. Fig. (**12**) shows the location of the gating residues of $A_{2A}AR$ [199, 201]. For compounds to be considered agonists, they bind to the A_{2A} in the open state or active conformation, while the antagonists in general can bind in either conformation open or closed, but keeps the receptor in the inactive state [199, 201]. Structural differences in the binding pocket are also believed to drive much of the differences between the $A_{2A}AR$ and the A_1AR crystal structures. Recently, the A_1AR was crystallized (Fig. **13**), and several key differences were noted, especially the larger secondary loop and the larger substrate cavity in the receptor [202].

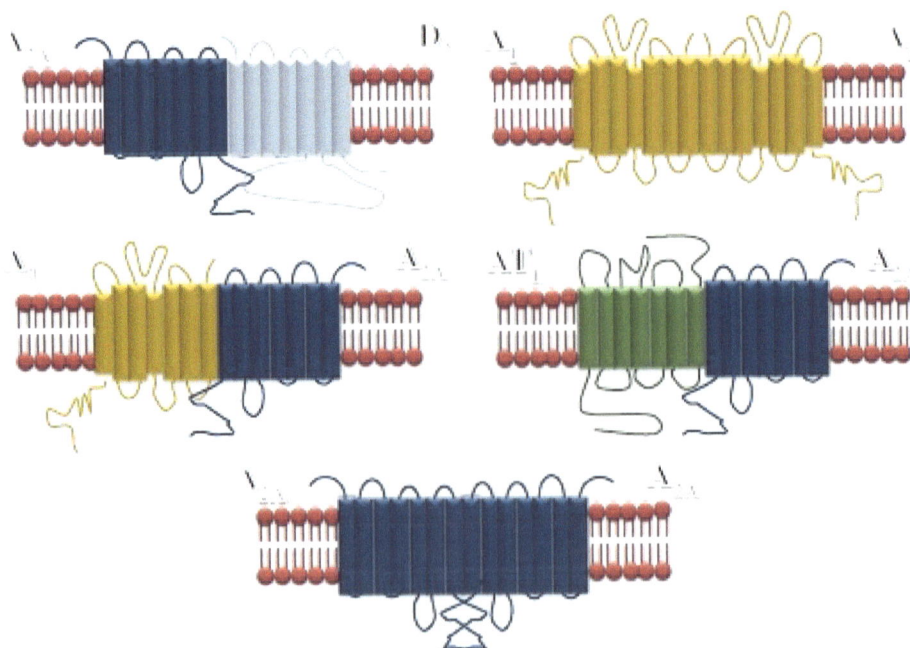

Fig. (9). Illustration of Adenosine Receptors Dimerization.

```
A₃AR    MPNNSTALSLANVTYITMEIFIGLCAIVGNVLVICVVKLNPSLQTTTFYFIVSLALADIA
A₁AR    ---MPPSISAFQAAYIGIEVLIALVSVPGNVLVIWAVKVNQALRDATFCFIVSLAVADVA
A₂ₐR    ------MPIMGSSVYITVELAIAVLAILGNVLVCWAVWLNSNLQNVTNYFVVSLAAADIA
A₂ᵦR    -----MLLETQDALYVALELVIAALSVAGNVLVCAAVGTANTLQTPTNYFLVSLAAADVA
                .  *: :*: *.  :: *****  .*     *:  *   *:**** **:*

A₃AR    VGVLVMPLAIVVSLGITIHFYSCLFMTCLLLIFTHASIMSLLAIAVDRYLRVKLTVRYKR
A₁AR    VGALVIPLAILINIGPQTYFHTCLMVACPVLILTQSSILALLAIAVDRYLRVKIPLRYKM
A₂ₐR    VGVLAIPFAITISTGFCAACHGCLFIACFVLVLTQSSIFSLLAIAIDRYIAIRIPLRYNG
A₂ᵦR    VGLFAIPFAITISLGFCTDFYGCLFLACFVLVLTQSSIFSLLAVAVDRYLAICVPLRYKS
        **  :.:*:** :. *     : **::* :*::*::**:.****:.***. : : :**:

A₃AR    VTTHRRIWLALGLCWLVSFLVGLTPMFGWNMKLTSEYH-------------RNVTFLSCQ
A₁AR    VVTPRRAAVAIAGCWILSFVVGLTPMFGWNNLSAVER----AWA---ANGSMGEPVIKCE
A₂ₐR    LVTGTRAKGIIAICWVLSFAIGLTPMLGWNN-------CGQPKEGKNHSQGCGEGQVACL
A₂ᵦR    LVTGTRARGVIAVLWVLAFGIGLTPFLGWNSKDSATNNCTEPWDGTTNESCC---LVKCL
        :.* *    :.  *::* :****::***                        : *

A₃AR    FVSVMRMDYMVYFSFLTWIFIPLVVMCAIYLDIFYIIRNKLSLNLSN---SKETGAFYGR
A₁AR    FEKVISMEYMVYFNFFVWVLPPLLLMVLIYLEVFYLIRKQLNKKVSAS--SGDPQKYYGK
A₂ₐR    FEDVVPMNYMVYFNFFACVLVPLLLMLGVYLRIFLAARRQLKQMESQPLPGERARSTLQK
A₂ᵦR    FENVVPMSYMVYFNFFGCVLPPLLIMLVIYIKIFLVACRQLQRTEL----MDHSRTTLQR
        * .*: *.*****.*:  ::  **::*    :*: :*    ..:*.             :

A₃AR    EFKTAKSLFLVLFLFALSWLPLSIINCIIYFNG----EVPQLVLYMGILLSHANSMMNPI
A₁AR    ELKIAKSLALILFLFALSWLPLHILNCITLFCPSC--HKPSILTYIAIFLTHGNSAMNPI
A₂ₐR    EVHAAKSLAIIVGLFALCWLPLHIINCFTFFCPDC-SHAPLWLMYLAIVLSHTNSVVNPF
A₂ᵦR    EIHAAKSLAMIVGIFALCWLPVHAVNCVTLFQPAQGKNKPKWAMNMAILLSHANSVVNPI
        *.: **** ::: :***.***:  :**.  *      . *     :.*.*:* ** :**:

A₃AR    VYAYKIKKFKETYLLILKACVVCHPSDSLDTSIEKNSE--------------------
A₁AR    VYAFRIQKFRVTFLKIWNDHFRCQPAPPIDEDLPEE--------------------
A₂ₐR    IYAYRIREFRQTFRKIIRSHVLRQQEPFKAAGTSARVLAAHGSDGEQVSLRLNGHPPGVW
A₂ᵦR    VYAYRNRDFRYTFHKIISRYLLCQADVKSGNGQ----------AGVQPALGVGL------
        :**:: :.*: *:  *    .  . :   .

A₃AR    --------------------------------------------------------
A₁AR    ----------RPDD------------------------------------------
A₂ₐR    ANGSAPHPERRPNGYALGLVSGGSAQESQGNTGLPDVELLSHELKGVCPEPPGLDDPLAQ
A₂ᵦR    --------------------------------------------------------

A₃AR    ------
A₁AR    ------
A₂ₐR    DGAGVS
A₂ᵦR    ------
```

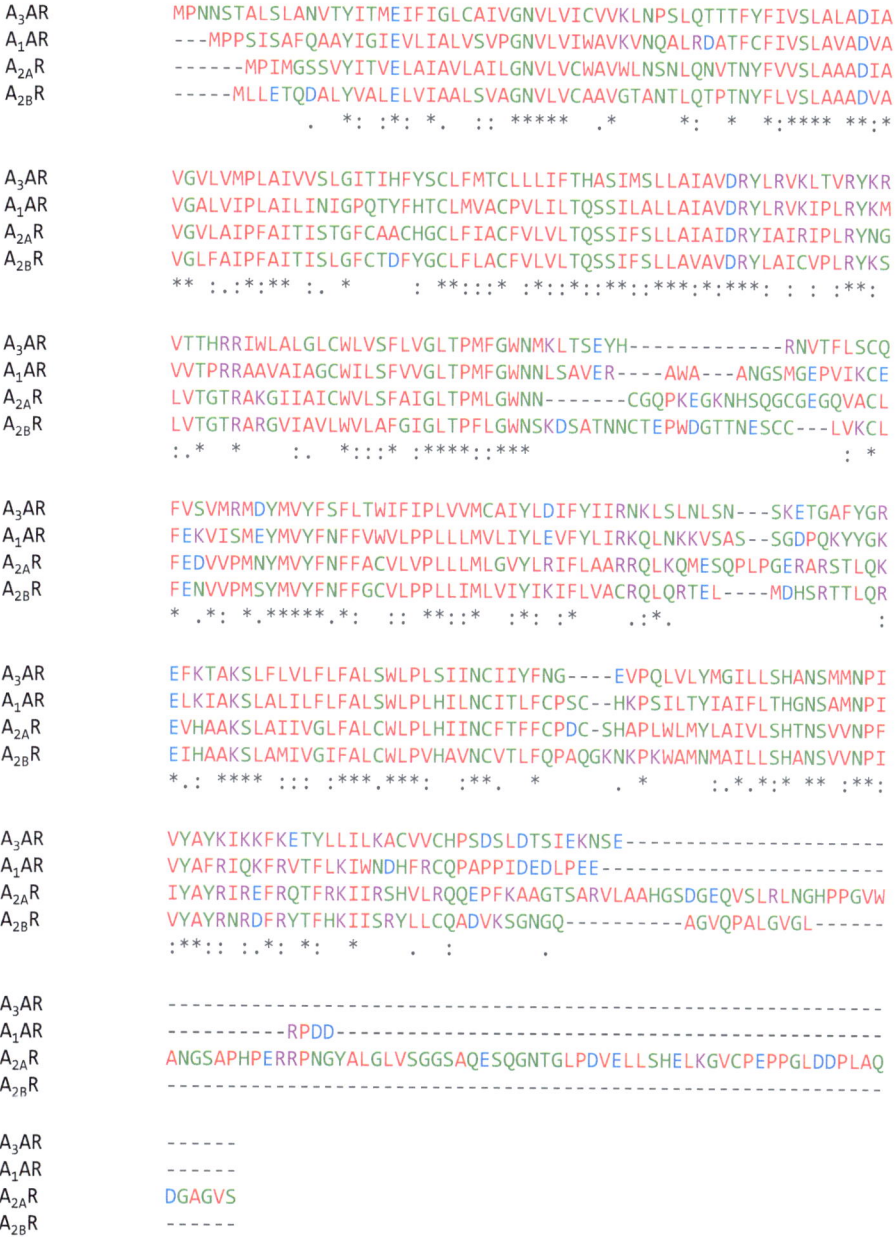

Fig. (10). Structural Alignment of Four Adenosine Receptors, A₁ᵣ, A₂ₐ, A₂ᵦ and A₃. Similar amino acids in the sequences are denoted by stars. Multiple sequence alignment was done with Clustal Omega.

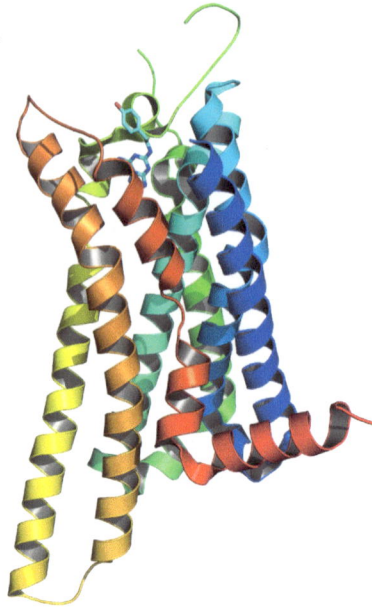

Fig. (11). Structure of the $A_{2A}AR$ Crystal with the Endogenous Agonist Adenosine (PDB ID: 2YDO).

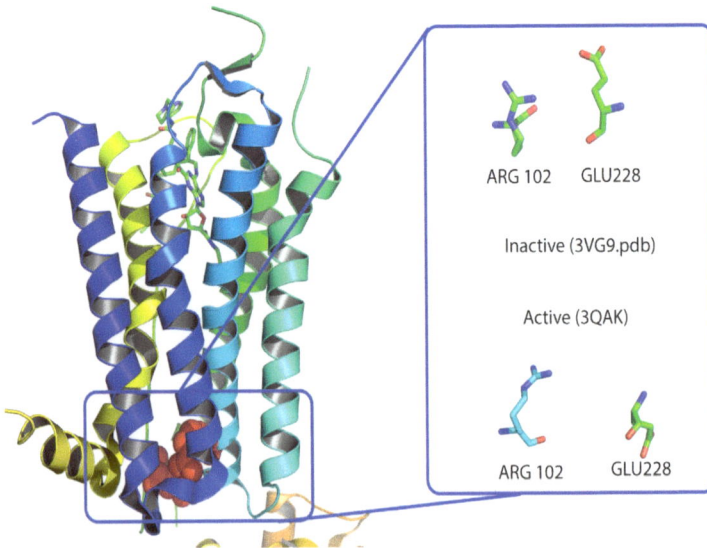

Fig. (12). $A_{2A}AR$ Structure in the Active (silver) and Inactive (green) Conformations. The agonist/antagonist structures are shown in atomic colors. Red spheres denote the position of the amino acids which play a role in the open and closed states during receptor signaling.

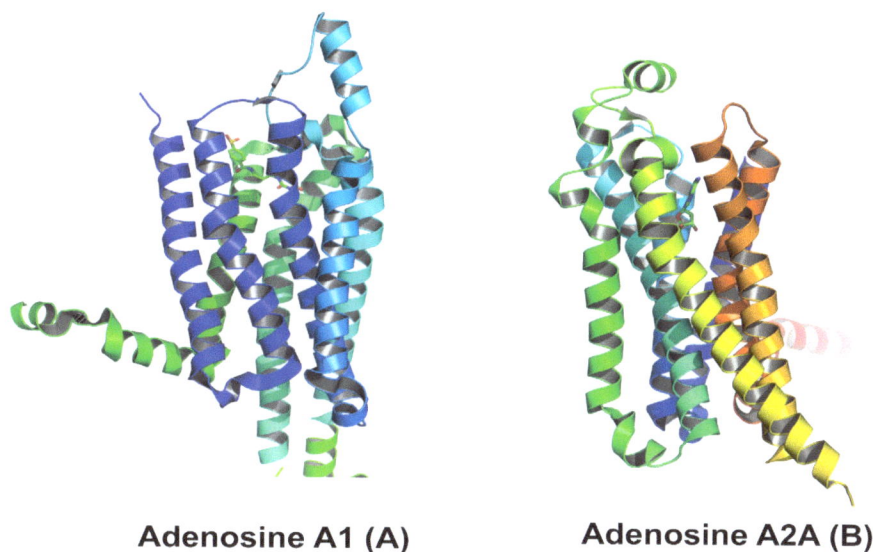

Adenosine A1 (A)   **Adenosine A2A (B)**

Fig. (13). Structure of the **A)** Adenosine A_1 receptor (left, 5uen.pdb) and **B)** Adenosine A_{2A} (right, 2ydo.pdb). The significant difference in pharmacology is speculated due to conformational differences in the binding pockets, in contrast to the differences in amino acid sequences [1].

Advancement in Developing New Adenosine Receptors Ligands

Currently, the approved clinical indications of adenosine include diagnostic imaging and supraventricular tachyarrhythmia, where intravenous adenosine is indicated for myocardial perfusion imaging in patients unable to exercise adequately [27]. Dipyridamole is also used in cardiac imaging by virtue of its nonselective activation of adenosine receptors [203]. Two A_{2A}AR-agonists, regadenoson and istradefylline, are approved for clinical use (see below). Clearly, there is a limited number of clinically available drugs targeting the adenosinergic system, which will be discussed later in the chapter. Here we will discuss and update the development progress of potent ARs ligands for the potential management of cardiovascular diseases.

A_{2A}AR Ligands

The nonselective activation of adenosine receptors by adenosine and dipyridamole is the reason behind the potentially serious side effects they may cause, including AV-block and bronchospasm [203]. In contrast, the relatively selective A_{2A}AR-agonist, regadenoson (Lexican®), is indicated for myocardial perfusion imaging and preferred over adenosine and dipyridamole because of a better safety profile [203]. While regadenoson is FDA-approved, the other selective A_{2A}AR-agonist, istradefylline, was denied FDA approval in 2008, but is approved in Japan for the treatment of Parkinson's disease [156]. Although there are structural similarities between regadenoson, CGS 21680, binodenoson, and apadenoson, the uniqueness of the pharmacological features of regadenoson makes it very successful in clinical use as stress agent. Regadenoson is potent, highly selective, and low-affinity agonist of $A_{2A}AR$ [204, 205] (Fig. **14A**, Table **3**). Regadenoson is potent, highly selective, and low-affinity agonist of $A_{2A}AR$ [204, 205] (Fig.**14A**, Table **3**). Regadenoson is highly selective to $A_{2A}AR$ (9 times selective) among other agonsts [203]. Once regadenoson binds to $A_{2A}AR$, it becomes for a short time (between 2-5 minutes), but enough for radionuclide intake and MPI procedure [203, 205]. Therefore, it induces coronary vasodilation and increases coronary blood flow (CBF) with resultant maximal hyperemia, which lasts for short duration [204, 205]. Binodenoson and apadenoson were investigated for the same indication, myocardial perfusion imaging, but were not approved by the FDA [112, 206] (Fig. **14A**). In a recent work by Fuentes *et al., in vitro* evaluation of new selective $A_{2A}AR$-agonists with antiplatelet activity, such as PSB 15826, PSB 12404, and PSB 16301, is in progress [207] (Fig. **14B**). Among those agonists, PSB 15826, is a highly potent inhibitor (EC_{50} 0.32 ± 0.05 μmol/L). Moreover, in comparison with CGS 21680 (EC_{50} 0.97 ± 0.07 μmol/L), this particular agonist was more active in preventing platelet aggregation, but it was comparable to NECA (EC_{50} 0.31 ± 0.05 μmol/L) [207]. The structural modifications among CGS 21680 and PBS derivatives will provide a framework that could lead to discovering more potent, and selective $A_{2A}AR$ agonists for antiplatelet aggregation. Bharate *et al.,* reported 7-(prolinol-Nyl)-2-phenylamino-thiazolo[5,4-d]pyrimidinesa as non-nucleoside A_{2A} partial agonists [208] (Fig. **14C**, Table **3**). This particular class was discovered *via* molecular modeling which proposed that the (*S*)-- -hydroxymethylene could resemble the ribose interaction in the binding site [208]. The binding affinity and selectivity were confirmed by functional assays [208] that indicates a potential lead for selective agonist of this class.

Table 3. Binding Interactions of $A_{2A}ARs$ Agonists.

Compound name	K_i (nM)			
	A_1	A_{2A}	A_{2B}	A_3
Regadenoson	>10,000 (h)[a]	290 (h)[a]	>10,000 (h)[a]	>10,000 (h)[a]
Binodenoson	48,000 (h)[a]	270 (h)[a]	430,000 (h)[a]	903 (h)[a]
Apadenoson	77 (h)[a]	0.5 (h)[a]	N.D	45 (h)[a]
38	974 (h)[b]	330 (h) [b]	N.D	1460 (h) [b]
39	555 (h) [b]	200 (h) [b]	N.D	978 (h) [b]
40	530 (h) [b]	153 (h) [b]	N.D	1070 (h) [b]

[a] Klotz *et al.*, 1998 [148].
[b] Bharate *et al.,* 2016 [208]

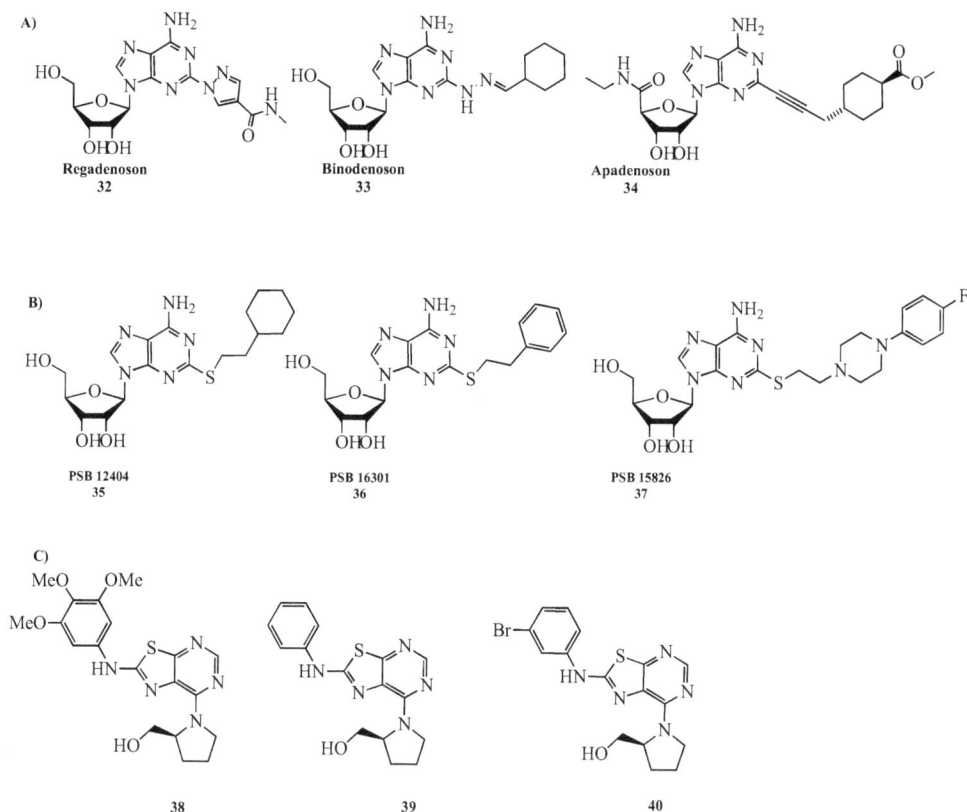

Fig. (14). Structures of $A_{2A}AR$ Agonists. **A)** Selective $A_{2A}AR$ agonists that reached clinical trials, **B)** $A_{2A}AR$ agonists with antiplatelet activity, and **C)** Non-nucleoside partial $A_{2A}AR$ agonists.

A_1AR Ligands

Adenosine's efficacy in terminating supraventricular tachyarrhythmia is due to activation of its A_1AR [27]. However, to avoid the potential for hypotensive and bronchoconstrictive side effects of adenosine through its effect on the other adenosine receptors, selective A_1AR-agonists have been developed, but none has reached clinical use yet [27]. Tecadenoson (CVT 510), a selective A_1AR-agonist, was synthesized for paroxysmal supraventricular tachycardia (PSVT), atrial flutter, and atrial fibrillation (AF) [209] (Fig. **15A**). Compared to adenosine, Tecadenoson, at low doses of tecadenoson, has minimal effect on blood pressure and AV nodal conduction [209], whereas at higher doses, it can cause AV block. Another A_1AR-agonist, selodenoson, has completed Phase II clinical trials for AF, was not associated with hypotension [110, 206] (Fig. **15A**, Table **4**).

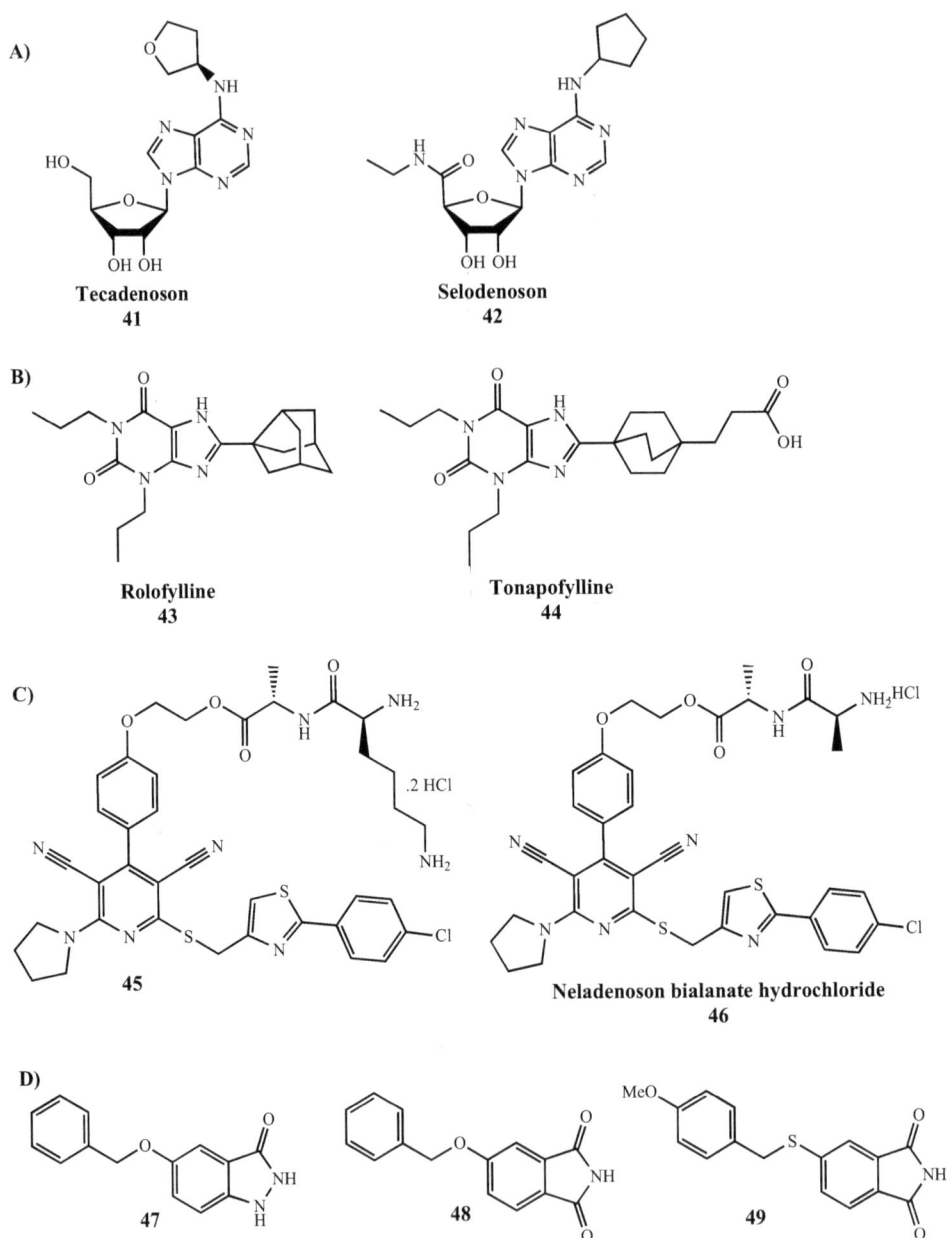

Fig. (15). Structues of A$_1$AR Ligands. **A**) Selective A$_1$AR agonists that reached clinical trials, **B**) A$_1$AR antagonist that failed in clinical trials, **C**) Prodrug of partial A$_1$AR agonist, and **D**) Sulfanylphthalimide analogs as dual antagonist for ARs and MOA.

Table 4. Binding Interactions of A_1ARs Ligands

Compound name	K_i (nM)			
	A_1	**A_{2A}**	**A_{2B}**	**A_3**
Tecadenoson	6.5 (p)[a]	2315 (h)[a]	N.D.	N.D.
Selodenoson	N.D.	N.D.	N.D.	N.D.
Rolofylline	0.72 (h)[b]	108 (h) [b]	296 (h) [b]	4390 (h) [b]
Tonapofylline	7.4 (h)	6,410 (h)	90 (h)	>10,000 (h)
47	9,790 (h) [c]	No affinity (h) [c]	N.D	N.D
48	4,670 (h) [c]	No affinity (h) [c]	N.D	N.D
49	369 (h) [c]	>100μM (h) [c]	N.D	N.D
50	1620 (h) [d]	2910 (h) [d]	N.D	1.8 (h)
51	480 (h) [d]	1080 (h) [d]	N.D	0.57 (h)

[a] Klotz *et al.*, 1998 [148].
[b] Chaparro *et al.*, 2008 [210].
[c] Van der Walt *et al.*, 2015 [216]
[d] Yu *et al.*, 2017 [217]

Rolofylline is an A_1AR-antagonist with a novel mechanism for congestive heart failure [112, 210] (Fig. **15B**, Table **4**). Congestive heart failure is associated with worsening in the renal function [211]. In renal dysfunction, adenosine production is increased [112]. Therefore, rolofylline was designed to enhance renal function [112] and to decrease the risk of renal failure [212]. Rolofylline's mechanism of action is byblocking A_1AR, which inhibits sodium reabsorption from the proximal tubule and enhances the blood flow and glomerular filtration leading to increased diuresis and natriuresis [210]. The antagonist as a new class for acute and chronic heart failure was very promising in early phases of clinical trials. Unfortunately, in Phase III trials, rolofylline failed to protect from persistent worsening of renal impairment and the results were disappointing [211].

Capadenoson, a non-nucleoside known by dicyanopyridine class, is a potent, selective partial A_1AR-agonist, and has acceptable metabolic and pharmacokinetic studies [213] (Fig. **2B**). In Phase II clinical trial, the total exercise time in patients with stable angina pectoris using capadenoson was improved without inducing AV block [121]. Moreover, this candidate drug had many beneficial effects, such as reduction of the infarct size in induced acute myocardial infarction in rodent model [214]. In addition, in a canine heart failure model, capadenoson enhanced left ventricular (LF) ejection fraction without adversely affecting the heart rate or blood pressure [215]. Unfortunately, capadenoson exerts some central side effects, such as dizziness and vertigo [121]. It also had low solubility and could not be used orally [121]. Therefore, Meibom *et al.* developed neladenoson bialanate hydrochloride (Fig. **15C**, Table **4**), a prodrug to overcome the solubility problem and has no cardiac AV blocks nor central effects such as sedative effects [213]. The addition of dipeptide ester group improved the solubility of the drug, more partial selective A_1AR agonist, and it is now in clinical trials for HF treatment [213].

Sulfanylphthalimide analogs were reported by Van der Walt that have dual antagonist effect on ARs (A_1 and A_{2A} subtypes) and monoamine oxidase (MAO) B [216]. Among these derivatives, 5-[(4-methoxybenzyl) sulfanyl]phthalimide was more selective for A_1AR than $A_{2A}AR$ and exerted inhibitory activity on MOA-B (Fig. **15D**, Table **4**) [216]. Considering the sulfanylphthalimides as lead molecule, it is likely to have potential for developing a new class with potent and selective A_1AR antagonists.

A_3AR Ligands

Most of ARs nucleoside agonists class have the ribose structure, which is also known as 4′-oxonucleosides. The concept of introducing new class such as 4′-selenonucleosides was started a decade ago [218]. Since then, the progress of developing and implementing this class in biological studies were successful that known as bioisostere [219]. Bioisostere is replacing a particular atom by another atom or an atom that have similar valiancy and biological activity. For instance, replacing the oxygen by selenium has solved a few problems, such as conformational dissimilarity of 4′-oxo-, 4′-thio-, and 4′-carbanucleosides, resistance, toxicity, chemical, and metabolic stability that occurred in the 4′-oxonucleosides [219]. In recent study by Yu *et al.*, they used 4′-selenonucleoside as a new class generation for A_3AR [217]. Among the 4′-selenonucleoside derivatives, compound **51**, was potent A_3AR-agonist and less selectivity to other ARs subtypes and three folds higher binding affinity than 4′-oxonucleosides **50** [217] (Fig. **16**, Table **4**). The study of the 4′-selenonucleoside analog is an indication of potential new class for developing selective A_3AR agonists and could be potential for other ARs subtypes with new scaffold.

Most of the drugs that reviewed above are have either failed in clinical trials or are still being investigated in clinical trials. However, undoubtedly drug discovery on adenosine and ARs is still ongoing.

Dual AR Ligands

In a recent work by Robinson group, they investigated the 2-aminopyrimidine derivatives as potential dual antagonists for A_1AR and $A_{2A}AR$ for motor disabilities improvements such as PD (2015 4,38-43). Among this series, compound **52** (4-(5-Methylfuran-2-yl)-6-[3-(piperidine-1-carbonyl)phenyl] pyrimidin-2-amine) had high affinity for both A_1AR and $A_{2A}AR$ (Fig. **17**). Moreover, *in vitro* studies, this compound had low toxicity profile and attenuated the catalepsy induced by haloperidol in an animal study on rats. This dual ARs antagonists could be promising for targeting the cardiovascular system, where both A_1AR and $A_{2A}AR$ have many physiologic effects.

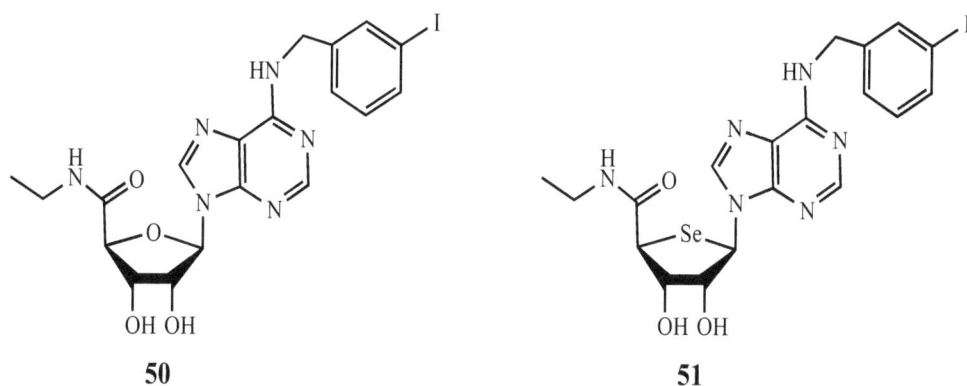

50   **51**

Fig. (16). Structures of A_3AR agonists, 4'-oxonucleosides (**50**) and 4'-selenonucleoside (**51**).

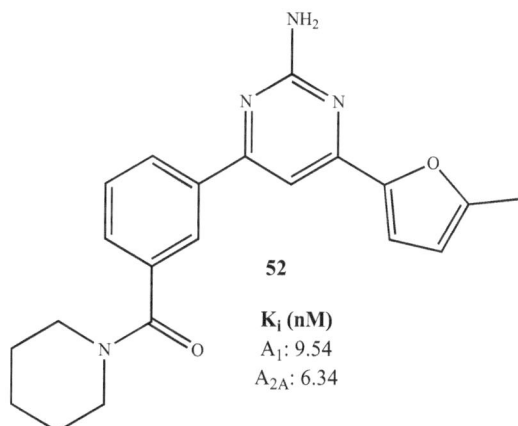

52

K_i (nM)
A_1: 9.54
A_{2A}: 6.34

Fig. (17). Structure of a dual antagonist of A_1AR and $A_{2A}AR$.

Challenges for the Therapeutic Application of the Adenosinergic System

As mentioned above, despite the fact that adenosine has been known and investigated for several decades, its clinical usefulness is comparatively limited with a few drugs whose mechanisms of action involve adenosine or its receptor including dipyridamole, regadenoson, istradefylline, and adenosine itself. This section discusses the challenges which hurdle the endeavor to find therapeutic applications for adenosine and adenosine receptors.

Receptor Distribution: the omnipresent nature of adenosine, are the extensive distribution of its receptors are probably the prime factors behind the limited clinical applicability for the adenosinergic system. For example, the discovery of the CGS 21680 between the late 1960s and 1970s, gave hope to developing an antihypertensive drug, but due to the non-selectivity *in vivo* experiments, the clinical studies were cancelled [110].

Adenosine's Pharmacokinetics: Adenosine's half-life is very short as it is rapidly degraded inside neighboring cells, especially circulating erythrocytes [220]. Intravenously administered adenosine cannot reach the interstitial space as the endothelial layer metabolizes it [221] on one hand, and IV adenosine would have serious adverse hemodynamic effects [222]. More focused application of adenosine, such as intracoronary administration, is considered for evaluating its effect in myocardial reperfusion to limit its systemic side effects.

Receptor Expression: The expression of adenosine receptors changes under some pathologic conditions as reported for $A_{2A}AR$ in Huntington disease [223], however, little is known about such changes in other disease states [112]. This is important to know as it would guide researchers to which adenosine receptors to be targeted for evaluation of the outcome of an intervention. Studies using *in vivo* imaging methods, such as positron emission tomography (PET) ligands, represent a useful and reliable method to measure receptor expression and distribution, and can potentially shed more light on how adenosine receptors' distribution may change in pathologic conditions [112].

Receptor Desensitization: Repeated or prolonged exposure to adenosine receptors ligands results in tolerance or desensitization, which is another issue. Receptor desensitization is defined as the limited or reduced ability of a ligand to binds to a receptor. In other words, the capacity to produce a cellular effect is dramatically reduced. This was observed with A_1AR-agonists and antagonists [224], and $A_{2A}AR$-agonists [225]. A study in rodents demonstrated that the acute administration of A_1AR-agonists has a preventive effect in brain injury, whereas their chronic administration aggravates ischemic brain injury [224, 226, 227]. In cultured cells, chronic $A_{2A}AR$-agonists treatment developed receptor desensitization. This desensitization or receptor internalization were not observed for $A_{2A}AR$-antagonists [228]. The underlying mechanism behind receptor desensitization is receptor internalization through coupling of α-actinin cross-linking protein to the carboxyl terminus of the receptor [225, 229]. Receptor desensitization is particularly important in cardiovascular diseases, which require chronic management plans.

One Tissue, Multiple Effects: Also, studies on tissues in the central nervous system revealed that adenosine, when acting on the same receptor, induces different effects in different cells of the same tissue [112], and that adenosine's effects are different in developing *versus* mature individuals [230, 231]. Whether or not these differences in adenosine's effects exist in the CV system is not known yet.

Receptor Dimerization: as mentioned above, adenosine receptors, like other GPCRs, are reported to dimerize to make hetero-, homo-, or oligodimers such as $A_{2A}AR$–dopamine D_2, $A_{2A}AR$–$A_{2B}AR$, and $A_{2A}AR$–A_1AR [112]. The extent and impact of this phenomenon on the CV function or pathology is not known. Also, the possibility of receptor dimerization challenges any conclusion of an outcome of an adenosine receptor ligand, unless dimerization is ruled out or its impact could be neglected.

Caffeine: The methylxanthine caffeine is widely consumed through drinking beverages, such as coffee, tea, and soda drinks [232]. At the regular doses people consume, caffeine's stimulant effect is partly attributed to antagonizing 25-50% of adenosine's effects at its $A_{2A}AR$ and A_1AR [233]. Moreover, caffeine's metabolites, paraxanthine and theophylline, are even more potent as adenosine inhibitors than caffeine [234]. Interaction of caffeine (in recently ingested two to four cups of coffee) with $A_{2A}AR$-agonists was confirmed by PK/PD analyses and affected the myocardial perfusion imaging [235]. Therefore, the consumption of caffeine-containing products should be taken into account when interpreting results of studies evaluating adenosine's ligands, which is yet another burden to consider when carrying out such studies.

Specific Issues: By the discovery of istradefylline, the 8-styrylxanthines derivatives have become very promising to develop very potent $A_{2A}AR$-antagonists. Unfortunately, due to the physicochemical properties, such as photosensitivity and poor water solubility, the development of these derivatives was remarkably obstructed [139, 236]. Moreover, the synthesis of 8-styrylxanthines derivatives poses challenges since they must be synthesized in light-restricted area to avoid cyclodimerization [158]. Also, since adenosine-agonists are mostly based on the scaffold of adenosine structure, the progress to develop new agonists is hampered by the limited possible modifications on this structure, as mentioned above.

FUTURE PERSPECTIVE

Our understanding of the biology of the adenosinergic system has tremendously increased over the years. Thanks to the advancement in experimental techniques, the effects of adenosine in physiology and pathology, in different tissues and organs, and in different species are better comprehended. This comes with more appreciation of the complexity of these effects. Still, the breadth and width of our understanding of the adenosinergic system has created even more unanswered questions. Several areas pertaining to this system still require further and more focused investigation. To mention few: the impact of AR dimerization, AR desensitization, AR expression change at different stages and pathologies, and AR interaction in the same organ or tissue. The discipline of medicinal chemistry is adding to our endeavor to translate all the knowledge we have accumulated so far into synthesizing better candidates for therapeutic applications in CVD through selective and may be tissue- or cell-specific adenosine ligands. We believe that adenosine and its receptors will remain a viable field for testing and evaluating potential drugs in many disease areas, including the CVDs.

CONSENT FOR PUBLICATION

Not applicable.

CONFLICT OF INTEREST

The author (editor) declares no conflict of interest, financial or otherwise.

ACKNOWLEDGEMENTS

This work was supported by National Institutes of Health (HL-114559) to M. A. Nayeem.

REFERENCES

[1] Sheth S, Brito R, Mukherjea D, Rybak LP, Ramkumar V. Adenosine receptors: expression, function and regulation. Int J Mol Sci 2014; 15(2): 2024-52.
[http://dx.doi.org/10.3390/ijms15022024] [PMID: 24477263]

[2] Zhou Y, Schneider DJ, Blackburn MR. Adenosine signaling and the regulation of chronic lung disease. Pharmacol Ther 2009; 123(1): 105-16.
[http://dx.doi.org/10.1016/j.pharmthera.2009.04.003] [PMID: 19426761]

[3] Headrick JP, Ashton KJ, Rose'meyer RB, Peart JN. Cardiovascular adenosine receptors: expression, actions and interactions. Pharmacol Ther 2013; 140(1): 92-111.
[http://dx.doi.org/10.1016/j.pharmthera.2013.06.002] [PMID: 23764371]

[4] de Mendonça A, Ribeiro JA. Adenosine and neuronal plasticity. Life Sci 1997; 60(4-5): 245-51.
[http://dx.doi.org/10.1016/S0024-3205(96)00544-9] [PMID: 9010479]

[5] Cunha RA. Adenosine as a neuromodulator and as a homeostatic regulator in the nervous system: different roles, different sources and different receptors. Neurochem Int 2001; 38(2): 107-25.
[http://dx.doi.org/10.1016/S0197-0186(00)00034-6] [PMID: 11137880]

[6] Sebastião AM, Ribeiro JA. Fine-tuning neuromodulation by adenosine. Trends Pharmacol Sci 2000; 21(9): 341-6.
[http://dx.doi.org/10.1016/S0165-6147(00)01517-0] [PMID: 10973087]

[7] Olsson RA, Pearson JD. Cardiovascular purinoceptors. Physiol Rev 1990; 70(3): 761-845.

[http://dx.doi.org/10.1152/physrev.1990.70.3.761] [PMID: 2194223]

[8]   Carroll MA, Doumad AB, Li J, Cheng MK, Falck JR, McGiff JC. Adenosine2A receptor vasodilation of rat preglomerular microvessels is mediated by EETs that activate the cAMP/PKA pathway. Am J Physiol Renal Physiol 2006; 291(1): F155-61.
[http://dx.doi.org/10.1152/ajprenal.00231.2005] [PMID: 16478979]

[9]   Feng MG, Navar LG. Afferent arteriolar vasodilator effect of adenosine predominantly involves adenosine A2B receptor activation. Am J Physiol Renal Physiol 2010; 299(2): F310-5.
[http://dx.doi.org/10.1152/ajprenal.00149.2010] [PMID: 20462966]

[10]   Hein TW, Belardinelli L, Kuo L, Adenosine A. Adenosine A(2A) receptors mediate coronary microvascular dilation to adenosine: role of nitric oxide and ATP-sensitive potassium channels. J Pharmacol Exp Ther 1999; 291(2): 655-64.
[PMID: 10525085]

[11]   Nayeem MA, Poloyac SM, Falck JR, *et al.* Role of CYP epoxygenases in A2A AR-mediated relaxation using A2A AR-null and wild-type mice. Am J Physiol Heart Circ Physiol 2008; 295(5): H2068-78.
[http://dx.doi.org/10.1152/ajpheart.01333.2007] [PMID: 18805895]

[12]   Nayeem MA, Ponnoth DS, Boegehold MA, Zeldin DC, Falck JR, Mustafa SJ. High-salt diet enhances mouse aortic relaxation through adenosine A2A receptor *via* CYP epoxygenases. Am J Physiol Regul Integr Comp Physiol 2009; 296(3): R567-74.
[http://dx.doi.org/10.1152/ajpregu.90798.2008] [PMID: 19109366]

[13]   Rivkees SA, Wendler CC. Regulation of cardiovascular development by adenosine and adenosine-mediated embryo protection. Arterioscler Thromb Vasc Biol 2012; 32(4): 851-5.
[http://dx.doi.org/10.1161/ATVBAHA.111.226811] [PMID: 22423036]

[14]   Fredholm BB, IJzerman AP, Jacobson KA, Linden J, Müller CE. International Union of Basic and Clinical Pharmacology. LXXXI. Nomenclature and classification of adenosine receptors--an update. Pharmacol Rev 2011; 63(1): 1-34.
[http://dx.doi.org/10.1124/pr.110.003285] [PMID: 21303899]

[15]   Schubert P, Komp W, Kreutzberg GW. Correlation of 5'-nucleotidase activity and selective transneuronal transfer of adenosine in the hippocampus. Brain Res 1979; 168(2): 419-24.
[http://dx.doi.org/10.1016/0006-8993(79)90186-0] [PMID: 87245]

[16]   Broch OJ, Ueland PM. Regional and subcellular distribution of S-adenosylhomocysteine hydrolase in the adult rat brain. J Neurochem 1980; 35(2): 484-8.
[http://dx.doi.org/10.1111/j.1471-4159.1980.tb06291.x] [PMID: 7452268]

[17]   Ueland PM. Pharmacological and biochemical aspects of S-adenosylhomocysteine and S-adenosylhomocysteine hydrolase. Pharmacol Rev 1982; 34(3): 223-53.
[PMID: 6760211]

[18]   Dunwiddie TV, Diao L, Proctor WR. Adenine nucleotides undergo rapid, quantitative conversion to adenosine in the extracellular space in rat hippocampus. J Neurosci 1997; 17(20): 7673-82.
[PMID: 9315889]

[19]   Baldwin SA, Beal PR, Yao SY, King AE, Cass CE, Young JD. The equilibrative nucleoside transporter family, SLC29. Pflugers Arch 2004; 447(5): 735-43.
[http://dx.doi.org/10.1007/s00424-003-1103-2] [PMID: 12838422]

[20]   Lloyd HG, Lindström K, Fredholm BB. Intracellular formation and release of adenosine from rat hippocampal slices evoked by electrical stimulation or energy depletion. Neurochem Int 1993; 23(2): 173-85.
[http://dx.doi.org/10.1016/0197-0186(93)90095-M] [PMID: 8369741]

[21]   Zetterström T, Vernet L, Ungerstedt U, Tossman U, Jonzon B, Fredholm BB. Purine levels in the intact rat brain. Studies with an implanted perfused hollow fibre. Neurosci Lett 1982; 29(2): 111-5.

[http://dx.doi.org/10.1016/0304-3940(82)90338-X] [PMID: 7088412]

[22]   Rudolphi KA, Schubert P, Parkinson FE, Fredholm BB. Adenosine and brain ischemia. Cerebrovasc Brain Metab Rev 1992; 4(4): 346-69.
[PMID: 1486019]

[23]   Spychala J, Datta NS, Takabayashi K, *et al.* Cloning of human adenosine kinase cDNA: sequence similarity to microbial ribokinases and fructokinases. Proc Natl Acad Sci USA 1996; 93(3): 1232-7.
[http://dx.doi.org/10.1073/pnas.93.3.1232] [PMID: 8577746]

[24]   Lloyd HG, Fredholm BB. Involvement of adenosine deaminase and adenosine kinase in regulating extracellular adenosine concentration in rat hippocampal slices. Neurochem Int 1995; 26(4): 387-95.
[http://dx.doi.org/10.1016/0197-0186(94)00144-J] [PMID: 7633332]

[25]   Sousa R, Serrano P, Gomes Dias J, Oliveira JC, Oliveira A. Improving the accuracy of synovial fluid analysis in the diagnosis of prosthetic joint infection with simple and inexpensive biomarkers: C-reactive protein and adenosine deaminase. The Bone & Joint Journal 2017; 99-b: 351-7.

[26]   Arslan G, Kull B, Fredholm BB. Signaling *via* A2A adenosine receptor in four PC12 cell clones. Naunyn Schmiedebergs Arch Pharmacol 1999; 359(1): 28-32.
[http://dx.doi.org/10.1007/PL00005319] [PMID: 9933147]

[27]   Riksen NP, Rongen GA. Targeting adenosine receptors in the development of cardiovascular therapeutics. Expert Rev Clin Pharmacol 2012; 5(2): 199-218.
[http://dx.doi.org/10.1586/ecp.12.8] [PMID: 22390562]

[28]   Swanson TH, Drazba JA, Rivkees SA. Adenosine A1 receptors are located predominantly on axons in the rat hippocampal formation. J Comp Neurol 1995; 363(4): 517-31.
[http://dx.doi.org/10.1002/cne.903630402] [PMID: 8847415]

[29]   McIntosh VJ, Lasley RD. Adenosine receptor-mediated cardioprotection: are all 4 subtypes required or redundant? J Cardiovasc Pharmacol Ther 2012; 17(1): 21-33.
[http://dx.doi.org/10.1177/1074248410396877] [PMID: 21335481]

[30]   Othman T, Yan H, Rivkees SA. Oligodendrocytes express functional A1 adenosine receptors that stimulate cellular migration. Glia 2003; 44(2): 166-72.
[http://dx.doi.org/10.1002/glia.10281] [PMID: 14515332]

[31]   Gebicke-Haerter PJ, Christoffel F, Timmer J, Northoff H, Berger M, Van Calker D. Both adenosine A1- and A2-receptors are required to stimulate microglial proliferation. Neurochem Int 1996; 29(1): 37-42.
[http://dx.doi.org/10.1016/0197-0186(95)00137-9] [PMID: 8808787]

[32]   Biber K, Klotz KN, Berger M, Gebicke-Härter PJ, van Calker D. Adenosine A1 receptor-mediated activation of phospholipase C in cultured astrocytes depends on the level of receptor expression. J Neurosci 1997; 17(13): 4956-64.
[PMID: 9185533]

[33]   Linden J. Structure and function of A1 adenosine receptors. FASEB J 1991; 5(12): 2668-76.
[PMID: 1916091]

[34]   Hansen PB, Schnermann J. Vasoconstrictor and vasodilator effects of adenosine in the kidney. Am J Physiol Renal Physiol 2003; 285(4): F590-9.
[http://dx.doi.org/10.1152/ajprenal.00051.2003] [PMID: 12954591]

[35]   Sebastião AM, Ribeiro JA. Adenosine A2 receptor-mediated excitatory actions on the nervous system. Prog Neurobiol 1996; 48(3): 167-89.
[http://dx.doi.org/10.1016/0301-0082(95)00035-6] [PMID: 8735876]

[36]   Li Q, Puro DG. Adenosine activates ATP-sensitive K(+) currents in pericytes of rat retinal microvessels: role of A1 and A2a receptors. Brain Res 2001; 907(1-2): 93-9.
[http://dx.doi.org/10.1016/S0006-8993(01)02607-5] [PMID: 11430889]

[37]   Melani A, Cipriani S, Vannucchi MG, *et al.* Selective adenosine A2a receptor antagonism reduces JNK activation in oligodendrocytes after cerebral ischaemia. Brain 2009; 132(Pt 6): 1480-95.
[http://dx.doi.org/10.1093/brain/awp076] [PMID: 19359287]

[38]   van Calker D, Müller M, Hamprecht B. Adenosine regulates *via* two different types of receptors, the accumulation of cyclic AMP in cultured brain cells. J Neurochem 1979; 33(5): 999-1005.
[http://dx.doi.org/10.1111/j.1471-4159.1979.tb05236.x] [PMID: 228008]

[39]   Abebe W, Makujina SR, Mustafa SJ. Adenosine receptor-mediated relaxation of porcine coronary artery in presence and absence of endothelium. Am J Physiol 1994; 266(5 Pt 2): H2018-25.
[PMID: 8203600]

[40]   Mustafa SJ, Askar AO. Evidence suggesting an Ra-type adenosine receptor in bovine coronary arteries. J Pharmacol Exp Ther 1985; 232(1): 49-56.
[PMID: 2981319]

[41]   Mustafa SJ, Morrison RR, Teng B, Pelleg A. Adenosine receptors and the heart: role in regulation of coronary blood flow and cardiac electrophysiology. Handb Exp Pharmacol 2009; (193): 161-88.
[http://dx.doi.org/10.1007/978-3-540-89615-9_6] [PMID: 19639282]

[42]   Ponnoth DS, Sanjani MS, Ledent C, Roush K, Krahn T, Mustafa SJ. Absence of adenosine-mediated aortic relaxation in A(2A) adenosine receptor knockout mice. Am J Physiol Heart Circ Physiol 2009; 297(5): H1655-60.
[http://dx.doi.org/10.1152/ajpheart.00192.2009] [PMID: 19749167]

[43]   Ralevic V, Burnstock G. Receptors for purines and pyrimidines. Pharmacol Rev 1998; 50(3): 413-92.
[PMID: 9755289]

[44]   Ramagopal MV, Chitwood RW Jr, Mustafa SJ. Evidence for an A2 adenosine receptor in human coronary arteries. Eur J Pharmacol 1988; 151(3): 483-6.
[http://dx.doi.org/10.1016/0014-2999(88)90548-1] [PMID: 3215272]

[45]   Ye D, Zhou W, Lu T, Jagadeesh SG, Falck JR, Lee HC. Mechanism of rat mesenteric arterial KATP channel activation by 14,15-epoxyeicosatrienoic acid. Am J Physiol Heart Circ Physiol 2006; 290(4): H1326-36.
[http://dx.doi.org/10.1152/ajpheart.00318.2005] [PMID: 16537788]

[46]   Hein TW, Yuan Z, Rosa RH Jr, Kuo L. Requisite roles of A2A receptors, nitric oxide, and KATP channels in retinal arteriolar dilation in response to adenosine. Invest Ophthalmol Vis Sci 2005; 46(6): 2113-9.
[http://dx.doi.org/10.1167/iovs.04-1438] [PMID: 15914631]

[47]   Kuo L, Chancellor JD. Adenosine potentiates flow-induced dilation of coronary arterioles by activating KATP channels in endothelium. Am J Physiol 1995; 269(2 Pt 2): H541-9.
[PMID: 7653618]

[48]   Mutafova-Yambolieva VN, Keef KD. Adenosine-induced hyperpolarization in guinea pig coronary artery involves A2b receptors and KATP channels. Am J Physiol 1997; 273(6 Pt 2): H2687-95.
[PMID: 9435605]

[49]   Arsyad A, Dobson GP. Adenosine relaxation in isolated rat aortic rings and possible roles of smooth muscle Kv channels, KATP channels and A2a receptors. BMC Pharmacol Toxicol 2016; 17(1): 23.
[http://dx.doi.org/10.1186/s40360-016-0067-8] [PMID: 27211886]

[50]   Ishibashi Y, Duncker DJ, Zhang J, Bache RJ. ATP-sensitive K+ channels, adenosine, and nitric oxide-mediated mechanisms account for coronary vasodilation during exercise. Circ Res 1998; 82(3): 346-59.
[http://dx.doi.org/10.1161/01.RES.82.3.346] [PMID: 9486663]

[51]   Fleming I. Cytochrome p450 and vascular homeostasis. Circ Res 2001; 89(9): 753-62.
[http://dx.doi.org/10.1161/hh2101.099268] [PMID: 11679404]

[52]   Harder DR, Campbell WB, Roman RJ. Role of cytochrome P-450 enzymes and metabolites of arachidonic acid in the control of vascular tone. J Vasc Res 1995; 32(2): 79-92.
       [http://dx.doi.org/10.1159/000159080] [PMID: 7537544]

[53]   Lapuerta L, Chacos N, Falck JR, Jacobson H, Capdevila JH. Renal microsomal cytochrome P-450 and the oxidative metabolism of arachidonic acid. Am J Med Sci 1988; 295(4): 275-9.
       [http://dx.doi.org/10.1097/00000441-198804000-00010] [PMID: 3364462]

[54]   Proctor KG, Falck JR, Capdevila J. Intestinal vasodilation by epoxyeicosatrienoic acids: arachidonic acid metabolites produced by a cytochrome P450 monooxygenase. Circ Res 1987; 60(1): 50-9.
       [http://dx.doi.org/10.1161/01.RES.60.1.50] [PMID: 3105909]

[55]   Ma YH, Harder DR, Clark JE, Roman RJ. Effects of 12-HETE on isolated dog renal arcuate arteries. Am J Physiol 1991; 261(2 Pt 2): H451-6.
       [PMID: 1908641]

[56]   Seger R, Krebs EG. The MAPK signaling cascade. FASEB J 1995; 9(9): 726-35.
       [http://dx.doi.org/10.1096/fasebj.9.9.7601337] [PMID: 7601337]

[57]   Faure M, Voyno-Yasenetskaya TA, Bourne HR. cAMP and beta gamma subunits of heterotrimeric G proteins stimulate the mitogen-activated protein kinase pathway in COS-7 cells. J Biol Chem 1994; 269(11): 7851-4.
       [PMID: 8132501]

[58]   Ponnoth DS, Nayeem MA, Tilley SL, Ledent C, Jamal Mustafa S. CYP-epoxygenases contribute to A2A receptor-mediated aortic relaxation *via* sarcolemmal KATP channels. Am J Physiol Regul Integr Comp Physiol 2012; 303(10): R1003-10.
       [http://dx.doi.org/10.1152/ajpregu.00335.2012] [PMID: 23019210]

[59]   Sexl V, Mancusi G, Höller C, Gloria-Maercker E, Schütz W, Freissmuth M. Stimulation of the mitogen-activated protein kinase *via* the A2A-adenosine receptor in primary human endothelial cells. J Biol Chem 1997; 272(9): 5792-9.
       [http://dx.doi.org/10.1074/jbc.272.9.5792] [PMID: 9038193]

[60]   Neary JT, McCarthy M, Kang Y, Zuniga S. Mitogenic signaling from P1 and P2 purinergic receptors to mitogen-activated protein kinase in human fetal astrocyte cultures. Neurosci Lett 1998; 242(3): 159-62.
       [http://dx.doi.org/10.1016/S0304-3940(98)00067-6] [PMID: 9530930]

[61]   Drury AN, Szent-Györgyi A. The physiological activity of adenine compounds with especial reference to their action upon the mammalian heart. J Physiol 1929; 68(3): 213-37.
       [http://dx.doi.org/10.1113/jphysiol.1929.sp002608] [PMID: 16994064]

[62]   Belardinelli L, Shryock JC, Song Y, Wang D, Srinivas M. Ionic basis of the electrophysiological actions of adenosine on cardiomyocytes. FASEB J 1995; 9(5): 359-65.
       [http://dx.doi.org/10.1096/fasebj.9.5.7896004] [PMID: 7896004]

[63]   Dobson JG Jr. Mechanism of adenosine inhibition of catecholamine-induced responses in heart. Circ Res 1983; 52(2): 151-60.
       [http://dx.doi.org/10.1161/01.RES.52.2.151] [PMID: 6297829]

[64]   Lorbar M, Chung ES, Nabi A, *et al.* Receptors subtypes involved in adenosine-mediated modulation of norepinephrine release from cardiac nerve terminals. Can J Physiol Pharmacol 2004; 82(11): 1026-31.
       [http://dx.doi.org/10.1139/y04-108] [PMID: 15644943]

[65]   Chandrasekera PC, McIntosh VJ, Cao FX, Lasley RD. Differential effects of adenosine A2a and A2b receptors on cardiac contractility. Am J Physiol Heart Circ Physiol 2010; 299(6): H2082-9.
       [http://dx.doi.org/10.1152/ajpheart.00511.2010] [PMID: 20935155]

[66]   Hove-Madsen L, Prat-Vidal C, Llach A, *et al.* Adenosine A2A receptors are expressed in human atrial myocytes and modulate spontaneous sarcoplasmic reticulum calcium release. Cardiovasc Res 2006; 72(2): 292-302.

[http://dx.doi.org/10.1016/j.cardiores.2006.07.020] [PMID: 17014834]

[67]   Tawfik HE, Schnermann J, Oldenburg PJ, Mustafa SJ. Role of A1 adenosine receptors in regulation of vascular tone. Am J Physiol Heart Circ Physiol 2005; 288(3): H1411-6.
[http://dx.doi.org/10.1152/ajpheart.00684.2004] [PMID: 15539423]

[68]   Wang J, Whitt SP, Rubin LJ, Huxley VH. Differential coronary microvascular exchange responses to adenosine: roles of receptor and microvessel subtypes. Microcirculation 2005; 12(4): 313-26.
[http://dx.doi.org/10.1080/10739680590934736] [PMID: 16020078]

[69]   Maczewski M, Beresewicz A. The role of adenosine and ATP-sensitive potassium channels in the protection afforded by ischemic preconditioning against the post-ischemic endothelial dysfunction in guinea-pig hearts. J Mol Cell Cardiol 1998; 30(9): 1735-47.
[http://dx.doi.org/10.1006/jmcc.1998.0736] [PMID: 9769229]

[70]   Zatta AJ, Matherne GP, Headrick JP. Adenosine receptor-mediated coronary vascular protection in post-ischemic mouse heart. Life Sci 2006; 78(21): 2426-37.
[http://dx.doi.org/10.1016/j.lfs.2005.09.035] [PMID: 16300799]

[71]   Teng B, Ledent C, Mustafa SJ. Up-regulation of A 2B adenosine receptor in A 2A adenosine receptor knockout mouse coronary artery. J Mol Cell Cardiol 2008; 44(5): 905-14.
[http://dx.doi.org/10.1016/j.yjmcc.2008.03.003] [PMID: 18423660]

[72]   Deussen A, Brand M, Pexa A, Weichsel J. Metabolic coronary flow regulation--current concepts. Basic Res Cardiol 2006; 101(6): 453-64.
[http://dx.doi.org/10.1007/s00395-006-0621-4] [PMID: 16944360]

[73]   Zatta AJ, Headrick JP. Mediators of coronary reactive hyperaemia in isolated mouse heart. Br J Pharmacol 2005; 144(4): 576-87.
[http://dx.doi.org/10.1038/sj.bjp.0706099] [PMID: 15655499]

[74]   Sharifi-Sanjani M, Zhou X, Asano S, *et al.* Interactions between A(2A) adenosine receptors, hydrogen peroxide, and KATP channels in coronary reactive hyperemia. Am J Physiol Heart Circ Physiol 2013; 304(10): H1294-301.
[http://dx.doi.org/10.1152/ajpheart.00637.2012] [PMID: 23525711]

[75]   Zhou X, Teng B, Tilley S, Mustafa SJ. A1 adenosine receptor negatively modulates coronary reactive hyperemia *via* counteracting A2A-mediated H2O2 production and KATP opening in isolated mouse hearts. Am J Physiol Heart Circ Physiol 2013; 305(11): H1668-79.
[http://dx.doi.org/10.1152/ajpheart.00495.2013] [PMID: 24043252]

[76]   Shepherd RK, Linden J, Duling BR. Adenosine-induced vasoconstriction *in vivo*. Role of the mast cell and A3 adenosine receptor. Circ Res 1996; 78(4): 627-34.
[http://dx.doi.org/10.1161/01.RES.78.4.627] [PMID: 8635220]

[77]   Guinzberg R, Cortés D, Díaz-Cruz A, Riveros-Rosas H, Villalobos-Molina R, Piña E. Inosine released after hypoxia activates hepatic glucose liberation through A3 adenosine receptors. Am J Physiol Endocrinol Metab 2006; 290(5): E940-51.
[http://dx.doi.org/10.1152/ajpendo.00173.2005] [PMID: 16352677]

[78]   Fain JN, Pointer RH, Ward WF. Effects of adenosine nucleosides on adenylate cyclase, phosphodiesterase, cyclic adenosine monophosphate accumulation, and lipolysis in fat cells. J Biol Chem 1972; 247(21): 6866-72.
[PMID: 4343159]

[79]   Epperson SA, Brunton LL, Ramirez-Sanchez I, Villarreal F. Adenosine receptors and second messenger signaling pathways in rat cardiac fibroblasts. Am J Physiol Cell Physiol 2009; 296(5): C1171-7.
[http://dx.doi.org/10.1152/ajpcell.00290.2008] [PMID: 19244482]

[80]   Dubey RK, Gillespie DG, Mi Z, Jackson EK. Exogenous and endogenous adenosine inhibits fetal calf serum-induced growth of rat cardiac fibroblasts: role of A2B receptors. Circulation 1997; 96(8): 2656-

66.
[http://dx.doi.org/10.1161/01.CIR.96.8.2656] [PMID: 9355907]

[81]   Kubota T, McTiernan CF, Frye CS, *et al.* Dilated cardiomyopathy in transgenic mice with cardiac-specific overexpression of tumor necrosis factor-alpha. Circ Res 1997; 81(4): 627-35.
[http://dx.doi.org/10.1161/01.RES.81.4.627] [PMID: 9314845]

[82]   Velot E, Haas B, Léonard F, *et al.* Activation of the adenosine-A3 receptor stimulates matrix metalloproteinase-9 secretion by macrophages. Cardiovasc Res 2008; 80(2): 246-54.
[http://dx.doi.org/10.1093/cvr/cvn201] [PMID: 18653544]

[83]   Adair TH. Growth regulation of the vascular system: an emerging role for adenosine. Am J Physiol Regul Integr Comp Physiol 2005; 289(2): R283-96.
[http://dx.doi.org/10.1152/ajpregu.00840.2004] [PMID: 16014444]

[84]   Auchampach JA. Adenosine receptors and angiogenesis. Circ Res 2007; 101(11): 1075-7.
[http://dx.doi.org/10.1161/CIRCRESAHA.107.165761] [PMID: 18040023]

[85]   Clark AN, Youkey R, Liu X, *et al.* A1 adenosine receptor activation promotes angiogenesis and release of VEGF from monocytes. Circ Res 2007; 101(11): 1130-8.
[http://dx.doi.org/10.1161/CIRCRESAHA.107.150110] [PMID: 17901362]

[86]   Feoktistov I, Goldstein AE, Ryzhov S, *et al.* Differential expression of adenosine receptors in human endothelial cells: role of A2B receptors in angiogenic factor regulation. Circ Res 2002; 90(5): 531-8.
[http://dx.doi.org/10.1161/01.RES.0000012203.21416.14] [PMID: 11909816]

[87]   Desai A, Victor-Vega C, Gadangi S, Montesinos MC, Chu CC, Cronstein BN. Adenosine A2A receptor stimulation increases angiogenesis by down-regulating production of the antiangiogenic matrix protein thrombospondin 1. Mol Pharmacol 2005; 67(5): 1406-13.
[http://dx.doi.org/10.1124/mol.104.007807] [PMID: 15673602]

[88]   Gessi S, Fogli E, Sacchetto V, *et al.* Adenosine modulates HIF-1alpha, VEGF, IL-8, and foam cell formation in a human model of hypoxic foam cells. Arterioscler Thromb Vasc Biol 2010; 30(1): 90-7.
[http://dx.doi.org/10.1161/ATVBAHA.109.194902] [PMID: 19834107]

[89]   Reiss AB, Rahman MM, Chan ES, Montesinos MC, Awadallah NW, Cronstein BN. Adenosine A2A receptor occupancy stimulates expression of proteins involved in reverse cholesterol transport and inhibits foam cell formation in macrophages. J Leukoc Biol 2004; 76(3): 727-34.
[http://dx.doi.org/10.1189/jlb.0204107] [PMID: 15197231]

[90]   Xaus J, Mirabet M, Lloberas J, *et al.* IFN-gamma up-regulates the A2B adenosine receptor expression in macrophages: a mechanism of macrophage deactivation. Journal of Immunology (Baltimore, Md: 1950) 1999; 162: 3607-14.

[91]   Barnholt KE, Kota RS, Aung HH, Rutledge JC. IFN-gamma-induced phosphorylation of STAT1 on serine 727 to reduce macrophage activation. Journal of immunology (Baltimore, Md : 1950) 2009; 183: 6767-77.

[92]   Koupenova M, Johnston-Cox H, Vezeridis A, *et al.* A2b adenosine receptor regulates hyperlipidemia and atherosclerosis. Circulation 2012; 125(2): 354-63.
[http://dx.doi.org/10.1161/CIRCULATIONAHA.111.057596] [PMID: 22144568]

[93]   Cohen MV, Downey JM. Ischemic postconditioning: from receptor to end-effector. Antioxidants & Redox Signaling 2011; 14: 821-31.

[94]   Headrick JP, Lasley RD. Adenosine receptors and reperfusion injury of the heart. Handb Exp Pharmacol 2009; (193): 189-214.
[http://dx.doi.org/10.1007/978-3-540-89615-9_7] [PMID: 19639283]

[95]   Peart JN, Headrick JP. Adenosinergic cardioprotection: multiple receptors, multiple pathways. Pharmacol Ther 2007; 114(2): 208-21.
[http://dx.doi.org/10.1016/j.pharmthera.2007.02.004] [PMID: 17408751]

[96]   Pang T, Gan XT, Freeman DJ, Cook MA, Karmazyn M. Compensatory upregulation of the adenosine system following phenylephrine-induced hypertrophy in cultured rat ventricular myocytes. Am J Physiol Heart Circ Physiol 2010; 298(2): H545-53.
[http://dx.doi.org/10.1152/ajpheart.00417.2009] [PMID: 19966059]

[97]   Burgdorf C, Richardt D, Kurz T, *et al.* Adenosine inhibits norepinephrine release in the postischemic rat heart: the mechanism of neuronal stunning. Cardiovasc Res 2001; 49(4): 713-20.
[http://dx.doi.org/10.1016/S0008-6363(00)00309-6] [PMID: 11230970]

[98]   Wagner DR, Kubota T, Sanders VJ, McTiernan CF, Feldman AM. Differential regulation of cardiac expression of IL-6 and TNF-alpha by A2- and A3-adenosine receptors. Am J Physiol 1999; 276(6 Pt 2): H2141-7.
[PMID: 10362698]

[99]   Koeppen M, Harter PN, Bonney S, *et al.* Adora2b signaling on bone marrow derived cells dampens myocardial ischemia-reperfusion injury. Anesthesiology 2012; 116(6): 1245-57.
[http://dx.doi.org/10.1097/ALN.0b013e318255793c] [PMID: 22531331]

[100]   Yitzhaki S, Huang C, Liu W, *et al.* Autophagy is required for preconditioning by the adenosine A1 receptor-selective agonist CCPA. Basic Res Cardiol 2009; 104(2): 157-67.
[http://dx.doi.org/10.1007/s00395-009-0006-6] [PMID: 19242639]

[101]   Ferdinandy P, Schulz R, Baxter GF. Interaction of cardiovascular risk factors with myocardial ischemia/reperfusion injury, preconditioning, and postconditioning. Pharmacol Rev 2007; 59(4): 418-58.
[http://dx.doi.org/10.1124/pr.107.06002] [PMID: 18048761]

[102]   Llach A, Molina CE, Prat-Vidal C, *et al.* Abnormal calcium handling in atrial fibrillation is linked to up-regulation of adenosine A2A receptors. Eur Heart J 2011; 32(6): 721-9.
[http://dx.doi.org/10.1093/eurheartj/ehq464] [PMID: 21177700]

[103]   Gan XT, Rajapurohitam V, Haist JV, Chidiac P, Cook MA, Karmazyn M. Inhibition of phenylephrine-induced cardiomyocyte hypertrophy by activation of multiple adenosine receptor subtypes. J Pharmacol Exp Ther 2005; 312(1): 27-34.
[http://dx.doi.org/10.1124/jpet.104.073122] [PMID: 15452191]

[104]   Wakeno M, Minamino T, Seguchi O, *et al.* Long-term stimulation of adenosine A2b receptors begun after myocardial infarction prevents cardiac remodeling in rats. Circulation 2006; 114(18): 1923-32.
[http://dx.doi.org/10.1161/CIRCULATIONAHA.106.630087] [PMID: 17043167]

[105]   Simonis G, Wiedemann S, Joachim D, Weinbrenner C, Marquetant R, Strasser RH. Stimulation of adenosine A2b receptors blocks apoptosis in the non-infarcted myocardium even when administered after the onset of infarction. Mol Cell Biochem 2009; 328(1-2): 119-26.
[http://dx.doi.org/10.1007/s11010-009-0081-x] [PMID: 19301100]

[106]   Funakoshi H, Chan TO, Good JC, *et al.* Regulated overexpression of the A1-adenosine receptor in mice results in adverse but reversible changes in cardiac morphology and function. Circulation 2006; 114(21): 2240-50.
[http://dx.doi.org/10.1161/CIRCULATIONAHA.106.620211] [PMID: 17088462]

[107]   Grden M, Podgorska M, Kocbuch K, Szutowicz A, Pawelczyk T. Expression of adenosine receptors in cardiac fibroblasts as a function of insulin and glucose level. Arch Biochem Biophys 2006; 455(1): 10-7.
[http://dx.doi.org/10.1016/j.abb.2006.08.022] [PMID: 17011509]

[108]   Grden M, Podgorska M, Szutowicz A, Pawelczyk T. Altered expression of adenosine receptors in heart of diabetic rat. Journal of Physiology and Pharmacology: An Official Journal of the Polish Physiological Society 2005; 56: 587-97.

[109]   Faulhaber-Walter R, Jou W, Mizel D, *et al.* Impaired glucose tolerance in the absence of adenosine A1 receptor signaling. Diabetes 2011; 60(10): 2578-87.

[http://dx.doi.org/10.2337/db11-0058] [PMID: 21831968]

[110] Jacobson KA, Gao ZG. Adenosine receptors as therapeutic targets. Nat Rev Drug Discov 2006; 5(3): 247-64.
[http://dx.doi.org/10.1038/nrd1983] [PMID: 16518376]

[111] Delacrétaz E. Clinical practice. Supraventricular tachycardia. N Engl J Med 2006; 354(10): 1039-51.
[http://dx.doi.org/10.1056/NEJMcp051145] [PMID: 16525141]

[112] Chen JF, Eltzschig HK, Fredholm BB. Adenosine receptors as drug targets--what are the challenges? Nat Rev Drug Discov 2013; 12(4): 265-86.
[http://dx.doi.org/10.1038/nrd3955] [PMID: 23535933]

[113] Seitun S, Castiglione Morelli M, Budaj I, *et al.* Stress Computed Tomography Myocardial Perfusion Imaging: A New Topic in Cardiology. Rev Esp Cardiol (Engl Ed) 2016; 69(2): 188-200.
[http://dx.doi.org/10.1016/j.rec.2015.10.018] [PMID: 26774540]

[114] Szentmiklósi AJ, Cseppento A, Harmati G, Nánási PP. Novel trends in the treatment of cardiovascular disorders: site- and event- selective adenosinergic drugs. Curr Med Chem 2011; 18(8): 1164-87.
[http://dx.doi.org/10.2174/092986711795029753] [PMID: 21291368]

[115] de Lera Ruiz M, Lim YH, Zheng J. Adenosine A2A receptor as a drug discovery target. J Med Chem 2014; 57(9): 3623-50.
[http://dx.doi.org/10.1021/jm4011669] [PMID: 24164628]

[116] Clarke DA, Davoll J, Philips FS, Brown GB. Enzymatic deamination and vasodepressor effects of adenosine analogs. J Pharmacol Exp Ther 1952; 106(3): 291-302.
[PMID: 13000625]

[117] Valls MD, Cronstein BN, Montesinos MC. Adenosine receptor agonists for promotion of dermal wound healing. Biochem Pharmacol 2009; 77(7): 1117-24.
[http://dx.doi.org/10.1016/j.bcp.2008.11.002] [PMID: 19041853]

[118] Jacobson KA. Introduction to adenosine receptors as therapeutic targets. Handb Exp Pharmacol 2009; (193): 1-24.
[PMID: 19639277]

[119] Beukers MW, Chang LC, von Frijtag Drabbe Künzel JK, *et al.* New, non-adenosine, high-potency agonists for the human adenosine A2B receptor with an improved selectivity profile compared to the reference agonist N-ethylcarboxamidoadenosine. J Med Chem 2004; 47(15): 3707-9.
[http://dx.doi.org/10.1021/jm049947s] [PMID: 15239649]

[120] Grenz A, Osswald H, Eckle T, *et al.* The reno-vascular A2B adenosine receptor protects the kidney from ischemia. PLoS Med 2008; 5(6): e137.
[http://dx.doi.org/10.1371/journal.pmed.0050137] [PMID: 18578565]

[121] Tendera M, Gaszewska-Żurek E, Parma Z, *et al.* The new oral adenosine A1 receptor agonist capadenoson in male patients with stable angina. Clin Res Cardiol 2012; 101(7): 585-91.
[http://dx.doi.org/10.1007/s00392-012-0430-8] [PMID: 22370739]

[122] Daly JW, Padgett WL, Secunda SI, Thompson RD, Olsson RA. Structure-activity relationships for 2-substituted adenosines at A1 and A2 adenosine receptors. Pharmacology 1993; 46(2): 91-100.
[http://dx.doi.org/10.1159/000139033] [PMID: 8441759]

[123] Bruns RF. Adenosine receptor activation in human fibroblasts: nucleoside agonists and antagonists. Can J Physiol Pharmacol 1980; 58(6): 673-91.
[http://dx.doi.org/10.1139/y80-110] [PMID: 6253037]

[124] van Galen PJ, van Bergen AH, Gallo-Rodriguez C, *et al.* A binding site model and structure-activity relationships for the rat A3 adenosine receptor. Mol Pharmacol 1994; 45(6): 1101-11.
[PMID: 8022403]

[125] Mueller CE, Stein B. Adenosine receptor antagonists: structures and potential therapeutic applications.

Curr Pharm Des 1996; 2: 501-30.

[126] Liang BT, Urso M, Zambraski E, Jacobson KA. Adenosine A3 Receptors in Muscle Protection.A3 Adenosine Receptors from Cell Biology to Pharmacology and Therapeutics. Dordrecht: Springer Netherlands 2010; pp. 257-80.
[http://dx.doi.org/10.1007/978-90-481-3144-0_13]

[127] Kuno A, Critz SD, Cui L, *et al.* Protein kinase C protects preconditioned rabbit hearts by increasing sensitivity of adenosine A2b-dependent signaling during early reperfusion. J Mol Cell Cardiol 2007; 43(3): 262-71.
[http://dx.doi.org/10.1016/j.yjmcc.2007.05.016] [PMID: 17632123]

[128] Auchampach JA, Kreckler LM, Wan TC, *et al.* Characterization of the A2B adenosine receptor from mouse, rabbit, and dog. J Pharmacol Exp Ther 2009; 329(1): 2-13.
[http://dx.doi.org/10.1124/jpet.108.148270] [PMID: 19141710]

[129] Slee DH, Zhang X, Moorjani M, *et al.* Identification of novel, water-soluble, 2-amino-N-pyrimid-n-4-yl acetamides as A2A receptor antagonists with *in vivo* efficacy. J Med Chem 2008; 51(3): 400-6.
[http://dx.doi.org/10.1021/jm070623o] [PMID: 18189346]

[130] Slee DH, Chen Y, Zhang X, *et al.* 2-Amino-N-pyrimidin-4-ylacetamides as A2A receptor antagonists: 1. Structure-activity relationships and optimization of heterocyclic substituents. J Med Chem 2008; 51(6): 1719-29.
[http://dx.doi.org/10.1021/jm701185v] [PMID: 18307292]

[131] Vu CB, Shields P, Peng B, *et al.* Triamino derivatives of triazolotriazine and triazolopyrimidine as adenosine A2a receptor antagonists. Bioorg Med Chem Lett 2004; 14(19): 4835-8.
[http://dx.doi.org/10.1016/j.bmcl.2004.07.048] [PMID: 15341934]

[132] Neustadt BR, Liu H, Hao J, *et al.* Potent and selective adenosine A2A receptor antagonists: 1,2,4-Triazolo[1,5-c]pyrimidines. Bioorg Med Chem Lett 2009; 19(3): 967-71.
[http://dx.doi.org/10.1016/j.bmcl.2008.11.075] [PMID: 19109019]

[133] Zhou G, Aslanian R, Gallo G, *et al.* Discovery of aminoquinazoline derivatives as human A(2A) adenosine receptor antagonists. Bioorg Med Chem Lett 2016; 26(4): 1348-54.
[http://dx.doi.org/10.1016/j.bmcl.2015.11.048] [PMID: 26781932]

[134] Francis JE, Cash WD, Psychoyos S, *et al.* Structure-activity profile of a series of novel triazoloquinazoline adenosine antagonists. J Med Chem 1988; 31(5): 1014-20.
[http://dx.doi.org/10.1021/jm00400a022] [PMID: 3361572]

[135] Neustadt BR, Hao J, Lindo N, *et al.* Potent, selective, and orally active adenosine A2A receptor antagonists: arylpiperazine derivatives of pyrazolo[4,3-e]-1,2,4-triazolo[1,5-c]pyrimidines. Bioorg Med Chem Lett 2007; 17(5): 1376-80.
[http://dx.doi.org/10.1016/j.bmcl.2006.11.083] [PMID: 17236762]

[136] Baraldi PG, Zappaterra L, Ongini E. 1,2,4-Triazolo[1,5-c]Pyrimidine Heterocyclic Analogues Having Antagonistic Activity on Adenosine A2 Receptor. Google Patents. 1995.

[137] Müller CE, Ferré S. Blocking striatal adenosine A2A receptors: a new strategy for basal ganglia disorders. Recent Patents CNS Drug Discov 2007; 2(1): 1-21.
[http://dx.doi.org/10.2174/157488907779561772] [PMID: 18221214]

[138] Shah U, Hodgson R. Recent progress in the discovery of adenosine A(2A) receptor antagonists for the treatment of Parkinson's disease. Curr Opin Drug Discov Devel 2010; 13(4): 466-80.
[PMID: 20597030]

[139] Preti D, Baraldi PG, Moorman AR, Borea PA, Varani K. History and perspectives of A2A adenosine receptor antagonists as potential therapeutic agents. Med Res Rev 2015; 35(4): 790-848.
[http://dx.doi.org/10.1002/med.21344] [PMID: 25821194]

[140] Jacobson KA, Ijzerman AP, Linden J. 1,3-Dialkylxanthine derivatives having high potency as antagonists at human A2b adenosine receptors. Drug Dev Res 1999; 47: 45-53.

[http://dx.doi.org/10.1002/(SICI)1098-2299(199905)47:1<45::AID-DDR6>3.0.CO;2-U]

[141] Abo-Salem OM, Hayallah AM, Bilkei-Gorzo A, Filipek B, Zimmer A, Müller CE. Antinociceptive effects of novel A2B adenosine receptor antagonists. J Pharmacol Exp Ther 2004; 308(1): 358-66.
[http://dx.doi.org/10.1124/jpet.103.056036] [PMID: 14563788]

[142] Borrmann T, Hinz S, Bertarelli DC, *et al.* 1-alkyl-8-(piperazine-1-sulfonyl)phenylxanthines: development and characterization of adenosine A2B receptor antagonists and a new radioligand with subnanomolar affinity and subtype specificity. J Med Chem 2009; 52(13): 3994-4006.
[http://dx.doi.org/10.1021/jm900413e] [PMID: 19569717]

[143] Kim SA, Marshall MA, Melman N, *et al.* Structure-activity relationships at human and rat A2B adenosine receptors of xanthine derivatives substituted at the 1-, 3-, 7-, and 8-positions. J Med Chem 2002; 45(11): 2131-8.
[http://dx.doi.org/10.1021/jm0104318] [PMID: 12014951]

[144] Grahner B, Winiwarter S, Lanzner W, Müller CE. Synthesis and structure-activity relationships of deazaxanthines: analogs of potent A1- and A2-adenosine receptor antagonists. J Med Chem 1994; 37(10): 1526-34.
[http://dx.doi.org/10.1021/jm00036a019] [PMID: 8182711]

[145] Daly JW, Hide I, Müller CE, Shamim M. Caffeine analogs: structure-activity relationships at adenosine receptors. Pharmacology 1991; 42(6): 309-21.
[http://dx.doi.org/10.1159/000138813] [PMID: 1658821]

[146] Bertarelli DC, Diekmann M, Hayallah AM, *et al.* Characterization of human and rodent native and recombinant adenosine A(2B) receptors by radioligand binding studies. Purinergic Signal 2006; 2(3): 559-71.
[http://dx.doi.org/10.1007/s11302-006-9012-4] [PMID: 18404493]

[147] Muller CE. Adenosine receptor ligands-recent developments part I. Agonists. Curr Med Chem 2000; 7(12): 1269-88.
[http://dx.doi.org/10.2174/0929867003374101] [PMID: 11032971]

[148] Klotz KN, Hessling J, Hegler J, *et al.* Comparative pharmacology of human adenosine receptor subtypes - characterization of stably transfected receptors in CHO cells. Naunyn Schmiedebergs Arch Pharmacol 1998; 357(1): 1-9.
[http://dx.doi.org/10.1007/PL00005131] [PMID: 9459566]

[149] Müller CE, Shi D, Manning M Jr, Daly JW. Synthesis of paraxanthine analogs (1,7-disubstituted xanthines) and other xanthines unsubstituted at the 3-position: structure-activity relationships at adenosine receptors. J Med Chem 1993; 36(22): 3341-9.
[http://dx.doi.org/10.1021/jm00074a015] [PMID: 8230124]

[150] Kase H, Aoyama S, Ichimura M, *et al.* KW-6002 US-001 Study Group. Progress in pursuit of therapeutic A2A antagonists: the adenosine A2A receptor selective antagonist KW6002: research and development toward a novel nondopaminergic therapy for Parkinson's disease. Neurology 2003; 61(11) (Suppl. 6): S97-S100.
[http://dx.doi.org/10.1212/01.WNL.0000095219.22086.31] [PMID: 14663020]

[151] Shimada J, Koike N, Nonaka H, *et al.* Adenosine A2A antagonists with potent anti-cataleptic activity. Bioorg Med Chem Lett 1997; 7: 2349-52.
[http://dx.doi.org/10.1016/S0960-894X(97)00440-X]

[152] Pretorius J, Malan SF, Castagnoli N Jr, Bergh JJ, Petzer JP. Dual inhibition of monoamine oxidase B and antagonism of the adenosine A(2A) receptor by (E,E)-8-(4-phenylbutadien-1-yl)caffeine analogues. Bioorg Med Chem 2008; 16(18): 8676-84.
[http://dx.doi.org/10.1016/j.bmc.2008.07.088] [PMID: 18723354]

[153] Jacobson KA, Gallo-Rodriguez C, Melman N, *et al.* Structure-activity relationships of 8-styrylxanthines as A2-selective adenosine antagonists. J Med Chem 1993; 36(10): 1333-42.
[http://dx.doi.org/10.1021/jm00062a005] [PMID: 8496902]

[154] Belardinelli L, Pelleg A, Eds. Adenosine and Adenine Nucleotides: From Molecular Biology to Integrative Physiology. Kluwer 1995.
[http://dx.doi.org/10.1007/978-1-4615-2011-5]

[155] Sauer R, Maurinsh J, Reith U, Fülle F, Klotz KN, Müller CE. Water-soluble phosphate prodrugs of 1-propargyl-8-styrylxanthine derivatives, A(2A)-selective adenosine receptor antagonists. J Med Chem 2000; 43(3): 440-8.
[http://dx.doi.org/10.1021/jm9911480] [PMID: 10669571]

[156] Dungo R, Deeks ED. Istradefylline: first global approval. Drugs 2013; 73(8): 875-82.
[http://dx.doi.org/10.1007/s40265-013-0066-7] [PMID: 23700273]

[157] Müller CE, Jacobson KA. Recent developments in adenosine receptor ligands and their potential as novel drugs. Biochim Biophys Acta 2011; 1808(5): 1290-308.
[http://dx.doi.org/10.1016/j.bbamem.2010.12.017] [PMID: 21185259]

[158] Hockemeyer J, Burbiel JC, Müller CE. Multigram-scale syntheses, stability, and photoreactions of A2A adenosine receptor antagonists with 8-styrylxanthine structure: potential drugs for Parkinson's disease. J Org Chem 2004; 69(10): 3308-18.
[http://dx.doi.org/10.1021/jo0358574] [PMID: 15132536]

[159] Mori Y, Tomonaga D, Kalashnikova A, *et al.* Effects of 3,3',5-triiodothyronine on microglial functions. Glia 2015; 63(5): 906-20.
[http://dx.doi.org/10.1002/glia.22792] [PMID: 25643925]

[160] Pinna A. Adenosine A2A receptor antagonists in Parkinson's disease: progress in clinical trials from the newly approved istradefylline to drugs in early development and those already discontinued. CNS Drugs 2014; 28(5): 455-74.
[http://dx.doi.org/10.1007/s40263-014-0161-7] [PMID: 24687255]

[161] Shook BC, Jackson PF, Adenosine A. Adenosine A(2A) Receptor Antagonists and Parkinson's Disease. ACS Chem Neurosci 2011; 2(10): 555-67.
[http://dx.doi.org/10.1021/cn2000537] [PMID: 22860156]

[162] Williams M, Francis J, Ghai G, *et al.* Biochemical characterization of the triazoloquinazoline, CGS 15943, a novel, non-xanthine adenosine antagonist. J Pharmacol Exp Ther 1987; 241(2): 415-20.
[PMID: 2883298]

[163] Gatta F, Del Giudice MR, Borioni A, Borea PA, Dionisotti S, Ongini E. Synthesis of imidazo[1,2-c]pyrazolo[4,3-e]pyrimidines, pyrazolo[4,3-e]1,2,4-triazolo[1,5-c]pyrimidines and 1,2,4-triazolo[5,-i]purines: new potent adenosine A2 receptor antagonists. Eur J Med Chem 1993; 28: 569-76.
[http://dx.doi.org/10.1016/0223-5234(93)90087-U]

[164] Baraldi PG, Cacciari B, Spalluto G, *et al.* Pyrazolo[4,3-e]-1,2,4-triazolo[1,5-c]pyrimidine derivatives: potent and selective A(2A) adenosine antagonists. J Med Chem 1996; 39(5): 1164-71.
[http://dx.doi.org/10.1021/jm950746l] [PMID: 8676354]

[165] Caulkett PW, Jones G, McPartlin M, Renshaw ND, Stewart SK, Wright B. Adenine isosteres with bridgehead nitrogen. Part 1. Two independent syntheses of the [1,2,4]triazolo[1,5-a][1,3,5]triazine ring system leading to a range of substituents in the 2, 5 and 7 positions. J Chem Soc, Perkin Trans 1 1995; 801-8.
[http://dx.doi.org/10.1039/p19950000801]

[166] Soudijn W, van Wijngaarden I, IJzerman AP. Allosteric modulation of G protein-coupled receptors. Curr Opin Drug Discov Devel 2002; 5(5): 749-55.
[PMID: 12630295]

[167] Soudijn W, Van Wijngaarden I, IJzerman AP. Allosteric modulation of G protein-coupled receptors: perspectives and recent developments. Drug Discov Today 2004; 9(17): 752-8.
[http://dx.doi.org/10.1016/S1359-6446(04)03220-9] [PMID: 15450241]

[168] May LT, Leach K, Sexton PM, Christopoulos A. Allosteric modulation of G protein-coupled

receptors. Annu Rev Pharmacol Toxicol 2007; 47: 1-51.
[http://dx.doi.org/10.1146/annurev.pharmtox.47.120505.105159] [PMID: 17009927]

[169] Lewis JA, Lebois EP, Lindsley CW. Allosteric modulation of kinases and GPCRs: design principles and structural diversity. Curr Opin Chem Biol 2008; 12(3): 269-80.
[http://dx.doi.org/10.1016/j.cbpa.2008.02.014] [PMID: 18342020]

[170] Göblyös A, Ijzerman AP. Allosteric modulation of adenosine receptors. Purinergic Signal 2009; 5(1): 51-61.
[http://dx.doi.org/10.1007/s11302-008-9105-3] [PMID: 18615273]

[171] Mohr K, Schmitz J, Schrage R, Tränkle C, Holzgrabe U. Molecular alliance-from orthosteric and allosteric ligands to dualsteric/bitopic agonists at G protein coupled receptors. Angew Chem Int Ed Engl 2013; 52(2): 508-16.
[http://dx.doi.org/10.1002/anie.201205315] [PMID: 23225228]

[172] Guo D, Heitman LH, IJzerman AP. Kinetic Aspects of the Interaction between Ligand and G Protein-Coupled Receptor: The Case of the Adenosine Receptors. Chem Rev 2017; 117(1): 38-66.
[http://dx.doi.org/10.1021/acs.chemrev.6b00025] [PMID: 27088232]

[173] Christopoulos A, Changeux JP, Catterall WA, *et al.* International Union of Basic and Clinical Pharmacology. XC. multisite pharmacology: recommendations for the nomenclature of receptor allosterism and allosteric ligands. Pharmacol Rev 2014; 66(4): 918-47.
[http://dx.doi.org/10.1124/pr.114.008862] [PMID: 25026896]

[174] Zhang R, Kavana M. Quantitative analysis of receptor allosterism and its implication for drug discovery. Expert Opin Drug Discov 2015; 10(7): 763-80.
[http://dx.doi.org/10.1517/17460441.2015.1041498] [PMID: 25927503]

[175] Melancon BJ, Hopkins CR, Wood MR, *et al.* Allosteric modulation of seven transmembrane spanning receptors: theory, practice, and opportunities for central nervous system drug discovery. J Med Chem 2012; 55(4): 1445-64.
[http://dx.doi.org/10.1021/jm201139r] [PMID: 22148748]

[176] Valant C, Robert Lane J, Sexton PM, Christopoulos A. The best of both worlds? Bitopic orthosteric/allosteric ligands of g protein-coupled receptors. Annu Rev Pharmacol Toxicol 2012; 52: 153-78.
[http://dx.doi.org/10.1146/annurev-pharmtox-010611-134514] [PMID: 21910627]

[177] Lane JR, Sexton PM, Christopoulos A. Bridging the gap: bitopic ligands of G-protein-coupled receptors. Trends Pharmacol Sci 2013; 34(1): 59-66.
[http://dx.doi.org/10.1016/j.tips.2012.10.003] [PMID: 23177916]

[178] Bruns RF, Fergus JH. Allosteric enhancement of adenosine A1 receptor binding and function by 2-amino-3-benzoylthiophenes. Mol Pharmacol 1990; 38(6): 939-49.
[PMID: 2174510]

[179] Tinney FJ, Sanchez JP, Nogas JA. Synthesis and pharmacological evaluation of 2,3-dihydro--H-thieno(2,3-e)(1,4)diazepines. J Med Chem 1974; 17(6): 624-30.
[http://dx.doi.org/10.1021/jm00252a011] [PMID: 4829942]

[180] Kollias-Baker C, Ruble J, Dennis D, Bruns RF, Linden J, Belardinelli L. Allosteric enhancer PD 81,723 acts by novel mechanism to potentiate cardiac actions of adenosine. Circ Res 1994; 75(6): 961-71.
[http://dx.doi.org/10.1161/01.RES.75.6.961] [PMID: 7955150]

[181] Jazayeri A, Andrews SP, Marshall FH. Structurally Enabled Discovery of Adenosine A2A Receptor Antagonists. Chem Rev 2017; 117(1): 21-37.
[http://dx.doi.org/10.1021/acs.chemrev.6b00119] [PMID: 27333206]

[182] Segala E, Errey JC, Fiez-Vandal C, Zhukov A, Cooke RM. Biosensor-based affinities and binding kinetics of small molecule antagonists to the adenosine A(2A) receptor reconstituted in HDL like

particles. FEBS Lett 2015; 589(13): 1399-405.
[http://dx.doi.org/10.1016/j.febslet.2015.04.030] [PMID: 25935416]

[183] Fawzi AB, Macdonald D, Benbow LL, *et al.* SCH-202676: An allosteric modulator of both agonist and antagonist binding to G protein-coupled receptors. Mol Pharmacol 2001; 59(1): 30-7.
[http://dx.doi.org/10.1124/mol.59.1.30] [PMID: 11125021]

[184] Andrews SP, Tehan B. Stabilised G protein-coupled receptors in structure-based drug design: a case study with adenosine A2A receptor. MedChemComm 2013; 4: 52-67.
[http://dx.doi.org/10.1039/C2MD20164J]

[185] Gao ZG, Ijzerman AP. Allosteric modulation of A(2A) adenosine receptors by amiloride analogues and sodium ions. Biochem Pharmacol 2000; 60(5): 669-76.
[http://dx.doi.org/10.1016/S0006-2952(00)00360-9] [PMID: 10927025]

[186] Giorgi I, Biagi G, Bianucci AM, *et al.* N6-1,3-diphenylurea derivatives of 2-phenyl-9-benzyladenines and 8-azaadenines: synthesis and biological evaluation as allosteric modulators of A2A adenosine receptors. Eur J Med Chem 2008; 43(8): 1639-47.
[http://dx.doi.org/10.1016/j.ejmech.2007.10.021] [PMID: 18045744]

[187] Ferré S, Baler R, Bouvier M, *et al.* Building a new conceptual framework for receptor heteromers. Nat Chem Biol 2009; 5(3): 131-4.
[http://dx.doi.org/10.1038/nchembio0309-131] [PMID: 19219011]

[188] Namba K, Suzuki T, Nakata H. Immunogold electron microscopic evidence of *in situ* formation of homo- and heteromeric purinergic adenosine A1 and P2Y2 receptors in rat brain. BMC Res Notes 2010; 3: 323.
[http://dx.doi.org/10.1186/1756-0500-3-323] [PMID: 21114816]

[189] Ciruela F, Casadó V, Mallol J, Canela EI, Lluis C, Franco R. Immunological identification of A1 adenosine receptors in brain cortex. J Neurosci Res 1995; 42(6): 818-28.
[http://dx.doi.org/10.1002/jnr.490420610] [PMID: 8847743]

[190] Canals M, Burgueño J, Marcellino D, *et al.* Homodimerization of adenosine A2A receptors: qualitative and quantitative assessment by fluorescence and bioluminescence energy transfer. J Neurochem 2004; 88(3): 726-34.
[http://dx.doi.org/10.1046/j.1471-4159.2003.02200.x] [PMID: 14720222]

[191] Ciruela F, Casadó V, Rodrigues RJ, *et al.* Presynaptic control of striatal glutamatergic neurotransmission by adenosine A1-A2A receptor heteromers. J Neurosci 2006; 26(7): 2080-7.
[http://dx.doi.org/10.1523/JNEUROSCI.3574-05.2006] [PMID: 16481441]

[192] Cristóvão-Ferreira S, Navarro G, Brugarolas M, *et al.* A1R-A2AR heteromers coupled to Gs and G i/0 proteins modulate GABA transport into astrocytes. Purinergic Signal 2013; 9(3): 433-49.
[http://dx.doi.org/10.1007/s11302-013-9364-5] [PMID: 23657626]

[193] Casadó V, Ferrada C, Bonaventura J, *et al.* Useful pharmacological parameters for G-protein-coupled receptor homodimers obtained from competition experiments. Agonist-antagonist binding modulation. Biochem Pharmacol 2009; 78(12): 1456-63.
[http://dx.doi.org/10.1016/j.bcp.2009.07.012] [PMID: 19643089]

[194] Oliveira PA, Dalton JA, López-Cano M, *et al.* Angiotensin II type 1/adenosine A 2A receptor oligomers: a novel target for tardive dyskinesia. Sci Rep 2017; 7(1): 1857.
[http://dx.doi.org/10.1038/s41598-017-02037-z] [PMID: 28500295]

[195] Agnati LF, Fuxe K, Zini I, Lenzi P, Hökfelt T. Aspects on receptor regulation and isoreceptor identification. Med Biol 1980; 58(4): 182-7.
[PMID: 6167826]

[196] Fuxe K, Agnati LF, Benfenati F, *et al.* Evidence for the existence of receptor--receptor interactions in the central nervous system. Studies on the regulation of monoamine receptors by neuropeptides. J Neural Transm Suppl 1983; 18: 165-79.

[PMID: 6192208]

[197] Jaakola VP, Griffith MT, Hanson MA, *et al.* The 2.6 angstrom crystal structure of a human A2A adenosine receptor bound to an antagonist. Science 2008; 322(5905): 1211-7.
[http://dx.doi.org/10.1126/science.1164772] [PMID: 18832607]

[198] Lebon G, Warne T, Edwards PC, *et al.* Agonist-bound adenosine A2A receptor structures reveal common features of GPCR activation. Nature 2011; 474(7352): 521-5.
[http://dx.doi.org/10.1038/nature10136] [PMID: 21593763]

[199] Martinelli A, Ortore G. Molecular modeling of adenosine receptors. Methods Enzymol 2013; 522: 37-59.
[http://dx.doi.org/10.1016/B978-0-12-407865-9.00003-0] [PMID: 23374179]

[200] Martinelli A, Ortore G. Molecular modeling of adenosine receptors. Methods Enzymol 2013; 522: 37-59.
[http://dx.doi.org/10.1016/B978-0-12-407865-9.00003-0] [PMID: 23374179]

[201] Li J, Jonsson AL, Beuming T, Shelley JC, Voth GA. Ligand-dependent activation and deactivation of the human adenosine A(2A) receptor. J Am Chem Soc 2013; 135(23): 8749-59.
[http://dx.doi.org/10.1021/ja404391q] [PMID: 23678995]

[202] Glukhova A, Thal DM, Nguyen AT, *et al.* Structure of the Adenosine A1 Receptor Reveals the Basis for Subtype Selectivity. Cell 2017; 168: 867-877 e813.

[203] Palani G, Ananthasubramaniam K. Regadenoson: review of its established role in myocardial perfusion imaging and emerging applications. Cardiol Rev 2013; 21(1): 42-8.
[http://dx.doi.org/10.1097/CRD.0b013e3182613db6] [PMID: 22643345]

[204] Gao Z, Li Z, Baker SP, *et al.* Novel short-acting A2A adenosine receptor agonists for coronary vasodilation: inverse relationship between affinity and duration of action of A2A agonists. J Pharmacol Exp Ther 2001; 298(1): 209-18.
[PMID: 11408544]

[205] Cerqueira MD. The future of pharmacologic stress: selective A2A adenosine receptor agonists. Am J Cardiol 2004; 94: 33D-40D. discussion 40D-42D.

[206] Gao Z-G, Jacobson KA. Emerging adenosine receptor agonists: an update. Expert Opin Emerg Drugs 2011; 16(4): 597-602.
[http://dx.doi.org/10.1517/14728214.2011.644786] [PMID: 22148938]

[207] Fuentes E, Fuentes M, Caballero J, *et al.* Adenosine A2A receptor agonists with potent antiplatelet activity. Platelets 2017; 1-9.
[http://dx.doi.org/10.1080/09537104.2017.1306043] [PMID: 28504052]

[208] Bharate SB, Singh B, Kachler S, *et al.* Discovery of 7-(Prolinol-N-yl)-2-phenylamino-thiazo-o[5,4-d]pyrimidines as Novel Non-Nucleoside Partial Agonists for the A2A Adenosine Receptor: Prediction from Molecular Modeling. J Med Chem 2016; 59(12): 5922-8.
[http://dx.doi.org/10.1021/acs.jmedchem.6b00552] [PMID: 27227326]

[209] Cheung JW, Lerman BB. CVT-510: a selective A1 adenosine receptor agonist. Cardiovasc Drug Rev 2003; 21(4): 277-92.
[http://dx.doi.org/10.1111/j.1527-3466.2003.tb00122.x] [PMID: 14647532]

[210] Chaparro S, Dittrich HC, Tang WW. Rolofylline (KW-3902): a new adenosine A1-receptor antagonist for acute congestive heart failure. Future Cardiol 2008; 4(2): 117-23.
[http://dx.doi.org/10.2217/14796678.4.2.117] [PMID: 19804290]

[211] Massie BM, O'Connor CM, Metra M, *et al.* Rolofylline, an adenosine A1-receptor antagonist, in acute heart failure. N Engl J Med 2010; 363(15): 1419-28.
[http://dx.doi.org/10.1056/NEJMoa0912613] [PMID: 20925544]

[212] Cotter G, Dittrich HC, Weatherley BD, *et al.* The PROTECT pilot study: a randomized, placebo-

controlled, dose-finding study of the adenosine A1 receptor antagonist rolofylline in patients with acute heart failure and renal impairment. J Card Fail 2008; 14(8): 631-40.
[http://dx.doi.org/10.1016/j.cardfail.2008.08.010] [PMID: 18926433]

[213] Meibom D, Albrecht-Küpper B, Diedrichs N, *et al.* Neladenoson Bialanate Hydrochloride: A Prodrug of a Partial Adenosine A1 Receptor Agonist for the Chronic Treatment of Heart Diseases. ChemMedChem 2017; 12(10): 728-37.
[http://dx.doi.org/10.1002/cmdc.201700151] [PMID: 28488817]

[214] Albrecht-Küpper BE, Leineweber K, Nell PG. Partial adenosine A1 receptor agonists for cardiovascular therapies. Purinergic Signal 2012; 8 (Suppl. 1): 91-9.
[http://dx.doi.org/10.1007/s11302-011-9274-3] [PMID: 22081230]

[215] Sabbah HN, Gupta RC, Kohli S, *et al.* Chronic therapy with a partial adenosine A1-receptor agonist improves left ventricular function and remodeling in dogs with advanced heart failure. Circ Heart Fail 2013; 6(3): 563-71.
[http://dx.doi.org/10.1161/CIRCHEARTFAILURE.112.000208] [PMID: 23564604]

[216] Van der Walt MM, Terre'Blanche G, Petzer A, Petzer JP. The adenosine receptor affinities and monoamine oxidase B inhibitory properties of sulfanylphthalimide analogues. Bioorg Chem 2015; 59: 117-23.
[http://dx.doi.org/10.1016/j.bioorg.2015.02.005] [PMID: 25746740]

[217] Yu J, Zhao LX, Park J, *et al.* N6-Substituted 5'-N-Methylcarbamoyl-4'-selenoadenosines as Potent and Selective A3 Adenosine Receptor Agonists with Unusual Sugar Puckering and Nucleobase Orientation. J Med Chem 2017; 60(8): 3422-37.
[http://dx.doi.org/10.1021/acs.jmedchem.7b00241] [PMID: 28380296]

[218] Jeong LS, Pal S, Choe SA, *et al.* Structure-activity relationships of truncated D- and l-4'-thioadenosine derivatives as species-independent A3 adenosine receptor antagonists. J Med Chem 2008; 51(20): 6609-13.
[http://dx.doi.org/10.1021/jm8008647] [PMID: 18811138]

[219] Sahu PK, Naik SD, Yu J, Jeong LS. 4'-Selenonucleosides as Next-Generation Nucleosides. Eur J Org Chem 2015; 2015: 6115-24.
[http://dx.doi.org/10.1002/ejoc.201500429]

[220] Möser GH, Schrader J, Deussen A. Turnover of adenosine in plasma of human and dog blood. Am J Physiol 1989; 256(4 Pt 1): C799-806.
[http://dx.doi.org/10.1152/ajpcell.1989.256.4.C799] [PMID: 2539728]

[221] Nees S, Herzog V, Becker BF, Böck M, Des Rosiers Ch, Gerlach E. The coronary endothelium: a highly active metabolic barrier for adenosine. Basic Res Cardiol 1985; 80(5): 515-29.
[http://dx.doi.org/10.1007/BF01907915] [PMID: 3000345]

[222] Smits P, Boekema P, De Abreu R, Thien T, van 't Laar A. Evidence for an antagonism between caffeine and adenosine in the human cardiovascular system. J Cardiovasc Pharmacol 1987; 10(2): 136-43.
[http://dx.doi.org/10.1097/00005344-198708000-00002] [PMID: 2441163]

[223] Cha JH, Kosinski CM, Kerner JA, *et al.* Altered brain neurotransmitter receptors in transgenic mice expressing a portion of an abnormal human huntington disease gene. Proc Natl Acad Sci USA 1998; 95(11): 6480-5.
[http://dx.doi.org/10.1073/pnas.95.11.6480] [PMID: 9600992]

[224] Jacobson KA, von Lubitz DK, Daly JW, Fredholm BB. Adenosine receptor ligands: differences with acute *versus* chronic treatment. Trends Pharmacol Sci 1996; 17(3): 108-13.
[http://dx.doi.org/10.1016/0165-6147(96)10002-X] [PMID: 8936347]

[225] Burgueño J, Blake DJ, Benson MA, *et al.* The adenosine A2A receptor interacts with the actin-binding protein alpha-actinin. J Biol Chem 2003; 278(39): 37545-52.
[http://dx.doi.org/10.1074/jbc.M302809200] [PMID: 12837758]

[226]   de Mendonça A, Sebastião AM, Ribeiro JA. Adenosine: does it have a neuroprotective role after all? Brain Res Brain Res Rev 2000; 33(2-3): 258-74.
[http://dx.doi.org/10.1016/S0165-0173(00)00033-3] [PMID: 11011069]

[227]   Von Lubitz DK, Lin RC, Melman N, Ji XD, Carter MF, Jacobson KA. Chronic administration of selective adenosine A1 receptor agonist or antagonist in cerebral ischemia. Eur J Pharmacol 1994; 256(2): 161-7.
[http://dx.doi.org/10.1016/0014-2999(94)90241-0] [PMID: 8050467]

[228]   Pinna A, Fenu S, Morelli M. Motor stimulant effects of the adenosine A2A receptor antagonist SCH 58261 do not develop tolerance after repeated treatments in 6-hydroxydopamine-lesioned rats. Synapse 2001; 39(3): 233-8.
[http://dx.doi.org/10.1002/1098-2396(20010301)39:3<233::AID-SYN1004>3.0.CO;2-K]   [PMID: 11284438]

[229]   Chern Y, Lai HL, Fong JC, Liang Y. Multiple mechanisms for desensitization of A2a adenosine receptor-mediated cAMP elevation in rat pheochromocytoma PC12 cells. Mol Pharmacol 1993; 44(5): 950-8.
[PMID: 8246918]

[230]   Chen JF, Huang Z, Ma J, *et al.* A(2A) adenosine receptor deficiency attenuates brain injury induced by transient focal ischemia in mice. J Neurosci 1999; 19(21): 9192-200.
[PMID: 10531422]

[231]   Adén U, Halldner L, Lagercrantz H, Dalmau I, Ledent C, Fredholm BB. Aggravated brain damage after hypoxic ischemia in immature adenosine A2A knockout mice. Stroke 2003; 34(3): 739-44.
[http://dx.doi.org/10.1161/01.STR.0000060204.67672.8B] [PMID: 12624301]

[232]   Yang JN, Bjorklund O, Lindstrom-Tornqvist K, *et al.* Mice heterozygous for both A1 and A(2A) adenosine receptor genes show similarities to mice given long-term caffeine. Journal of applied physiology (Bethesda, Md : 1985) 2009; 106: 631-9.

[233]   Lazarus M, Chen JF, Huang ZL, Urade Y, Fredholm BB. Adenosine and Sleep. Handb Exp Pharmacol 2017.
[http://dx.doi.org/10.1007/164_2017_36] [PMID: 28646346]

[234]   Arnaud MJ. Pharmacokinetics and metabolism of natural methylxanthines in animal and man. Handb Exp Pharmacol 2011; (200): 33-91.
[http://dx.doi.org/10.1007/978-3-642-13443-2_3] [PMID: 20859793]

[235]   Tejani FH, Thompson RC, Iskandrian AE, McNutt BE, Franks B. Effect of caffeine on SPECT myocardial perfusion imaging during regadenoson pharmacologic stress: rationale and design of a prospective, randomized, multicenter study. Journal of Nuclear Cardiology: Official publication of the American Society of Nuclear Cardiology 2011; 18: 73-81.

[236]   Nonaka Y, Shimada J, Nonaka H, *et al.* Photoisomerization of a potent and selective adenosine A2 antagonist, (E)-1,3-Dipropyl-8-(3,4-dimethoxystyryl)-7-methylxanthine. J Med Chem 1993; 36(23): 3731-3.
[http://dx.doi.org/10.1021/jm00075a031] [PMID: 8246243]

[237]   Chen W, Guéron M. AMP degradation in the perfused rat heart during 2-deoxy-D-glucose perfusion and anoxia. Part II: The determination of the degradation pathways using an adenosine deaminase inhibitor. J Mol Cell Cardiol 1996; 28(10): 2175-82.
[http://dx.doi.org/10.1006/jmcc.1996.0209] [PMID: 8930812]

[238]   Deussen A. Metabolic flux rates of adenosine in the heart. Naunyn Schmiedebergs Arch Pharmacol 2000; 362(4-5): 351-63.
[http://dx.doi.org/10.1007/s002100000318] [PMID: 11111829]

CHAPTER 3

Platelet Reactivity in Patients with Coronary Stenting Treated with Dual Antiplatelet Therapy and after Withdrawal of Clopidogrel: Impact of Bioactive Titanium Stent *versus* Everolimus-coated Stent

Amparo Hernándiz[1,*], José Luis Díez[3], Antonio Moscardó[2], Ana Latorre[2], Maria Dolores Domenech[4], Maria Teresa Santos[2] and Juana Vallés[2]

[1] *Cardiology Research Unit, Health Research Institute La fe, Torre A lab 5.04 Avda. Fernando Abril Martorell nº 106, 46026 Valencia, Spain*

[2] *Hemostasis, Thrombosis, Atherosclerosis, and Vascular Biology Unit, Health Research Institute La Fe, 46026 Valencia, Spain*

[3] *Department of Cardiology, University and Polytechnic Hospital La Fe, Valencia, Spain*

[4] *Cardiology Department Dr Peset Aleixandre Hospital, Valencia, Spain*

Abstract:

Objective: To study platelet reactivity at different times while on dual antiplatelet therapy (DAPT) with aspirin (ASA) and clopidogrel in patients treated with bioactive stents (TITAN$_2$®) or everolimus-coated stents (XIENCE V®) and one month after clopidogrel cessation.

Background: Coronary intervention damages the endothelium and causes platelet response leading to thrombotic occlusion, which is prevented with DAPT.

Methods: We studied 20 patients with bioactive stent and stable ischemia (BAS-SI group); 31 patients with bioactive stent and acute coronary syndrome (BAS-ACS group) and 31 patients with stable ischemia and everolimus-coated stent (EVE group). DAPT was administered (ASA 100 mg/day and clopidogrel 75 mg/day) for one year in BAS-ACS and EVE groups and for 1 month in BAS-SI group. Platelet aggregation induced by different agonists and platelet recruitment were analyzed at different times of DAPT and 1 month after clopidogrel cessation.

Results: After one month of DAPT, platelet aggregation showed no difference between groups; at 12 months of DAPT, the response to collagen and ADP increased in EVE

* **Corresponding author Amparo Hernándiz:** Cardiology Research Unit, Health Research Institute La Fe, Torre A lab 5.04 Avda. Fernando Abril Martorell nº 106, 46026 Valencia, Spain; Tel: 0034961246686; E-mail: hernandiz_amp@gva.es

Atta-ur-Rahman & M. Iqbal Choudhary (Eds.)

group. Platelet recruitment at 1 month was higher in the BAS-ACS than the other groups; after 12 months, recruitment increased in the EVE group with respect to BAS-ACS. Platelet aggregation and recruitment in diabetics were significantly higher in all situations than in non-diabetic patients. Clopidogrel withdrawal increased ADP-induced aggregation and collagen-induced aggregation and recruitment.

Conclusion: Platelet reactivity in patients with DAPT varies with time, depending on the subset of patients, the type of the stent implanted and the time after implantation.

Keywords: Platelet Activity, Stent, Recruitment, Aggregation, Dual Antiplatelet Therapy, Clopidogrel Withdrawal.

INTRODUCTION

Coronary stents are used in over 90% of percutaneous coronary interventions (PCI) due to their effectiveness in reducing the incidence of early complications and diminishing restenosis as compared with balloon angioplasty [1, 2]. Implanting a stent involves endothelial injury and a subsequent inflammatory response. The mechanical action of expansion and the following stent implantation cause endothelial denudation, damage to the structure of the vessel wall and atherosclerotic plaque rupture that lead to platelet adhesion, activation, aggregation and platelet recruitment to the forming thrombus that could produce a thrombotic coronary occlusion. In addition, impaired response to antiplatelet therapy or suppression of the anti-aggregants confers an important risk [3, 4]. In this context, the knowledge of platelet reactivity at different times after stent imposition could help to avoid the possible appearance of new vascular events. For this reason, the administration of dual antiplatelet therapy with ASA and P_2Y_{12} receptor antagonists (DAPT) is necessary when a stent is implanted [5]. It is recognized that bare metal stents (BMS) have an endothelization period lasting approximately one month [6], therefore current clinical guidelines recommend the administration of DAPT for at least four weeks to prevent stent thrombosis and other coronary events [5].

The advent of drug-eluting stents (DES) has been a step forward in terms of lower rates of restenosis and repeat revascularization of the target lesion [7]. Since the publication of the first clinical trials, the use of DES has spread worldwide. However, several alarming developments in relation to its safety have been published since then [8 - 10]. One of the most significant is the incidence of stent thrombosis, a phenomenon associated with the delay or even absence of endothelization of the meshes of the DES, particularly in those of the first generation [8]. This complication, although rare, could be catastrophic as it results in acute occlusion of the artery, leading to myocardial infarction or even death. While this problem affects both coated and non-coated stents, particularly in the first year after implantation [11 - 13], studies have found that some patients may suffer a very late DES-related thrombosis, beyond the first year of implantation, a fact rarely observed with BMS [14, 15].

BMS remains a commonly used alternative treatment strategy to DES, particularly for patients who present with the acute coronary syndrome and increased bleeding risk [5]. Recently, a bare metal and bioactive stent, the titanium nitride oxide-coated stent (TITAN$_2$®) constructed of stainless steel, a titanium alloy and nitric oxide, which completely prevent the release of nickel, chromium and molybdenum have been introduced. This, and the fact that they are not carriers of polymer makes them less proinflammatory and less pro-aggregatory in experimental animal models than coated stents and even than those of conventional metal [16, 17]. Also, their effectiveness has been demonstrated in various clinical scenarios [16, 18]. Among DES, the everolimus-eluting stent (XIENCE V®), a cobalt chromium stent eluting polymer and everolimus as an immunosuppressive agent have proven its superiority to others [19].

For most stable and acute coronary syndrome, patients treated with either DES or BMS, in whom surgery is not anticipated and the bleeding risk is not excessive, DAPT is recommended for a minimum 6 to 12 months. Rates of stent thrombosis are highest shortly after stent placement and remain significantly high until endothelization has occurred [5, 20].

As indicated above, platelet reactivity plays an important role in the development of stent thrombosis. Our goal has been to study platelet reactivity at different times of DAPT and after discontinuation of clopidogrel (P$_2$Y$_{12}$ ADP receptor blocker) in patients with bare metal bioactive stents and patients with everolimus-coated stents.

STUDY DESIGN AND METHODS

Ethics Statement

The study conformed to the ethical guidelines for human research defined by the Declaration of Helsinki and was approved by the Institutional Review Board of the University Hospital La Fe. All patients gave their written informed consent as approved by the Institutional Review Board.

Study Subjects

A prospective, observational, double-blind study was designed to examine platelet function in patients with ischemic heart disease undergoing PCI, according to standard clinical practice. Two types of stents were implanted: the bare metal bioactive stent TITAN$_2$® (Hexacath, Paris, France), (BAS group) and the everolimus-coated stent XIENCEV® (Abbott Vascular, Santa Clara, California, USA) (EVE group). Two cohorts with BAS were analyzed, patients with stable ischemic heart disease (BAS-SI group) undergoing DAPT (ASA 100 mg/day; clopidogrel 75 mg/day) for one month; and patients with acute coronary syndrome (BAS-ACS group) receiving DAPT for one year. In the EVE group, patients with stable ischemia requiring DAPT for one year were included. The indication and choice of the stent were made by the cardiologist, taking into account the clinical and anatomical criteria. The time-course of platelet function studies in the protocol is shown in Fig. (**1**). Compliance of patients with the antiplatelet therapy was closely followed by a personal interview with one of the researchers at each visit of the patients.

Exclusion criteria

Patients with allergy and/or intolerance to ASA and/or clopidogrel, a need for oral anticoagulation, diagnosis of infectious diseases, chronic inflammation, cancer diagnosis, indication for implantation of a new stent to treat restenosis, or implanted stents different from those studied. Patients who did not follow through with antiplatelet therapy correctly (non-compliant) were also excluded, as were those who suffered from an adverse cardiovascular event that forced the restart of dual antiplatelet therapy. Also patients with platelet counts $< 100 \times 10^3/\mu L$, anemia (hemoglobin<10g/dL), and renal insufficiency (creatinine >2.5mg/dL) were excluded.

Study Protocols

After inclusion and initiation of DAPT, all patients underwent an extraction of a peripheral venous blood sample a month after stent implantation to conduct studies of platelet function and baseline hematological and biochemical profiles (month 1). In the BAS-SI cohort, one month after implantation and with DAPT, clopidogrel was withdrawn after first blood sampling; a second sample was extracted in month 2, with only ASA as antiplatelet treatment; then in month 13, this cohort underwent another extraction after 12 months on ASA (Fig. **1**). In the BAS-ACS cohort and the EVE group, dual antiplatelet therapy was maintained for 1 year: a first extraction was performed in month 1; a second at month 12 before suspending clopidogrel; and another one in month 13, when only receiving ASA (Fig. **1**).

Blood Cell Collection and Processing

Citrate-anticoagulated (3.2%) venous blood was collected from patients into siliconized glass tubes (Vacutainer; Becton Dickinson, Madrid, Spain). Platelet-rich plasma (PRP) and platelet-poor plasma were prepared by differential centrifugation [21, 22]. The PRP samples were capped and stored at 22°C under 5% CO_2-air for use in the platelet aggregation and recruitment studies within 4 h of venipuncture.

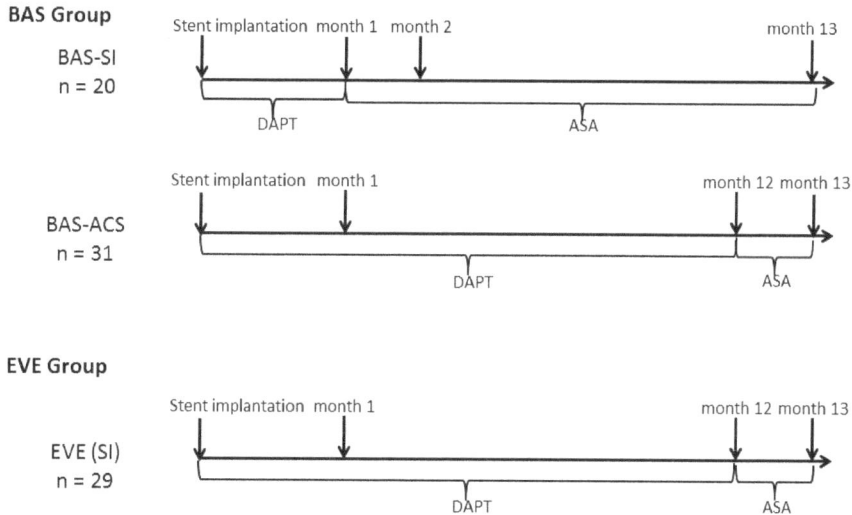

Fig. (1). Time course of study protocol for the evaluation of platelet reactivity. Month indicate the sequence of platelet function analysis.

Platelet Aggregation

Platelet aggregation induced with arachidonic acid (AA, 1 mM), adenosine diphosphate (ADP3 μM), thrombin-receptor-activating peptide (TRAP 15 μM), epinephrine (5 μM) (all from Sigma-Aldrich, Madrid, Spain), 1 μg/mL collagen (Nycomed Pharma GmbH, Munich, Germany) and 1 μM U46619, a stable analog of thromboxane A_2 (Cayman Chemicals, Ann Harbor, MI, USA) was determined by optical aggregometry (Chrono-Log 540, Havertown, PA, USA) as the change in light transmission. After the addition of the different platelet agonists to PRP, maximum platelet aggregation was measured and expressed as a percentage of aggregation.

Measurement of Platelet Recruitment

Platelet recruitment was evaluated as previously described (21-23). Collagen (1 μg/ml was added as the primary platelet agonist to whole blood (WB); the tube contents were mixed by inversion for 10 seconds and rapidly centrifuged (13,000g for 60 seconds) to obtain a cell-free release. An aliquot of this was immediately transferred as an inducer of platelet aggregation in an autologous platelet-rich plasma assay system (recruitment).

Statistical Analysis

The results for quantitative variables are presented as a mean and standard deviation and categorical variables are presented as absolute and relative frequencies (number of patients and percentage). The normality of the distribution was analyzed with the Kolmogorov-Smirnov test. To compare means in the variables with normal distribution, the Student's t-test was used for paired samples for intragroup comparisons and for unpaired samples in the comparison between groups. When the distribution was not normal the Mann-Whitney U test was used to compare two means, and Chi-square test to compare proportions. A p-value <0.05 was considered significant.

RESULTS

In one year, 80 patients were included in the study. However, for the evaluation of platelet function, a number of patients had to be excluded. Figs. (**2** and **3**) show the flow chart of the patients included in the study, patients excluded, the motive, and those who eventually underwent the platelet function testing. Noncompliance was an important factor to exclude patients for the platelet function studies; along with the study, 13.8% of patients included in the EVE group and a 31.4% of the BAS group were non-compliant for antiplatelet treatment. All results presented in this work come from compliant patients in which the platelet study was possible.

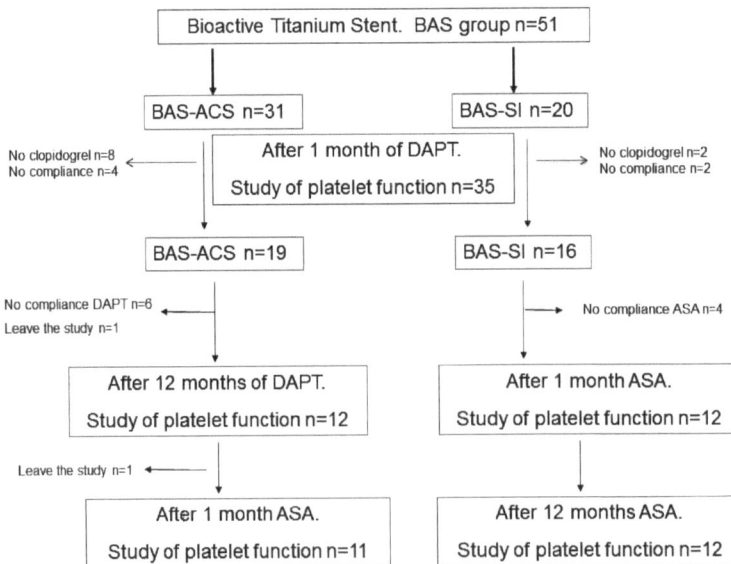

Fig. (2). Flow diagram of study protocol in patients with bioactive nitric oxide-coated stent implanted (Titan$_2$®).

```
┌─────────────────────────────────────────────┐
│   Everolimus-coated stent. EVE group  n=29    │
└─────────────────────────────────────────────┘
                    │          No clopidogrel n=1
                    ▼
        ┌───────────────────────────────────┐
        │  DAPT: Clopidogrel + ASA n=28     │
        └───────────────────────────────────┘
No compliance DAPT n=1 ◄────────────┤
                                     │
                    ┌────────────────────────────┐
                    │      1 month of DAPT.       │
                    │  Study of platelet function  n=27 │
                    └────────────────────────────┘
                            │             Leave the study n=4
                            │             No compliance DAPT n=3
                            ▼
                    ┌────────────────────────────┐
                    │   After 12 months of DAPT   │
                    │  Study of platelet function  n=20 │
                    └────────────────────────────┘
                            │
                            ▼
                    ┌────────────────────────────┐
                    │      After 1 month ASA      │
                    │  Study of platelet function n=20 │
                    └────────────────────────────┘
```

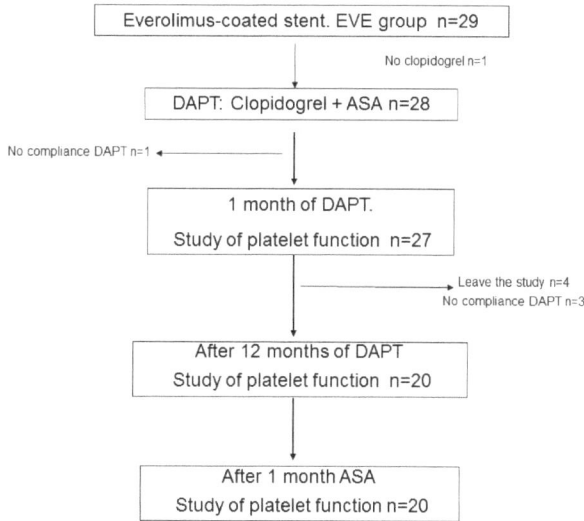

Fig. (3). Flow diagram of study protocol in patients with everolimus-coated stent implanted (XienceV®).

Baseline Characteristics

Anthropometric characteristics, biochemical and hematological profiles and cardiovascular risk factors of patients with platelet function studies are shown in Table **1**. Age, gender and biochemical and hematological profiles were similar in the three groups (Table **1**). With regard to cardiovascular risk factors, there were more smokers and greater presence of peripheral arterial disease in the BAS-ACS cohort (Table **1**). As expected, there was a higher percentage of diabetics in the EVE group, so more patients in this group were taking oral antidiabetic agents and/or insulin. There were no differences between groups with reference to other treatments with cardiovascular activity. The total length of implanted stents was significantly higher in the EVE group (32.4±19.1 mm *vs.* 17.8±6.7 mm BAS-SI, p<0.001; and 18.2±4.9 mm BAS-ACS, p<0.001).

Platelet Aggregation

After one month of stent implantation and DAPT, platelet aggregation induced by different agonists tested, showed no differences between groups, acute and stable patients with everolimus or bioactive stent (Table **2**). After twelve months of maintaining DAPT, a trend to increase platelet aggregation was observed in the EVE group when using ADP, collagen or U46619 as platelet agonists, being significant for TRAP-induced aggregation when compared to one month of DAPT. These results are in contrast with those obtained in the BAS-ACS group, in which after 12 months of DAPT, a decrease in platelet aggregation to collagen was found with respect to one month without changes in the presence of other agonists. Furthermore, after 12 months of DAPT, the platelet aggregation to collagen was significantly lower in the BAS-ACS group when compared with the EVE group (17.8±10.6 *vs.* 30.5±17.8%; p<0.05) (Table **2**).

Table 1. Clinical Characteristics and Cardiovascular Risk Factors in Patients with Platelet Function Study.

	EVE (n27)	**BAS-SI (n16)**	**BAS-ACS(n19)**	**P value**
Age (years)	63.6 ±11.1	66.7±11.4	62.2±12.6	ns
BMI	31.6 ± 4.8	28.5 ± 4.1*	30.0±4.2	*p<0.05
Gender (men)	(19) 70.4%	(11) 69.8%	(15) 78.9%	ns
PAD (clinical).	0%	(1) 6.3%	(3) 15.8%*	*p<0.05
Diabetes (DMT2)	(14) 52%	(6) 37.5%	(6) 31.6%	ns
Hypertension	(20) 74.1%	(12) 75%	(11) 57.9%	ns
Dyslipemia	(17) 63%	(9) 56.3%	(11) 57.9%	ns
CVD Familiar history	(17) 63%	(10) 62.5%	(12) 63.2%	ns
Smoking≤1 year	(6) 22.2%	(3) 18.8%	(12) 63.2%**[A]	**p<0.01[A]p<0.01
Clycemia (mg/dL)	124.1 ± 51.2	110.6 ± 30.3	106.9 ±17.6	ns
HbA1c (%)	6.7±1.4	6.5±1.2	6.2±0.7	ns
Total Cholest.(mg/dL)	168.6± 34.6	176 ± 50.1	148.7±39.3	ns
TGL(mg/dL)	151 ± 55.1	169.5 ± 150.3	114.4 ± 50.6*	*p<0.05
Creatinine (mg/dL)	0.89 ± 0.18	0.86± 0.21	0.82±0.21	ns
CRP (mg/L)	3.9 ± 4.1	5.3 ± 4.9	3.6 ± 2.4	ns
Hematocrit (%)	41.5 ± 3.5	41.9 ± 4.4	42.3±2.9	ns
Platelets (x10³/μL)	222.6 ± 57.5	209.1± 73.2	218.7±40.9	ns
Platelets vol. (fL)	12.2 ±5.1	11.2±0.9	11.1±0.9	ns
Leukocytes (x10³/μL)	7.4 ± 2.01	7.2 ± 2.7	7.6 ± 1.7	ns
ACEI/ARA II	(17) 62.4%	(11) 68.8%	(11) 57.6%	ns
ß Blocker	(21) 77.8%	(11) 68.8%	(14) 73.7%	ns
Ca Antagonist	(8) 29.6%	(3) 18.8%	(4) 21.1%	ns
Diuretic	(5) 18.5%	(4) 25%	(2) 10.5%	ns
Oral antidiabetic	(11) 40.7%	(4) 25%*	(6) 31.6%**	*p<0.05**p<0.01
Insulin	(8) 29.6%	(3) 18.8%	(1) 5.3%*	*p<0.05
Statin	(24) 88.4%	(15) 93.9%	(18) 94.7%	ns

BMI: body mass index; PAD: peripheral arterial disease; CVD: cardiovascular disease; HbA1c: glycated hemoglobin. TGL: triglycerides; CRP: C reactive protein.
*p<0.05; **p≤0.01 comparing EVE *vs.* BAS-SI or comparing EVE *vs.* BAS-ACS; [A] p<0.01 comparing BAS-SI *vs.* BAS-ACS.

Table 2. Platelet Aggregation by Optical Aggregometry in Patients with EVE or BAS Stent.

% max. I.	EVE			BAS-ACS			BAS-SI		
	Month1 DATP n=27	Month 12 DAPT n=20	Month 13 ASA n=20	Month 1 DAPT n=19	Month 12 DAPT n=12	Month 13 ASA n=11	Month 1 DAPT n=16	Month 2 ASA n=12	Month 13 ASA n=12
AA (1μM)	12.03±17	6.4±5.7	13.0±20.2	5.1±4.2	3.3±4.9	9.8±14.9	7.3±4.3	7.5±3.6	7.9±6.9
ADP (3 μM)	48.1±10	50.9±9.6	62.4±6.4*	48.6±10.1	46.6±6.4	63.2±8.7*	47.4±3.8	58.9±17.5*	68.2±9.6*
Coll (1μg/ml)	24.1±14.1	30.5±17.8	43.6±17.9*	24.3±12.7	17.8±10.6 a	41.2±21.9*	25.8±14.3	36.3±12.2	36.4±15.3
Epi (5μM)	34.02±13.1	31.6±12.4	33.02±10.6	36.4±11.1	38.3±11.6	37.7±14.9	36.2±11	38.8±16.1	40.8±10.5
U (1μM)	66.2±17.6	70.3±7.4	71.4±14.1	67.9±13.1	62.3±14.2	70.3±19.1	65.9±12	71.6±8.1	73.9±10.7
TRAP (15 μM)	67.7±6.1	72.1±7.5*	74.3±5.7	71.5±8.6	74.1±6.2	77.4±7.1	72.8±17	74.8±6.6	79.4±6.4

AA: arachidonic acid; ADP: adenosine diphosphate; Coll: collagen; Epi: epinephrine; U: U46619; TRAP: thrombin receptor activator. Max. I: maximum intensity of aggregation. DAPT: ASA and clopidogrel (P_2Y_{12} inhibitor); * $p<0.05$; intragroup comparisons *vs.* previous value; a $p<0.05$ comparing EVE *vs.* BAS-ACS month 12; Mean and standard deviation of % max. Intensity of platelet aggregation.

Platelet Recruitment

The maximal intensity of the pro-aggregatory activity of cell-free releasates from collagen stimulating whole blood (recruitment, mm) is shown in Fig. (**4**). After one month of stent implantation and DAPT, a significantly higher recruiting activity in WB was observed in BAS-ACS group (56.7±22.7 mm) when compared with the EVE (44.03±19.8 mm; $p<0.05$) (Fig. **4A**) and BAS-SI groups (50.3±24.3 mm) (Fig. **4B**), However, after 12 months of DAPT, patients in the EVE group showed a significant increase in the platelet recruiting activity (60.2±23.6 mm; $p<0.05$) when compared to one month of treatment, while in the BAS-ACS group, the opposite was observed; recruitment decreased with the time of DAPT treatment (56.7±22.7mm *vs.* 50.4±16.9 mm) (Fig. **4B**). This suggests that similar to data on collagen-induced aggregation, a time-dependent increase in collagen-induced platelet recruitment takes place in patients in the EVE group.

Effect of Clopidogrel Withdrawal on Platelet Aggregation and Platelet Recruitment in WB

Platelet Aggregation

After clopidogrel withdrawal, a significant increase in platelet aggregation in the presence of ADP and collagen was observed in all cases, with no differences between groups (Table **2**). Also no differences were observed in the aggregation induced by the other platelet agonists tested in any of the groups of patients after clopidogrel withdrawal (Table **2**).

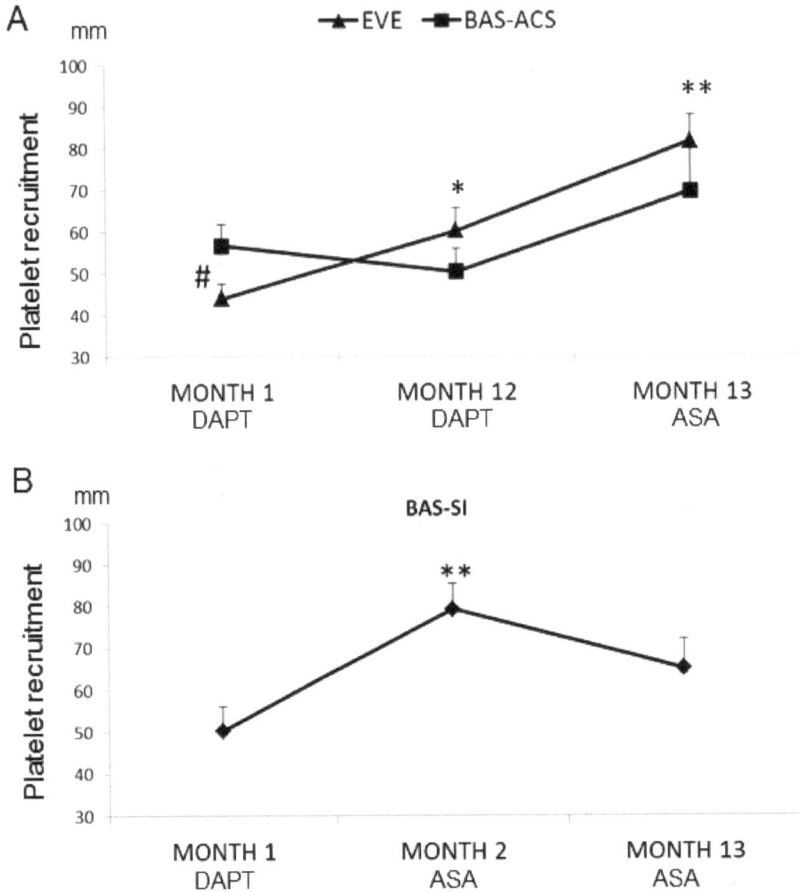

Fig. (4). Platelet recruitment in whole blood in the different groups of patients. Graph A represents BAS-ACS group and EVE group values at one and 12 months of DAPT after stent imposition and after clopidogrel withdrawal (month 13); Graph B represents BAS-SI group values at one month of DAPT after stent imposition and at month 2 and month 13 after clopidogrel withdrawal (only ASA). Data is mean ± SEM Statistical significance: * $p<0.05$; ** $p<0.01$ intragroup comparison *vs.* previous value; # $p<0.05$ BAS-ACS *vs.* EVE comparison. The BAS-ACS group showed higher platelet recruitment at one month of DAPT than the other groups; at 12 months the EVE group showed an increase in platelet reactivity respect to one month values and the BAS-ACS group. After clopidogrel withdrawal all groups presented an increase of platelet recruitment.

Platelet Recruitment

One month after clopidogrel withdrawal, an increase in platelet recruiting activity with respect to the previous value on DAPT was observed in the 3 groups of patients, month 13 on ASA alone: in the EVE group (81.6 ± 28.5 *vs*. 60.2 ± 23.6 mm; $p < 0.01$) and BAS-ACS (69.6 ± 34.7 *vs*. 50.4 ± 16.9 mm) and month 2 after 1 month of DAPT in the BAS-SI group (79.2 ± 23.4 *vs*. 50.3 ± 24.3; $p < 0.01$) (Fig. **4A, B**).

Influence of Cardiovascular Risk Factors

When we compared the three groups of patients concerning their cardiovascular risk factors, only two of them showed differences: smoking was present in more BAS-ACS patients (63.2%) and diabetes (DMT2) in more EVE group patients (52%) (Table **1**).

Diabetes is a recognized risk factor for stent thrombosis. When we analyzed the influence of diabetes on the profile of platelet reactivity in patients from the different groups, we observed that after 1 month of stent implantation and DAPT, comparing diabetic (n=26) with non-diabetic patients (n=36), diabetics had a higher maximal intensity of platelet aggregation (%) induced by ADP (44.6 ± 11.4 non-diabetics *vs*. 53.3 ± 9.9 diabetics; $p < 0.05$); collagen (19.8 ± 11.4 non-diabetics *vs*. 31.5 ± 13.6 diabetics; $p < 0.001$); epinephrine (32.3 ± 9.6 non-diabetics *vs*. 39.6 ± 13.6 diabetics; $p < 0.05$) and arachidonic acid (7.9 ± 9.9 non-diabetics *vs*. 10.04 ± 14.9 diabetics; $p < 0.01$). The recruiting activity was also significantly higher in diabetic patients (57.2 ± 24.8) than non-diabetic patients (44.2 ± 18.9; $p < 0.05$).

When different groups of patients were evaluated separately (Fig. **5**), the increase in platelet recruiting activity was significantly higher in BAS-ACS diabetic patients in the first month after stent implantation and DAPT, which was also significantly higher when compared with diabetic patients from the other studied groups at the first month of treatment. After 12 months of DAPT, platelet recruiting activity decreased in the BAS-ACS diabetics and increased in EVE diabetics with respect to month 1 values. Clopidogrel withdrawal also produced a similar increase in platelet recruiting activity in both diabetic and non-diabetic patients in all groups when data on DAPT *vs*. ASA alone were compared. Non-diabetic patients showed a similar profile of the recruiting activity with no differences between groups.

DISCUSSION

Platelet activation plays an important role in the development of restenosis and thrombosis after stent implantation. In this context, the present study was performed because, in our knowledge, no data are available concerning platelet reactivity at different times after stenting, comparing patients with one or more everolimus-coated stents and bare metal bioactive stents. In addition, the time-course of the effect of DAPT (one moth *vs.* one year) in patients treated with these two types of stents has not been previously evaluated. Furthermore, there are controversial data in the literature concerning the effect of clopidogrel suppression on platelet reactivity after a time of dual antiplatelet treatment with aspirin plus clopidogrel.

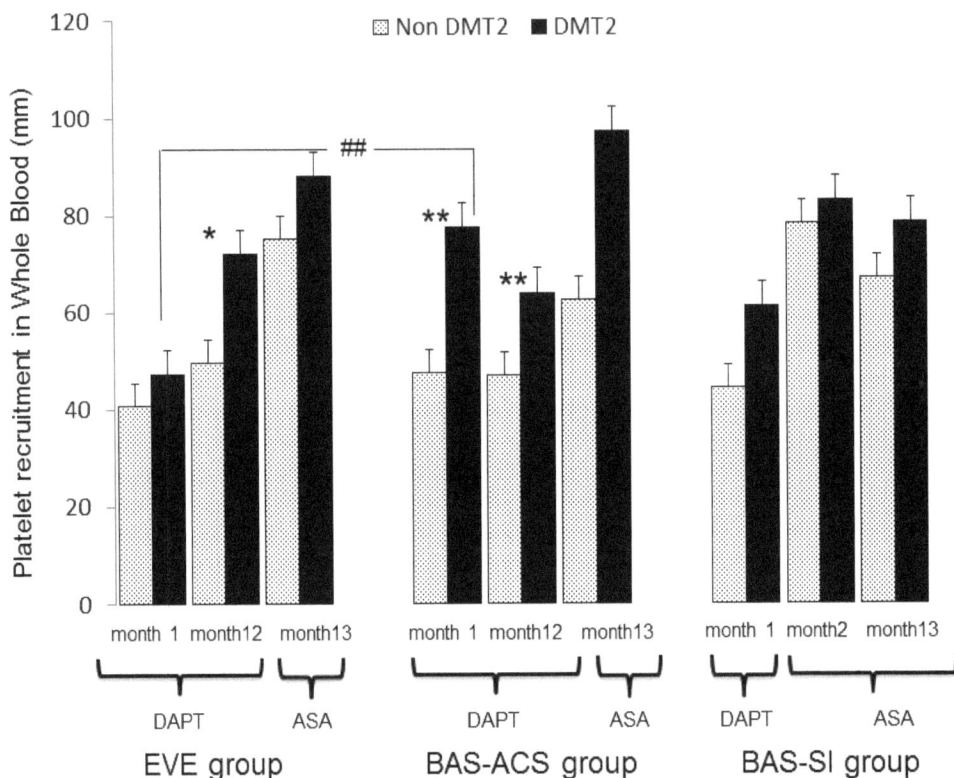

Fig. (5). Platelet recruitment in diabetic and non-diabetic patients from the different groups. BAS-SI: diabetics n=6; non-diabetics n=10; BAS-ACS: diabetics n=6; non-diabetics n=13; and EVE: diabetics n=14; non-diabetics n=1. Values at one and 12 months of DAPT after stent imposition and one month after clopidogrel withdrawal in BAS-ACS and EVE groups; BAS-SI group values at one month of DAPT after stent imposition and at month 2 and month 13 after clopidogrel withdrawal (only ASA). Statistical significance: * $p<0.05$; ** $p<0.01$ intragroup comparison DMT2 *vs.* non-DMT2; # $p<0.01$ DMT2 BAS-ACS patients *vs.* DMT2 EVE patients.

The results obtained in this study show that there is a different profile of platelet aggregation in patients on DAPT after the implantation of an everolimus-coated stent (XIENCE V®) or bioactive stents (TITAN$_2$®).

Advances in interventional cardiology techniques and stent technology have significantly developed in the last years. Currently, a new-generation of DES is the standard device for stenting in stable and unstable coronary artery disease patients. However, the need for extended dual antiplatelet therapy following DES implantation can be complicated in particular subsets of patients with an increased risk of bleeding [5]. The fact that dual antiplatelet therapy is needed for no more than one month following implantation of $TITAN_2^®$ presents these stents as eligible candidates in these subsets of patients [17, 18].

While a month after stent implantation and DAPT, platelet aggregation was similar in the EVE and BAS groups (both SI and ACS), platelet aggregation tended to increase after 12 months in the EVE group compared with one month of treatment, and to decrease in the BAS-ACS, patients with the $TITAN_2^®$ stent and acute coronary syndrome (Table **2**). After one month of DAPT and stent implantation, a similar response in WB platelet recruitment in both the EVE group and BAS-SI group was detected; while higher platelet recruitment in the BAS-ACS group was observed. However, after 12 months, this response changed, increasing in the EVE group *vs.* BAS-ACS group (Fig. **4**).

The results of this study were obtained by concordantly using two different methods for platelet function testing. We analyzed platelet aggregation in PRP with light transmission aggregometry, which remains the gold standard technique in this setting, but we also evaluated the collagen-induced platelet recruitment in WB, where a cell-free release obtained within 1 minute by centrifugation (13,000xg) is used as an inducer of platelet aggregation of an autologous PRP assay system (recruitment). Platelet recruitment is an essential step for thrombus growth, which in WB is influenced by cell-cell interactions between platelets and other cells in blood, thus giving a more physiological measure than the study in PRP [21 - 23].

Although platelet reactivity showed similar tendencies over time with both methods used after the imposition of each type of stent (Table **2**, Fig. **4**), we observed some differences in platelet response at short times (one month) when we measured platelet recruitment depending on the clinical situation. This result could be explained by the participation of other blood components that may modulate platelet function [21 - 23]. In the BAS-ACS patients, the high platelet recruitment might be related to a possible early stent thrombosis, described in the acute coronary syndrome [24].

The increase in platelet function seen in the EVE group at 12 months with respect to one month after the stent implantation may be explained by the absence of endothelization of their meshes and may support, in part, the presence of a late stent thrombosis in patients with DES stent [25, 26].

Diabetes is a recognized risk factor for stent thrombosis; our results obtained from diabetic patients after stenting showed an increase in the platelet response when compared with non-diabetic patients in all situations of the study. These results agree with other studies that show higher platelet aggregation and recruitment in diabetics [27, 28]. However, this response differs depending on the patient's condition (stable or ACS) and the type of stent implanted, as does the time of DAPT. Diabetic BAS-ACS patients showed higher platelet activity after a short time (one month) of DAPT than stable diabetic patients (BAS-SI and EVE groups), this recognizes the increase in platelet function in acute coronary syndrome, and these results are in line with other studies in patients with diabetes mellitus (TITANIC XV study [29]). This situation was reversed at 12 months of DAPT, where patients with stable heart disease, diabetes and with XIENCEV® stents increased their platelet function, while in the acute patients with TITAN$_2$® it decreased.

Different studies have suggested an increased risk of recurrent cardiovascular events after stopping clopidogrel therapy [4]. It has been proposed that it could be due to a "rebound" of platelet reactivity after clopidogrel cessation [30]. However, other studies indicate that platelet response remained stable over time after stopping clopidogrel therapy [31]. Our results after one month of withdrawal indicate an increase in platelet aggregation in response to ADP as expected after cessation of the inhibition of the P_2Y_{12} receptor pathway; independently of the stent implanted and the duration of DAPT. When we used different platelet agonists, only collagen showed a significant increase, which indicates that ADP mediates the platelet aggregation to collagen, demonstrated in "*in vitro*" studies. The platelet recruitment in WB showed a similar response after clopidogrel cessation in the different groups.

STUDY LIMITATIONS

This study has some limitations partly due to the inclusion of real-world patients in a clinical setting. Platelet function studies require compliance with daily antiplatelet medication; the patient sample is less than in the inclusion mainly due to the incorrect compliance in antiplatelet therapy. To make comparisons of duration of DAPT possible, we included patients who suffered an ACS, but because of their characteristics needed a bioactive stent and DAPT for 12 months, and ischemic stable patients who needed an everolimus stent and 12 months of DAPT; and for comparing the degree of cardiac ischemia patients with stable ischemic heart disease and bioactive stent implantation but with one month of DAPT.

CONCLUSION

Our results show that the platelet reactivity measured with two different methods used in this study, platelet aggregation in PRP and platelet recruitment in WB; showed a different profile of platelet activation depending on the subset of patient studied, the type of stent, and the time after stent implantation and DAPT.

ABBREVIATIONS

AA	Arachidonic Acid
ACS	Acute Coronary Syndrome
ADP	Adenosine Diphosphate
ASA	Acetylsalicylic Acid, Aspirin
BAS	Bioactive Stent Group
BMS	Bare Metal Stent
DAPT	Dual Antiplatelet Therapy
DES	Drug-eluting Stent
EVE	Everolimus Stent Group
PCI	Percutaneous Coronary Intervention
PRP	Platelet-rich Plasma
SI	Stable Ischemia
TRAP	Thrombin Receptor Activator Peptide
U	U46619 Stable Analog of Thromboxane A_2
WB	Whole Blood

ETHICS APPROVAL AND CONSENT TO PARTICIPATE

Not applicable.

HUMAN AND ANIMAL RIGHTS

No Animals/Humans were used for studies that are the basis of this research.

CONSENT FOR PUBLICATION

Not applicable.

CONFLICT OF INTEREST

The authors declare no conflict of interest, financial or otherwise.

ACKNOWLEDGEMENTS

This study has been supported in part by FISS 13/00016 Fondos FEDER una forma de hacer Europa.

REFERENCES

[1]   Fischman DL, Leon MB, Baim DS, *et al.* A randomized comparison of coronary-stent placement and balloon angioplasty in the treatment of coronary artery disease. N Engl J Med 1994; 331(8): 496-501.
[http://dx.doi.org/10.1056/NEJM199408253310802] [PMID: 8041414]

[2]   Serruys PW, de Jaegere P, Kiemeneij F, *et al.* A comparison of balloon-expandable-stent implantation with balloon angioplasty in patients with coronary artery disease. N Engl J Med 1994; 331(8): 489-95.
[http://dx.doi.org/10.1056/NEJM199408253310801] [PMID: 8041413]

[3]   McFadden EP, Stabile E, Regar E, *et al.* Late thrombosis in drug-eluting coronary stents after discontinuation of antiplatelet therapy. Lancet 2004; 364(9444): 1519-21.
[http://dx.doi.org/10.1016/S0140-6736(04)17275-9] [PMID: 15500897]

[4]   Ford I. Coming safely to a stop: a review of platelet activity after cessation of antiplatelet drugs. Ther Adv Drug Saf 2015; 6(4): 141-50.
[http://dx.doi.org/10.1177/2042098615588085] [PMID: 26301068]

[5]   Levine GN, Bates ER, Bittl JA, *et al.* 2016 ACC/AHA Guideline Focused Update on Duration of Dual Antiplatelet Therapy in Patients With Coronary Artery Disease: A Report of the American College of Cardiology/American Heart Association Task Force on Clinical Practice Guidelines. J Am Coll Cardiol 2016; 68(10): 1082-115.
[http://dx.doi.org/10.1016/j.jacc.2016.03.513] [PMID: 27036918]

[6]   Nath FC, Muller DW, Ellis SG, *et al.* Thrombosis of a flexible coil coronary stent: frequency, predictors and clinical outcome. J Am Coll Cardiol 1993; 21(3): 622-7.
[http://dx.doi.org/10.1016/0735-1097(93)90093-G] [PMID: 8436743]

[7]   Kastrati A, Mehilli J, Pache J, *et al.* Analysis of 14 trials comparing sirolimus-eluting stents with bare-metal stents. N Engl J Med 2007; 356(10): 1030-9.
[http://dx.doi.org/10.1056/NEJMoa067484] [PMID: 17296823]

[8]   Virmani R, Liistro F, Stankovic G, *et al.* Mechanism of late in-stent restenosis after implantation of a paclitaxel derivate-eluting polymer stent system in humans. Circulation 2002; 106(21): 2649-51.
[http://dx.doi.org/10.1161/01.CIR.0000041632.02514.14] [PMID: 12438288]

[9]   Joner M, Finn AV, Farb A, *et al.* Pathology of drug-eluting stents in humans: delayed healing and late thrombotic risk. J Am Coll Cardiol 2006; 48(1): 193-202.
[http://dx.doi.org/10.1016/j.jacc.2006.03.042] [PMID: 16814667]

[10] Nilsen DW, Melberg T, Larsen AI, Barvik S, Bonarjee V. Late complications following the deployment of drug eluting stents. Int J Cardiol 2006; 109(3): 398-401.
[http://dx.doi.org/10.1016/j.ijcard.2005.05.029] [PMID: 16102858]

[11] Wenaweser P, Rey C, Eberli FR, *et al.* Stent thrombosis following bare-metal stent implantation: success of emergency percutaneous coronary intervention and predictors of adverse outcome. Eur Heart J 2005; 26(12): 1180-7.
[http://dx.doi.org/10.1093/eurheartj/ehi135] [PMID: 15728650]

[12] Moreno R, Fernández C, Hernández R, *et al.* Drug-eluting stent thrombosis: results from a pooled analysis including 10 randomized studies. J Am Coll Cardiol 2005; 45(6): 954-9.
[http://dx.doi.org/10.1016/j.jacc.2004.11.065] [PMID: 15766835]

[13] Kereiakes DJ, Yeh RW, Massaro JM. Discoll- Shempp P, Cutlip DE, Steg PG, Gershlick AH, Darius H, Meredith IT, Ormiston J, Tanguay JF, Windecker S, Garratt KN, Kandzari DE, Lee DP, Simon DI, Iancu AC, Trebacz J, Mauri L, DAPT Study Investigators. Stent thrombosis in drug-eluting or bare-

metal stents in patients receiving dual antiplatelet therapy. J Am Coll Cardiol 2015; 8: 1552-62.
[http://dx.doi.org/10.1016/j.jcin.2015.05.026]

[14]   Bavry AA, Kumbhani DJ, Helton TJ, Borek PP, Mood GR, Bhatt DL. Late thrombosis of drug-eluting
       stents: a meta-analysis of randomized clinical trials. Am J Med 2006; 119(12): 1056-61.
       [http://dx.doi.org/10.1016/j.amjmed.2006.01.023] [PMID: 17145250]

[15]   Bavry AA, Kumbhani DJ, Helton TJ, Bhatt DL. What is the risk of stent thrombosis associated with
       the use of paclitaxel-eluting stents for percutaneous coronary intervention?: a meta-analysis. J Am Coll
       Cardiol 2005; 45(6): 941-6.
       [http://dx.doi.org/10.1016/j.jacc.2004.11.064] [PMID: 15766833]

[16]   Karjalainen PP, Ylitalo A, Airaksinen JK, Nammas W. Titanium-nitride-oxide-coated Titan-$_2$ bioactive
       coronary stent: a new horizon for coronary intervention. Expert Rev Med Devices 2010; 7(5): 599-
       604.
       [http://dx.doi.org/10.1586/erd.10.44] [PMID: 20822383]

[17]   Windecker S, Mayer I, De Pasquale G, *et al.* Stent coating with titanium-nitride-oxide for reduction of
       neointimal hyperplasia. Circulation 2001; 104(8): 928-33.
       [http://dx.doi.org/10.1161/hc3401.093146] [PMID: 11514381]

[18]   Tuomainen PO, Sia J, Nammas W, *et al.* Pooled analysis of two randomized trials comparing
       titanium-nitride-oxide-coated stent *versus* drug-eluting stent in STEMI. Rev Esp Cardiol (Engl Ed)
       2014; 67(7): 531-7.
       [http://dx.doi.org/10.1016/j.rec.2014.01.024] [PMID: 24952392]

[19]   Serruys PW, Ruygrok P, Neuzner J, *et al.* A randomised comparison of an everolimus-eluting
       coronary stent with a paclitaxel-eluting coronary stent:the SPIRIT II trial. EuroIntervention 2006; 2(3):
       286-94.
       [PMID: 19755303]

[20]   Cutlip D, Nicolau JC. Long term antiplatelet therapy after coronary artery stenting in stable
       patients.UptoDate Saperic GM. , 2017. [accesed July 25, 2017];

[21]   Santos MT, Vallés J, Marcus AJ, *et al.* Enhancement of platelet reactivity and modulation of
       eicosanoid production by intact erythrocytes. A new approach to platelet activation and recruitment. J
       Clin Invest 1991; 87(2): 571-80.
       [http://dx.doi.org/10.1172/JCI115032] [PMID: 1991840]

[22]   Vallés J, Santos MT, Aznar J, *et al.* Erythrocytes metabolically enhance collagen-induced platelet
       responsiveness *via* increased thromboxane production, adenosine diphosphate release, and recruitment.
       Blood 1991; 78(1): 154-62.
       [PMID: 1712639]

[23]   Vallés J, Santos MT, Aznar J, *et al.* Erythrocyte promotion of platelet reactivity decreases the
       effectiveness of aspirin as an antithrombotic therapeutic modality: the effect of low-dose aspirin is less
       than optimal in patients with vascular disease due to prothrombotic effects of erythrocytes on platelet
       reactivity. Circulation 1998; 97(4): 350-5.
       [http://dx.doi.org/10.1161/01.CIR.97.4.350] [PMID: 9468208]

[24]   Ong AT, Hoye A, Aoki J, *et al.* Thirty-day incidence and six-month clinical outcome of thrombotic
       stent occlusion after bare-metal, sirolimus, or paclitaxel stent implantation. J Am Coll Cardiol 2005;
       45(6): 947-53.
       [http://dx.doi.org/10.1016/j.jacc.2004.09.079] [PMID: 15766834]

[25]   Finn AV, Nakazawa G, Joner M, *et al.* Vascular responses to drug eluting stents: importance of
       delayed healing. Arterioscler Thromb Vasc Biol 2007; 27(7): 1500-10.
       [http://dx.doi.org/10.1161/ATVBAHA.107.144220] [PMID: 17510464]

[26]   Byrne RA, Joner M, Kastrati A. Stent thrombosis and restenosis: what have we learned and where are
       we going? The Andreas Grüntzig Lecture ESC 2014. Eur Heart J 2015; 36(47): 3320-31.
       [http://dx.doi.org/10.1093/eurheartj/ehv511] [PMID: 26417060]

[27] Kukula K, Klopotowski M, Kunicki PK, *et al.* Platelet aggregation and risk of stent thrombosis or bleeding in interventionally treated diabetic patients with acute coronary syndrome. BMC Cardiovasc Disord 2016; 16(1): 252-60.
[http://dx.doi.org/10.1186/s12872-016-0433-x] [PMID: 27931181]

[28] Vallés J, Santos MT, Aznar J, Velert M, Barberá G, Carmena R. Modulatory effect of erythrocytes on the platelet reactivity to collagen in IDDM patients. Diabetes 1997; 46(6): 1047-53.
[http://dx.doi.org/10.2337/diab.46.6.1047] [PMID: 9166678]

[29] López-Minguez JR, Nogales-Asensio JM, Doncel-Vecino LJ, *et al.* on behalf of the members of the TITANIC XV Working Group. A randomized study to compare bioactive Titanium stents and Everolimus-eluting stents in diabetic patients (TITANIC XV): 1-year results. Rev Esp Cardiol 2014; 67: 511-3.
[PMID: 24952388]

[30] Ho PM, Peterson ED, Wang L, *et al.* Incidence of death and acute myocardial infarction associated with stopping clopidogrel after acute coronary syndrome. JAMA 2008; 299(5): 532-9.
[http://dx.doi.org/10.1001/jama.299.5.532] [PMID: 18252883]

[31] Sibbing D, Stegherr J, Braun S, *et al.* A double-blind, randomized study on prevention and existence of a rebound phenomenon of platelets after cessation of clopidogrel treatment. J Am Coll Cardiol 2010; 55(6): 558-65.
[http://dx.doi.org/10.1016/j.jacc.2009.09.038] [PMID: 20152561]

CHAPTER 4

Immunosuppressive Drugs in Heart Transplantation

Sule Apikoglu-Rabus[1,*], **Murat B. Rabus**[2] and **Rashida Muhammad Umar**[1]

[1] *Marmara University Faculty of Pharmacy, Clinical Pharmacy Department, Istanbul, Turkey*

[2] *Kartal Kosuyolu Higher Specialization Training and Research Hospital, Cardiovascular Surgery Department, Istanbul, Turkey*

Abstract: Congestive heart failure affects 23 million people worldwide [1]. Cardiac transplantation provides a lifesaving treatment for patients with end-stage heart disease. It offers a longer life with a higher quality to those who have no other treatment alternative. Although cardiac transplantation offers a relief from heart immunosuppression. The goal of immunosuppression immediately following surgery is to prevent hyperacute and acute rejections. Transplantation immunosuppression must be balanced in order to prevent rejection while minimizing the serious adverse effects of therapy including life-threatening infections and malignancies. Immunosuppressive regimens are classified as induction, maintenance, or anti-rejection regimens. Induction regimens consist of intense early post-operative immunosuppression while maintenance regimens are used indefinitely for prevention of acute and chronic rejection. This chapter will review the induction and maintenance immunosuppressive regimens used in heart transplantation with summaries of selected literature as well as the most common complications of these therapies and significant drug-drug interactions.

Keywords: Heart transplantation, Immunosuppression, Interactions, Pharmacotherapy.

INTRODUCTION

Congestive heart failure affects 23 million people worldwide [1]. Cardiac transplantation provides a lifesaving treatment for patients with end-stage heart disease. It offers a longer life with a higher quality to those who have no other treatment alternative. Although cardiac transplantation offers a relief from heart failure problems, new problems may arise due to the unwanted effects of failure

---

* **Corresponding author Sule Apikoglu-Rabus:** Marmara University Faculty of Pharmacy, Clinical Pharmacy Department, Istanbul, Turkey; Tel: +90.216.3464060; Fax: +90.216.3452952 ; E-mail: sulerabus@yahoo.com, sule.rabus@marmara.edu.tr

Atta-ur-Rahman & M. Iqbal Choudhary (Eds.)

problems, new problems may arise due to the unwanted effects of immunosuppression.

According to the Registry of International Society for Heart and Lung Transplantation (ISHLT) data a total of 4,477 heart transplants (including 3,817 adult transplants) from 252 centers were performed in 2013 and reported to the ISHLT [2]. As the population gets older, the demand for cardiac transplantation increases. However, the number of cadaveric donors has been relatively stable during the last decades. It was reported that for each year number of the patients on the waiting list is 1.5 – 3 times more than the number of donors [3]. The annual mortality rate while on the waiting list in 2001 was 17%. This rate has gradually declined over the last decade to 13.7% in 2009 [4] as left ventricular assist devices are now being used more commonly as a bridge to transplantation.

Survival after transplantation has improved significantly over the past three decades. This is a result of improvements in surgical techniques, postoperative patient management and advances in pharmacotherapy. The ISHLT 2015 report states that for all 112,521 pediatric and adult heart transplants (excluding heart-lung) performed between 1982 and June 2013, 1-year survival was 82% and 5-year survival was 69%, with median survival of 11 years for all patients and 13 years for those surviving the first year. Survival was better in the pediatric population with median survival of 15.3 years for all patients and 20 years for those surviving the first year [2]. The ISHLT 2015 report shows incremental improvement of unadjusted 1-year survival in the most recent era (2009 to 2013), when compared with that of the 2002 to 2008 era (86% *vs.* 84%) [2].

Acute rejection is a major determinant of survival after cardiac transplantation. More than half of the cardiac transplant recipients will experience at least one episode of acute rejection. On the other hand chronic rejection is a major cause of late graft loss. According to the ISHLT data, the leading causes of death were graft failure, infection and multiple-organ failure. Death due to graft failure was most prominent in the acute and long term, while infection was the prominent cause in the first year, and cardiac allograft vasculopathy (CAV), malignancy and renal failure were more frequent causes of death over time [2]. Acute rejection accounted for 8% of deaths in years 1 to 3 [2].

The goal of immunosuppression immediately following surgery is to prevent hyperacute and acute rejections. Therefore, higher doses of immunosuppressive agents are required to achieve this goal. If these higher doses are continued for long term, serious complications such as nephrotoxicity, infections, thrombocytopenia and diabetes may arise. Transplantation immunosuppression must be balanced in order to prevent rejection while minimizing the serious adverse effects of therapy including life-threatening infections and malignancies. In the period between discharge and end of the postoperative first year the rate of rejection, which was 30% in 2004 - 2006, has decreased to 25% in 2010 - 2012 due to the improvements in immunosuppression [2].

Immunosuppressive regimens are classified as induction, maintenance, or anti-rejection regimens. Induction regimens consist of intense early post-operative immunosuppression while maintenance regimens are used indefinitely for prevention of acute and chronic rejection. This chapter will review the induction and maintenance immunosuppressive regimens used in heart transplantation with summaries of selected literature as well as the most common complications of these therapies and significant drug-drug interactions.

Induction Immunosuppressive Therapy

Rejection episodes most frequently happen during the first months following cardiac transplantation. The main reason for this is the increased immune response of the recipient shortly after transplantation due to factors such as surgical trauma, ischemia/reperfusion and donor brain death. Therefore, almost half of the heart transplantation centers are applying induction therapy for the heart transplant recipients [5, 6].

Induction therapy is an intensive perioperative immunosuppressive therapy. The aim of the induction therapy is to deplete T lymphocytes or to prevent lymphocyte proliferation during this most immunoreactive phase. The overall utility of induction therapy has remained controversial for more than 20 years. Induction therapy reduces the rejection rate in the early post-transplant period and allows the late introduction of calcineurin inhibitors, thus avoiding renal dysfunction exacerbation. On the other hand, rate of late rejection as well as the potential for infection and malignancy is increased [7 - 9].

Induction therapy is clearly indicated in those with severe renal dysfunction (avoiding the initiation of calcineurin inhibitors within the first two days after transplantation) and in significantly presensitized patients such as patients who received blood transfusion, transplantation or those who used to receive ventricular assist device support with high levels of pre-formed antibodies. Also, rabbit antithymocyte globulin (RATG)'s potential of inhibiting CAV makes induction therapy considerable [10]. Besides, those with higher risk for fatal rejection such as the African-American patients, younger patients and patients having a high number of HLA mismatches may benefit from induction therapy [11].

Induction consists of the use of monoclonal or polyclonal antibodies for 7-14 days postoperatively. Today, interleukin-2 receptor (IL-2R) antagonists have been more frequently used for induction therapy. When compared with rATG, induction with IL-2R antagonists has an excellent safety profile [10].

Summary of Selected Literature

Whitson *et al.* [12] utilizing the United Network for Organ Sharing (UNOS) data, evaluated the effect of induction immunosuppression agents following heart transplantation with the primary endpoint of survival. They included all adult (≥18 yr) patients receiving heart transplantation between 1987 and 2011, and followed the patients for at least 12 months post-transplantation. Patients were reported to have received either: no antibody-based induction (NONE) or the induction agents (INDUCED) of either: anti-thymocyte globulin (ATG)/anti-lymphocyte globulin (ALG)/thymoglobulin, alemtuzumab or basiliximab/daclizumab (IL-2R antibody). During the follow-up period, 4635 (26%) of the 17857 heart transplant recipients that were included in the study were reported to have died. Forty-six percent (n=8216) of the patients were INDUCED. Of the INDUCED agents, 40% were ALG/ATG/thymoglobulin, 4% were alemtuzumab and 55% were IL-2R antibody. The authors reported that while ALG/ATG/thymoglobulin appeared to have a beneficial effect on survival compared to IL-2R antibody in the univariable model, this difference was no longer statistically significant once adjusted for clinically relevant covariates. The authors concluded that when compared with no induction immunosuppression, induction agents did not appear to affect survival [12].

In another study, Mazimba *et al.* [13] analyzed data from Cardiac Transplant Research Database (CTRD) from 1999 to 2006 to examine the effects of different induction strategies at the time of cardiac transplantation. A total of 2090 primary heart transplants were included in the study and categorized by induction agent as no induction (NI), ATG or IL-2R blocker. Infection and rejection probabilities were estimated using parametric time-related models. Two theoretical patient profiles were assumed: Profile 1, had lower risk of rejection and higher risk of infection and Profile 2, had higher risk of rejection and lower risk of infection. Hazard was calculated for these two models. Of the 2090 transplants, 49.8% (1095) did not receive induction, while 18.0% (396) received ATG and 27.3% (599) received IL-2R blocker. Profile 1 patients had lower hazard for rejection with IL-2R blocker compared to ATG and NI (p<0.01), but at the cost of increased risk of infection (5.0 *vs.* 1.8 *vs.* 1.6, respectively, at four wk, p<0.01). Profile 2 patients experienced a fivefold decreased hazard for rejection when treated with IL-2R blocker compared with ATG and NI (p<0.01). In patients at high risk of infection, IL-2R blockers reduced risk of rejection but at the expense of increased hazard for infection [13].

In a Cochrane review performed by Penninga *et al.* [14] 22 randomized clinical trials with a total of 1427 heart-transplant recipients were assessed for the effectiveness of immunosuppressive T-cell antibody induction for heart transplant recipients. All relevant trials between 1946 and 2012 were included. They included the trials where all participants of each individual trial were receiving the same maintenance immunosuppressive therapy. Five trials (n=606) compared any kind of T-cell antibody induction *versus* no antibody induction; four trials (n=576) compared IL-2R antagonist *versus* no induction; one trial (n=30) compared monoclonal antibody (other than IL-2R antagonist) *versus* no antibody induction; two trials (n=159) compared IL-2R antagonist *versus* monoclonal antibody (other than IL-2R antagonist) induction; four trials (n=185) compared IL-2R antagonist *versus* polyclonal antibody induction; seven trials (n=315) compared monoclonal antibody (other than IL-2R antagonist) *versus* polyclonal antibody induction; and four trials (n=162) compared polyclonal antibody induction *versus* another kind, or dose of polyclonal antibodies. When the analysis were conducted for the outcomes of mortality, CAV, post-transplantation lymphoproliferative disorder (PTLD), cancer, adverse events, renal function, infection, cytomegalovirus (CMV) infection, diabetes mellitus, hypertension or hyperlipidemia, significant difference was found for any of the comparisons. The authors concluded that acute rejection might be reduced by IL-2R antagonist compared with no induction, and by polyclonal antibody induction compared with IL-2R antagonist. This review did not show other clear benefits or harms associated with the use of any kind of T-cell antibody induction compared with no induction, or when one type of T-cell antibody was compared with another type of antibody. The authors noted that the included trials were at a high risk of bias [14].

Muromonab-CD3 (OKT3)

OKT3 is a murine monoclonal anti-CD3 antibody. It binds to the CD3 antigen of the T-cell receptor complex, which is present on the surface of activated T lymphocytes in the circulation. It demonstrates its effects through multiple mechanisms, such as T cell depletion from the peripheral circulation by opsonization in the spleen and liver and modulation of the T cell receptor-CD3 antigen recognition complex, which results in the blockage of the immunologic function of these cells [15, 16].

OKT3 is used as induction therapy at a dose of 5 mg/day for a total of 5-10 days following transplantation. In pediatric patients (<30 kg body weight) initial dose may be 2,5 mg per day. Concentrations above 0,9 mcg/mL are considered to be therapeutic. Another target is a concentration of ≥0,8 mcg/mL together with a

CD3-positive (activated) T-cell count of <25 cells/mL. It is administered intravenously. If given repeatedly or used for a long time there will be some efficacy loss and a risk of antibody-mediated rejection due to the production of anti-mice antibodies in the body [17, 18].

Following a course of OKT3, there is an immediate increase in CD3-positive T-lymphocyte counts that may lead to acute cellular or humoral rejection. T-cell depletion is achieved within minutes of administration and CD3+ T cells are undetectable during the OKT3 course. After cessation of OKT3 therapy, CD3+ T cells appear again in circulation within 12-24 hours, while the normalization of T cell function takes a week [19]. In order to overcome this situation, many programs prophylactically increase the steroid dose while weaning from OKT3.

The most specific adverse effects of OKT3 include cytokine-release syndrome, aseptic meningitis, pulmonary edema, encephalopathy, nephrotoxicity, lymphoproliferative disorder and opportunistic viral infections (particularly with cytomegalovirus). The first several doses of OKT3 are associated with a cytokine-release syndrome, which is characterized by fever, chills, rigors, chest pain, dyspnea and alterations in blood pressure. This begins 30-60 minutes following the administration of an OKT3 dose and may continue for several hours. This syndrome, which is caused by the initial activation of T cells and release of cytokines, can be alleviated by premedication with methylprednisolone, paracetamol and antihistamines.

In order to prevent pulmonary edema it is recommended that patients be within 3% of their dry weight and their chest radiograph evaluated prior to administration. OKT3-treated patients have a higher risk for PTLD and lymphoma with a cumulative dose >75 mg.

Summary of Selected Literature

Delgado *et al.* [20] reported their experience in their center with 2 consecutive cohorts, treated with basiliximab and OKT3. These cohorts suggested that the use of basiliximab displayed a similar immunosuppressive efficacy with a better safety profile than OKT3, and a simpler patient management during the initial hospital stay that could have been associated with a reduction in post-transplant costs [20].

Two retrospective studies comparing the use of an IL-2 receptor antagonist with OKT3 showed conflicting results as less allograft rejection in the IL-2 receptor blocker group in one and no difference in rejection between groups in the other [21, 22]. On the other hand, in two prospective trials with daclizumab and basiliximab, survival and rejection incidence were similar in IL-2 receptor blocker- and OKT3- treated groups; while, safety was significantly better with IL2-receptor antagonists [23, 24].

Due to all of these adverse effects and concerns, induction treatment with OKT3 has significantly declined and now OKT3 is used in less than 1% of heart transplant patients. OKT3 or intensive lymphocyte-depleting regimen use has largely been substituted by modern induction protocols using interleukin-2 receptor antagonist agents and antithymocyte globulins.

Polyclonal Anti-Lymphocyte Antibodies

Polyclonal antibodies are derived by immunization of horses or rabbits with human thymocytes and then collecting the serum of the animals. Antithymocyte Globulin Equine (ATG/lymphocyte immune globulin) is horse based, while Antithymocyte Globulin Rabbit (RATG/thymoglobulin) is rabbit based. These antibodies are directed against various targets on the surface of B- and T-cells and cause rapid depletion of T-lymphocytes by inducing complement-mediated cytolysis and cell-mediated opsonization in the spleen and liver. This antilymphocytic effect is believed to alter the function of lymphocytes, which are responsible in part for cell medicated immunity and are involved in humoral immunity [25].

The recommended dose of ATG is 15 mg/kg per day while it is 1.5 mg/kg per day for thymoglobulin. They are usually used for 7-10 days [3]. Antibodies against the animal component of these products can form in up to 78% of patients on ATG and 68% of patients on thymoglobulin [26].

The main acute adverse effect of these drugs is serum sickness reaction, which is characterized by fever, chills, alterations in blood pressure, tachycardia and rash. Premedication with methylprednisolone, antihistamines and antipyretics may help to prevent or attenuate the symptoms. The reaction can be encountered during the administration of the first or the second dose. As the treatment, the infusion may be temporarily stopped and restarted at a lower rate. Serum sickness is more frequently reported for ATG than thymoglobulin. Likewise, infusion-related febrile reactions most frequently occur with the several first doses and premedication with paracetamol, diphenhydramine and corticosteroids may be helpful.

Further adverse effects are dose-dependent thrombocytopenia (30-40%), dose-dependent leucopenia (30-50%) and anemia. Cessation of therapy may be needed for severe cases (platelet count <50,000 cells/mm^3 or WBC <2,000 cells/mm^3). It is recommended to dose rATG depending on lymphocyte count as it reduces cumulative dose without negatively affecting efficacy.

Patients receiving ATG and thymoglobulin are at increased risk (30%) of opportunistic infections. This may necessitate the routine prophylactic administration of ganciclovir for preventing CMV infection. Other adverse effects include PTLD, lymphoma and nephrotoxicity (which is rare in the absence of serum sickness).

Summary of Selected Literature

In a study aiming to assess the impact for immune monitoring in induction prophylaxis in pediatric heart recipients conducted by Thrush *et al.* [27], tailoring rATG induction with CD3 monitoring resulted in similar rejection, while reduced costs and less infection. They retrospectively reviewed heart transplant recipients receiving rATG induction. Control cases received 'usual' rATG dosing (1.5 mg/kg/day typically × 5 days). Study cases received absolute CD3 monitoring (target <25 cells/mm^3) guided rATG dosing. Study cases (n=32) received fewer doses of rATG (median 4 *vs.* 5, p<0.001) and less total rATG (median 3.2 *vs.* 7.4 mg/kg, p<0.001) when compared with control cases (n=17). Rates of infection, rejection or patient survival during the first year after transplantation were similar. One early death occurred in each group and there was one late case of PTLD in the control group. Significant drug savings (median drug cost per patient was $2718 *vs.* $4756, p<0.001) were achieved. CD3-tailored rATG induction in heart transplant recipients was associated with similar rates of rejection/infection, with reduced drug costs [27].

Czer *et al.* [28] conducted a study on the efficacy of ATG induction therapy adjusted for immunologic risk after heart transplantation. They included all patients who received ATG induction in their clinic from January 2000 through January 2010 and categorized these patients into two groups according to their risk of rejection. A higher-risk group (age <60 years, multiparous females, African Americans, panel-reactive antibody >10% or positive cross-match) received ATG (1.5 mg/kg) for 7 days (ATG7), and the remaining lower-risk group received ATG for 5 days (ATG5), all followed by calcineurin inhibitor, mycophenolate, and prednisone. Endomyocardial biopsies were performed based a standard protocol for up to 3 years after heart transplantation, and for suspected rejection. Of 253 heart transplant recipients, 87 received ATG5 and 166 received ATG7. Absolute lymphocyte count <200/microliter was achieved within 10 days in 88% of ATG5 and 86% of ATG7. Baseline creatinine was 1.3 ± 0.8 mg/dL pre-transplantation, 1.8 ± 0.9 mg/dL post-transplantation and 1.0 ± 0.4 mg/dL at discharge (mean ± standard deviation [SD]; p<0.001, compared with pre-transplantation). Of 3667 biopsies, 33 (0.90%) had ≥3A/2R cellular rejection (CR). Of 3599 biopsies, 16 (0.44%) had definite antibody-mediated rejection (AMR). At 5 years, freedom from ≥3A/2R CR and freedom from AMR were similar between ATG5 and ATG7. Survival for ATG5 and ATG7 was comparable at one year (94% ± 2.5% *vs* 93% ± 2.0%), and at 8 years (61% ± 6.9% and 61% ± 4.7%; p=0.88). At 5 years, ATG5 and ATG7 were similar in freedom from CMV infection (92.3% *vs* 94.3%; p=not significant), freedom from pneumonia (83.8% *vs* 82.1%; p=not significant), and in rate of malignancy (excluding skin cancer; 8.0% *vs* 6.0%; p=not significant). It was concluded that ATG induction therapy (prospectively dose-adjusted for immunologic risk) in low- and high-risk patients resulted in excellent and equivalent short- and long-term survival rates, with a low incidence of CR and AMR. The use of ATG did not increase CMV infection rates with appropriate prophylaxis [28].

In their study Rafiei *et al.* [29] evaluated the effect of ATG in preventing post transplant antibody production. . They reviewed their patients who received rATG induction therapy against those who did not receive therapy for post-transplant de novo antibody production. They assessed 196 non-sensitized heart transplant recipients and categorized them into two groups as: those who received 3 to 5 days of rATG induction therapy mostly due to renal insufficiency (n=35) and patients who did not receive therapy (n=161). All patients received tacrolimus, mycophenolate mofetil, and corticosteroids. At 1, 3, 6, and 12 months after heart transplantation, circulating antibodies were routinely monitored. The rATG-treated group was found to have a significantly higher 12-month freedom from de novo antibody production compared with the patients who did not receive rATG induction (89% *vs* 71%, log-rank p=0.043). Treated rejection rates in the first-year were comparable in both groups; 3-year actuarial survival, freedom from CAV and freedom from non-fatal major adverse cardiac events were also similar between both groups. They concluded that rATG induction therapy appeared to reduce the production of de novo circulating antibodies in non-sensitized patients during the first year after heart transplantation [29].

Ansari *et al.* [30] aiming to evaluate the effect of basiliximab *vs* ATG induction on long-term survival after heart transplantation utilized data from the ISHLT Registry. A total of 9,324 transplantations were performed between 2000 and 2011 whose recipients received either ATG (n=6,144) or basiliximab (n−3,180). The ATG group had a higher panel reactive antibody class 1 (7.5% *vs* 6.1%; p<0.018) and class 2 (6.6% *vs* 3.7%; p<0.001), respectively, whereas the basiliximab group was less likely to have non-ischemic cardiomyopathy but more likely to be in the intensive care unit pre-transplant. One-year survival was similar for both groups, 90% *vs* 91% (p=0.858). Basiliximab use led to less-favorable long-term survival when compared with ATG at 5 years (77% *vs* 82%, p=0.005) and at 10 years (64% *vs* 67%, p=0.007). In multivariable Cox model, basiliximab use was found to be associated with increased mortality over a median follow-up of 3.0 years (range, 0-12 years), with a hazard ratio of 1.22 (95% confidence interval, 1.09-1.37; p<0.001). They concluded that in the ISHLT Registry experience, use of ATG rather than basiliximab as induction therapy appeared to be associated with better long-term survival [30].

In their retrospective single-center study on thymoglobulin induction after heart transplantation, Goland *et al.* [31] compared lymphocyte depletion in 144 heart transplant recipients using two different induction protocols with thymoglobulin. Thymoglobulin (1.5 mg/kg) was given to 105 patients for 7 days (Thymo7) and 39 patients for 5 days (Thymo5). Patient clinical characteristics were similar except that the Thymo7 group had a higher prevalence of women (33% *vs* 15%, p 0.04), gender mismatch (35% *vs* 19%, p=0.07), donor African American race (19% *vs* 2%, p=0.008), older donor age (35 ± 13 *vs* 31 ± 12, p=0.08), and higher pre-transplant creatinine (1.43 ± 0.67 *vs* 1.25 ± 0.48 mg/dl, p=0.095). Seventy-five percent of the Thymo7 group and 42% of the Thymo5 group reached target (absolute lymphocyte count < or = 200) at 21 days (p=0.002). Thymo7 patients had significantly lower rejection rates within the first year than the Thymo5 patients (7% *vs* 22%, p=0.02). There was no humoral rejection. At 1 year, freedom from rejection was 93% in the Thymo7 group *vs* 80% in the Thymo5 group (p=0.007), and cytomegalovirus disease (9% and 5%, p=0.5) and bacterial infection (26% *vs* 32%, p=0.5) were similar. One-year actuarial survival was 92% ± 3% in the Thymo7 and 100% in the Thymo5 group (p=0.07), and at 3 years, 85 ± 4% and 90 ± 6%, respectively (p=0.4). They concluded that while both thymoglobulin regimens were well tolerated, the 7-day treatment led to more efficient and prolonged lymphocyte depletion and significantly less rejection at 1 year, without an increase in cytomegalovirus infection rate [31]. Shorter duration of ATG therapy was associated with higher rejection rates [31]. In contrast, adjustment of ATG doses according to T- cell counts was associated with lower rejection rates as well as lower or fewer ATG doses [32].

Cantarovich *et al.* [33] suggested that prolonged induction time with ATG permitted safe delay in CYC initiation in cardiac transplant patients with postoperative renal dysfunction.

The results of 5 trials comparing thymoglobuline with basiliximab showed less rejection episodes in thymoglobuline groups, while the infection rates were lower in the basiliximab groups and survival was similar between groups [34, 35 - 38].

Monoclonal Antibodies (Interleukin-2 Receptor Antagonists)

IL-2R antagonists basiliximab and daclizumab are humanized monoclonal anti CD-25 antibodies that selectively bind to the IL-2 receptor of T-lymphocytes. Therefore, they block binding of IL-2 to the receptor complex and exhibit their immunosuppressive effects by inhibiting IL-2 mediated T-lymphocyte proliferation which is a critical pathway in the cellular immune response involved in allograft rejection. Basiliximab is a chimeric monoclonal antibody (25% murine). Daclizumab is marketed in the US, but not in Europe. Daclizumab as a humanized monoclonal antibody (90% human, 10% murine) is thought to be less immunogenic than basiliximab.

Both basiliximab and daclizumab should be given intravenously in 2-14 hours following transplantation. The administration should be repeated within 4 days for basiliximab or 2 weeks for daclizumab. The usual basiliximab dose is 20 mg. The two (Day 0 and Day 4) intravenous administrations of basiliximab will result in IL-2 receptor saturation for 30-45 days. The approved daclizumab dose is 1 mg/kg every 2 weeks from the time of transplantation for a total of 5 doses. This regimen maintains IL-2 receptor saturation for 90-120 days. For attaining this level of receptor saturation as measured by ELISA, the recommended serum levels are 0,2 mcg/mL for basiliximab and 5-10 mcg/mL for daclizumab.

IL-2R antagonist induction has a favorable safety profile. Fewer adverse effects have been reported with basiliximab and daclizumab due to the specific blockade of IL-2 receptor, preventing global immunosuppression. Unlike OKT3 and polyclonal antibody preparations, basiliximab and daclizumab have not been associated with infusion-related reactions. Allergic reactions are among serious adverse effects of these preparations. Increased risk of opportunistic infections and a higher risk of lymphomas still exist for these drugs. Other side effects include nausea, vomiting, diarrhea, tremor, flu symptoms and peripheral edema.

Summary of Selected Literature

A randomized controlled trial by Mullen *et al.* [39] aimed to test the efficacy and safety of daclizumab (DAC) *versus* anti-thymocyte globulin (ATG) as a component of induction therapy in heart transplant recipients. They randomized 30 heart transplant patients to receive either ATG or DAC during induction therapy. Patients in the DAC group received an initial dose of 2 mg/kg intravenous (IV) at the time of transplant and 1 mg/kg iv on postoperative day 4. Recipient, donor, and intraoperative variables did not differ significantly between groups. The cost of induction therapy, total drug cost, and hospital ward costs were significantly less for the DAC group. Average absolute lymphocyte and platelet counts were significantly higher in the DAC group. There were no significant differences in the incidence of rejection, infection, malignancy, or steroid-induced diabetes. One-year survival was excellent in both groups (87%, p=0.1). The authors concluded that daclizumab was a safe component of induction therapy in heart transplantation [39].

As a result of their prospective, randomized, open-label pilot trial with daclizumab, conducted on 55 patients, Beniaminovitz *et al.* [40] reported that rejection was decreased during the post-transplant 3 months, while the rejection and survival rates did not differ at year one. A multicenter trial conducted on 434 patients in a prospective, randomized and double-blinded manner demonstrated significantly less acute rejection episodes with daclizumab at one year after cardiac transplantation. The risk of death from infection was higher in the daclizumab group [41].

A multicenter, prospective, double-blind, randomized trial of basiliximab induction *versus* placebo in 56 patients failed to show significant differences between treatment groups in terms of adverse events and time to acute rejection [42].

MAINTENANCE IMMUNOSUPPRESSIVE REGIMENS

Most maintenance immunosuppressive protocols use a three-drug regimen consisting of a calcineurin-inhibitor (cyclosporine or tacrolimus), an antimetabolite (mycophenolate mofetil or azathioprine) and corticosteroids (with tapering doses over the first-year following transplantation). According to the current ISHLT data [43], the most frequently prescribed (89%) calcineurin inhibitor in heart transplantation patients is tacrolimus. As the antimetabolite, mycophenolate is the drug of choice for 91% of the patients. Antiproliferative agents have been used at smaller rates both at one year (8%) and at five years (19%). On the other hand 80% of the patients receive some amount of corticosteroid during the first post-transplant year.

The drug combination tacrolimus plus mycophenolate mofetil with or without corticosteroids during the first year following transplantation was most common (41%) and this is followed by cyclosporine plus mycophenolate mofetil with or without corticosteroids (36%) [43].

Main features of immunosuppressive agents used as maintenance therapy in cardiac transplantation are summarized in Table **1** and their mechanisms of action are schematized in Fig. (**1**).

Summary of recommendations on the principles of immunosuppressive regimens in heart transplant recipients published in the "International Society of Heart and Lung Transplantation Guidelines for the care of heart transplant recipients" [44] is presented in Table **2**.

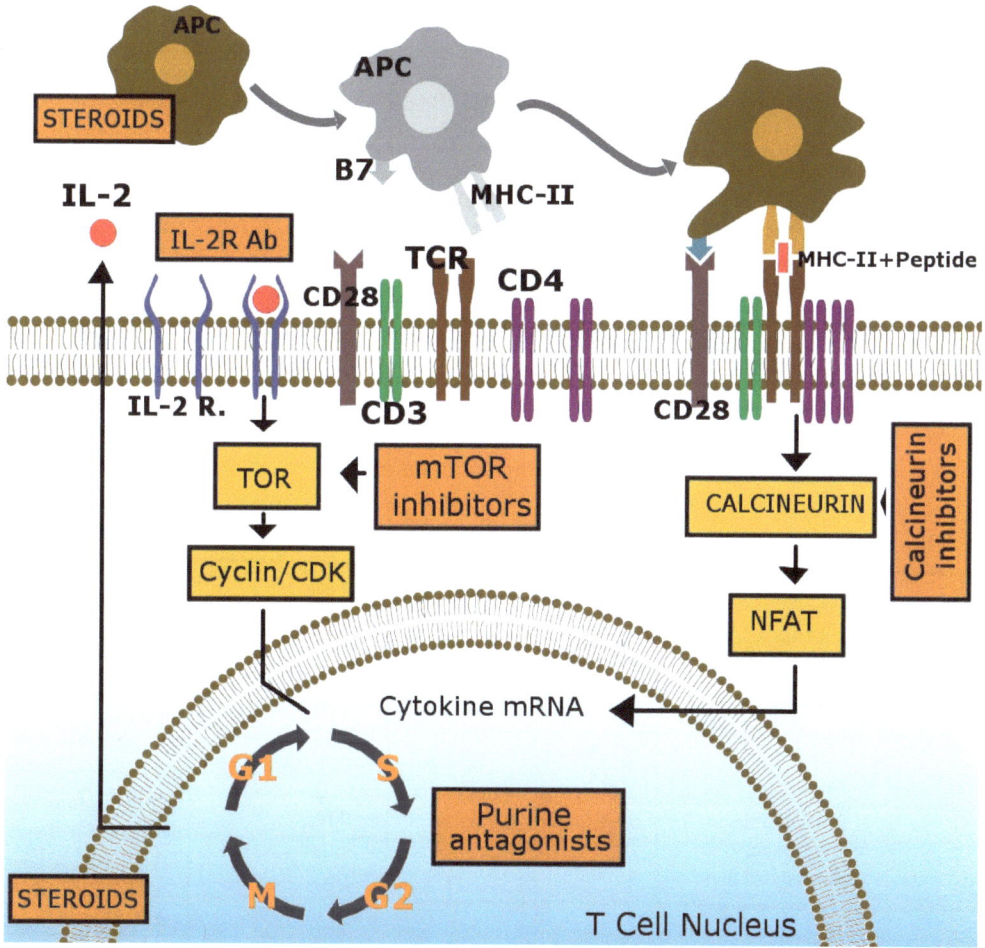

Fig. (1). Mechanisms of action of immunosuppressive drugs. Antigen-presenting cells present donor antigens resulting in T-cell proliferation. Calcineurin is activated through B7 complex and major histocompatibility complex class II leading to IL-2 production. The mammalian target of rapamycin is activated by the IL-2 stimulation of the T-cell IL-2 receptor. Unlike calcineurin inhibitors, which inhibit the production of cytokines, mTOR inhibitors which block the response to these cytokines by causing cell cycle arrest at the G1 to S phase. Purine antagonists interfere with the nucleic acid synthesis and inhibit T-cell proliferation. Steroids binding to nuclear receptors prevent the expression of several cytokines and impair the activation and proliferation of T-cells. Phases of the cell cycle: G1 (first phase of cell growth), S (DNA synthesis), G2 (second phase of cell growth) and M (mitotic phase). *APC: antigen presenting cell; CDK: cyclin-dependent kinase; IL-2: interleukin-2; IL-2R: interleukin-2 receptor; IL-2R Ab: interleukin-2 receptor antibody; mTOR: mammalian target of rapamycin; MHC: major histocompatibility complex; NFAT: nuclear factor of activated T cells; TCR: T-cell receptor.*

Table 1. Summary of immunosuppressive agents used as maintenance therapy in cardiac transplantation.

Drug	Mechanism of Action	Dose*	Target Drug Levels*	Adverse Effects	Important Drug-Drug Interactions
Cyclosporine	Binds to the intracellular immunophilin named cyclophilin forming a complex that inhibits the phosphatase activity of the calcineurin and therefore, activation of the T-cells.	4-8 mg/kg/day in 2 divided doses	12- hr trough levels: 0-6 months: 250-350 ng/mL 6-12 months: 200-250 ng/mL >12 months: 100-200 ng/mL	Nephrotoxicity, neurotoxicity (headache, tremors, seizures), hypertension, new-onset diabetes, hypertrichosis, hirsutism, gingival hyperplasia, osteoporosis	Antifungal drugs (ketoconazole, posaconazole, itraconazole, fluconazole, voriconazole); calcium channel blockers (verapamil, diltiazem, nifedipine, nicardipine); macrolide antibiotics; metoclopramide; ciprofloxacin; amiodarone and anti-HIV protease inhibitors increase CYC and TAC levels. Phenobarbital, phenytoin, rifampin and octreotide decrease CYC and TAC levels. Amphotericin B, aminoglycoside antibiotics, colchicine and non-steroidal anti-inflammatory agents synergistically cause nephrotoxicity when used with CYC or TAC.
Tacrolimus	Binds to another immunophilin, which is FK506-binding protein 12, forming a complex that inhibits the phosphatase activity of the calcineurin and therefore, activation of the T-cells.	0.05-0.1 mg/kg/day in 2 divided doses	12- hr trough levels: 0-6 months: 10-15 ng/mL 6-12 months: 5-10 ng/mL >12 months: 5-10 ng/mL	Nephrotoxicity, neurotoxicity (tremors, headache, paresthesias), new-onset diabetes mellitus, hypertension, anemia, alopecia	

(Table 1) cont.....

Drug	Mechanism of Action	Dose*	Target Drug Levels*	Adverse Effects	Important Drug-Drug Interactions
Azathioprine	Antagonises purine nucleotide synthesis and metabolism, and inhibits the synthesis and function of RNA and DNA.	1.5-3.0 mg/kg/day titrated to keep white blood cell count to remain >4000/mm³	-	Myelosuppression (leucopenia, anemia), nausea, vomiting, alopecia, hepatotoxicity, pancreatitis	Allopurinol slows metabolism by inhibiting xanthine oxidase. This prolongation of AZA activity may result in pancytopenia.
Mycophenolate mofetil	Selectively, noncompetitively and reversibly inhibits inosine monophosphate dehydrogenase (IMPDH); thus inhibits the de novo biosynthesis of guanine nucleotide.	1000-3000 mg/day in 2 divided doses	Mycophenolic acid (MPA): 2- 5 ng/ml	Leukopenia, nausea, vomiting, diarrhea, gastrointestinal bleeding, peptic ulcer disease	AZA and mTOR inhibitors may cause excessive myelosuppression. Antacids, cholestyramine and oral ferrous sulfate decrease intestinal absorption of MMF. CYC may decrease MMF concentrations.
Sirolimus	mTOR inhibitors block the response to cytokines such as IL-2 by causing cell cycle arrest at the G1 to S phase. The result of this is the inhibition of T- and B-cell proliferation.	1-3 mg/day	24-hr trough levels: 5-10 ng/mL	Oral ulcerations, peripheral edema, hypertension, hyperlipidemia, thrombocytopenia, neutropenia, anemia, delayed would healing, dehiscence, pulmonary toxicity	Azole antifungals; calcium channel blockers; macrolide antibiotics; metoclopramide; ciprofloxacin; amiodarone and protease inhibitors increase sirolimus levels. Phcnobarbital, phenytoin, rifampin and octreotide decrease sirolimus levels.
Everolimus		0,75 mg twice daily.	Blood trough level: 3-8 ng/mL.		Clarithromycin, telithromycin, nefazodone, ketoconazole, itraconazole, voriconazole, protease inhibitors

(Table 1) cont.....

Drug	Mechanism of Action	Dose*	Target Drug Levels*	Adverse Effects	Important Drug-Drug Interactions
Corticosteroids	Prevent the expression of several cytokines; thus, impair the activation and proliferation of B- and T-cells.	1 mg/kg/day in 2 divided doses; tapered to 0.05 mg/kg/day by 6- 12 months	-	Hypercorticism, mood changes, depression, cataracts, hypertension, hyperglycemia, osteopenia, bruising, peptic ulcer	Multiple drug interactions, majority is not clinically significant

*CYC: cyclosporine; TAC: tacrolimus; AZA: azathioprine; mTOR: mammalian target of rapamycin; MMF: mycophenolate mofetil. *http://www.uptodate.com/contents/induction-and-maintenance-of-immunosuppress-ive-therapy-in-cardiac-transplantation*

Corticosteroids

Corticosteroids have potent immunosuppressive and anti-inflammatory properties. Their use as immunosuppressive agents depends on a complex mechanism. Steroids binding to nuclear receptors prevent the expression of several cytokines such as IL-1, IL-2, IL-3, IL-6, γ-interferon and tumor necrosis factor-α; thus, impair the activation and proliferation of B- and T-cells [3]. This effect on B- and T-lymphocytes seems to be mediated by inhibition of activator protein-1 and nuclear factor (NF) kappaB [45, 46]. Steroids also have anti-inflammatory features and suppress macrophage activity. They decrease the production of vasoactive and chemoattractant factors resulting in inhibition of neutrophil adhesion to endothelial cells and prevention of macrophage differentiation [45, 46].

Steroid therapy is a standard component of induction, maintenance and antirejection therapy in cardiac transplantation. Corticosteroids are used in higher doses in the early postoperative period; however they are tapered to lower doses or discontinued after the first 6-12 months following transplantation. Some low-risk patients may discontinue corticosteroids as early as one-two months following transplantation without long-term problems. Recent studies on corticosteroid-free immunosuppression with newer, more specific immunosuppresants may suggest that corticosteroids have a less important role in maintenance immunosuppression.

Prednisone is converted to its active form prednisolone in liver. Prednisone and prednisolone are 4-5 times more potent compared to hydrocortisone (cortisol). The bioavailability of oral prednisone is 70%. It has a long half-life; therefore it can be dosed once daily [26, 47].

Steroid protocols may vary from one center to another. Before bringing the patient to the operating room high dose (500-1000 mg) IV methylprednisolone is administered. This is followed by a total of three more doses each 125-150 mg administered every 8 hours. If the patient is extubated, oral prednisolone is started generally at divided (one to four) doses of 0.05 to 2 mg/kg/day [47]. Generally a dose of 1 mg/kg/day is preferred. Then this dose is tapered to 0.3 mg/kg/day at 3-6 months and to 0.1 mg/kg/day at 6 months. Some weaning protocols decrease the daily prednisolone dosage by 1 mg each month starting at the 6th month following cardiac transplantation [48]. These weaning protocols are guided by daily cortisol measurements in order to prevent adrenal insufficiency (*i.e.* >8 μg/dL continue weaning, otherwise continue steroid therapy).

It is advisable to administer corticosteroids between 7AM and 8AM mimicking the body's diurnal cortisol release. After conversion to alternate-day regimens, corticosteroids can be withdrawn in stable patients by some transplantation centers. But others still prefer to put their patients on corticosteroids (2,5 to 5 mg/day prednisone) for the lifetime [26]. It was reported that 85% of the centers reporting to the ISHLT keep on using corticosteroids within the first year after cardiac transplantation and this figure remains to be 50% after 5 years [5, 49].

Besides induction therapy, steroids are also used to treat acute cellular rejection episodes in 'pulses'. If the patient with acute graft rejection has hemodynamic compromise then, 1000 mg methylprednisolone daily is administered for 3 days. Cytolytic therapy, plasmapheresis or both may also be administered. If the patient with acute graft rejection is hemodynamically stable, treatment with oral prednisone (100-200 mg) for three days is usually adequate. After that, doses of oral prednisone are tapered over 5 days to 20 mg/day. Corticosteroids should not be discontinued abruptly due to the potential of suppression of the hypothalamic pituitary adrenal axis. As corticosteroids impair growth in children; clinicians usually use alternate-day dosing or withhold corticosteroids until a rejection episode ensues.

Prednisone use may cause hypercorticism or hypothalamic pituitary adrenal (HPA) axis suppression. Therefore, withdrawal and discontinuation should be done carefully and slowly. Patients receiving >20 mg per day of prednisone (or equivalent) may be most susceptible. Secondary infections may develop due to prolonged corticosteroid use; while acute infections (including the fungal ones) may be masked and viral infections may be prolonged or exacerbated.

The most common (that occur in more that 10% of patients) adverse effects of prednisone include increased appetite, indigestion, insomnia and mood changes. Corticosteroid use may cause psychiatric derangements including mood swings, depression, euphoria, insomnia and personality changes besides other central nervous system effects such as increase in intracranial pressure, seizures and vertigo. Pre-existing psychiatric conditions may worsen.

Adverse effects that occur less often and particularly associated with higher doses and prolonged treatment include cataracts, glaucoma, hyperglycemia, new-onset diabetes, hirsutism, bruising, acne, sodium and water retention, hypertension, congestive heart failure in susceptible subjects, osteopenia, growth retardation in children, ulcerative esophagitis and peptic ulcer (with possible perforation and hemorrhage), avascular necrosis of the femoral head [26, 50].

Summary of Selected Literature

While corticosteroids are still the main medications used in rescue, induction and maintenance immunosuppression in heart transplantation, they cause significant side effects generally related with the dose and duration of the therapy. Alternating ways to avoid or eliminate the need for long-term steroid treatment can minimize these side effects. These regimens are named as steroid-free or steroid withdrawal protocols (early within the first 3–6 months after heart transplantation or late between 6–12 months and beyond post- transplant) [51].

According to the ISHLT Guidelines, corticosteroid avoidance, early corticosteroid weaning or very low-dose maintenance corticosteroid therapy are all acceptable therapeutic approaches with level of evidence B [44].

Faulhaber *et al.* [52], as the result of their study on steroid withdrawal and reduction of cyclosporine A under mycophenolate mofetil after heart transplantation concluded that corticosteroid-free immunosuppression comprising reduced cyclosporine levels and addition of mycophenolate mofetil in long-term heart transplant recipients was safe and improved the cardiovascular risk profile, carbohydrate metabolism and renal function [52].

In a recent review conducted by Baraldo *et al.* [51] on steroid-free and steroid withdrawal protocols in heart transplantation it was concluded that steroid-free therapy should be advisable and sometimes mandatory in pediatric age, in cases of active infection, insulin dependent diabetes mellitus, familial metabolic disorders/obesity, severe osteoporosis, and in elderly patients. In all heart transplant patients, steroid withdrawal seems to be feasible (any age, sex, and race; at present, a success rate of 50–80%) and safe (does not increase rejection-related mortality and has no adverse impact on survival) and maybe more practicable when combined with the new drugs [51].

Calcineurin Inhibitors

Calcineurin inhibitors (CNIs) [cyclosporine (CYC) and tacrolimus (TAC)] consists the most commonly used immunosuppressive drugs. They are routinely used for immunosuppression following heart transplantation. The advantage of these drugs over cytotoxic immunosuppressants is that they act specifically on the immune system not affecting other rapidly proliferating cells [53].

They produce their immunosuppressive effects through blocking the production of pro-inflammatory cytokines such as IL-2, INF-γ, TNF-α and inhibiting T cell activation and proliferation. They inactivate calcineurin, which is a calcium-dependent protein phosphatase and a critical factor of cell signaling in immune cells. Calcineurin inhibition completely blocks the adaptive immune response. Calcineurin dephosphorylates a wide range of proteins; including the critical transcription factors of the 'nuclear factor of activated T cells (NFATc)' family [54, 55]. NFATc regulates the expression of cytokines such as IFNγ, IL-2 and IL-4 or some surface proteins (CD40L and CD95L) [56 - 58].

Calcineurin inhibitors are the keystones of immunosuppressive therapy. As a part of the maintenance therapy in heart transplantation, they lead to excellent short-term outcomes as well as increased medium-term life expectancy, but only limited impact on long-term outcomes. However, their long-term use results in nephrotoxicity (which is characterized by a progressive decline in the glomerular filtration rate, progressive tubulointerstitial damage and glomerulosclerosis), cardiovascular side effects (such as hypertension and hyperlipidemia) and new-onset diabetes after transplantation.

Summary of Selected Literature

The cumulative chronic renal failure incidences at 1, 5, and 10 years after transplantation were reported to be 26%, 33% and 39%, respectively at ISHLT Registry Report. According to the same report 2.5% of patients required dialysis at 5 years, while 0.5% of patients required a renal transplantation [59]. In order to overcome this issue CNI dose reduction is suggested. In the literature there is a wide variety of studies of various designs, including various drug regimens and evaluating various outcomes showing that overall CNI reduction or minimization is effective in improving renal function, while maintaining the positive clinical outcomes such as freedom-from biopsy-proven rejection episodes and survival.

Groetzner *et al.* [60] in their prospective, randomized, multi-center trial, investigated the impact of immunosuppressive conversion toward CNI-free (mycophenolate mofetil and sirolimus) or a CNI-reduced immunosuppressive regimen on renal function, efficacy, and safety. They included 63 heart transplant patients (0.5-18.4 years after transplantation) with CNI-based immunosuppression and reduced creatinine clearance (less than 60 mL/min) (39 ± 15 mL/min). Patients in the CNI-free-Group (Group 1) were converted to sirolimus that was started with 2 mg/day until target trough levels (8-14 ng/mL) were achieved. Subsequently, CNIs were withdrawn. In CNI-reduction-Group (Group 2), CNI target trough levels were reduced by 40%. In both groups mycophenolate mofetil was continued and trough level adjusted (1.5-4 microg/mL). Patient demographics and survival (mean follow-up time: 16.7 ± 9 months) was equal (100%). Renal function improved significantly after complete CNI withdrawal while remaining unchanged with CNI-reduction (creatinine clearance after 12 months: 53 ± 24 mg/dL [Group 1] *vs.* 38 ± 20 mg/dL [Group 2], p=0.01). End-stage renal failure (hemodialysis) was avoided by CNI-withdrawal and occurred only after CNI reduction (n=6; p=0.01). Acute rejection episodes were more common in Group 2 (4 *vs.* 2). Graft function remained stable (echocardiography) within both groups. Adverse events were more common in Group 1 (65%) than in Group 2 (n=40%) and were responsible for discontinuation in 4 and 0 cases, respectively. The authors concluded that conversion toward a CNI-free immunosuppression (mycophenolate, sirolimus) is superior to CNI-reduced immunosuppression in improving renal failure in late heart transplantation recipients. However, the increased incidence and severity of sirolimus/ mycophenolate mofetil-associated side effects should be kept in mind [60].

Recently, Cornu *et al.* [61] conducted a systematic review and meta-analysis on the impact of the reduction of calcineurin inhibitors on renal function in heart transplant patients. They aimed to identify, appraise, select and analyse all high-quality research evidence relevant to the question of the clinical impact of CNI-sparing strategies in heart transplantation patients. As a result of their meta-analysis, they could not conclude without a doubt that CNI reduction after a heart transplant led to improved kidney function. They reported that the incidence of acute rejection did not increase in the CNI reduction group; while other safety criteria, such as graft loss, mortality, adverse events and infections, did not differ between CNI-reduction and standard groups. This meta-analysis did not confirm unambiguously that early CNI reduction might be more beneficial than delayed CNI reduction. The hypothesis that patients with impaired renal function may benefit more from CNI reduction was confirmed by this meta-analysis. They concluded that the risk/benefit ratio of reducing CNI after heart transplantation had not been demonstrated, even though there seemed to be a favorable effect on kidney function without an increase in the risk of acute rejection [61].

In a trial comparing regimens of TAC/mycophenolate mofetil (MMF), TAC/sirolimus and CYC/MMF, patients receiving any of the TAC-based regimens had significantly lower rates of rejection at 6-months than those receiving CYC/MMF regimen. TAC/MMF treated patients had the best renal function and the lowest triglyceride levels and the TAC/sirolimus-treated patients suffered from poor wound healing and higher insulin requirements [62]. The TICTAC Trial demonstrated that rejection rates were similar for TAC monotherapy recipients and TAC/MMF recipients [63].

As a result of the trials comparing TAC with CYC, it was shown that patients receiving CYC suffered more frequently from hypertension, gingival hyperplasia, cholelithiasis and hirsutism, and had higher cholesterol and triglyceride levels than those receiving TAC; while, TAC-treated patients experienced tremor, diabetes mellitus and anemia more frequently [64 - 66].

Cyclosporine

Cyclosporine is a prodrug that binds to the intracellular immunophilin named cyclophilin. The complex so formed inhibits the phosphatase activity of the calcineurin and therefore, activation of the T-cells. Cyclosporine and modified cyclosporine are used for the treatment and prophylaxis of cardiac transplant rejection in combination with corticosteroids.

The older cyclosporin formulation, which is an oil-based one, has variable and incomplete absorption. The modified formulation, which is a microemulsion, has an improved drug absorption and consistent bioavailability. The results of a study comparing these formulations in de novo heart transplant recipients show that the use of the newer microemulsion formulation was associated with fewer rejection episodes at 24 months (7% *vs* 18%, p=0,002); however, graft and patient survival were similar [67].

In adult and pediatric patients (6 months or older), the initial dose of cyclosporine is 15 mg/kg [range 14-18 mg/kg) orally or 5 to 6 mg/kg IV infused over 2-6 hours as a single daily dose. The first dose is to be administered 4 to 12 hours before transplantation or may be given postoperatively. The daily starting dose should be continued for 1 to 2 weeks. The iv administration should be switched to oral as soon as possible postoperatively. As maintenance therapy, the oral dose is decreased by 5% per week to 5 to 10 mg/kg/day and continued based on clinical response, predefined blood concentrations, and tolerability. When patient is unable to tolerate oral formulation, iv dose is at one-third the oral maintenance dose administered as two infusions 12 hours apart or as continuous infusion over 24 hours. Children have required and tolerated higher doses than those used in adults.

Due to the inter-patient differences in cyclosporine bioavailability and the narrow therapeutic range of the drug, dosing should be based on drug through levels. The dose should be titrated to reach a therapeutic 12-hour trough level of 200-350 ng/mL during the first year following transplantation; it can later be lowered to 100-200 ng/mL at the subsequent years.

Cyclosporine is not bioequivalent to modified cyclosporine and cannot be used interchangeably. The total daily dose of modified cyclosporine for microemulsion capsules or solution should always be administered in 2 divided doses [68]. Conversion from cyclosporine to modified cyclosporine can be done as follows: start modified cyclosporine at same daily dose as previously used cyclosporine; adjust modified cyclosporine dose to attain pre-conversion cyclosporine blood trough concentration with monitoring every 4 to 7 days after conversion and more frequently (at least twice weekly) with doses greater than 10 mg/kg/day [69]. Higher doses are used more commonly in two-drug regimens, while lower doses are preferred in triple-drug regimens.

Nephrotoxicity is the most important adverse effect of cyclosporine and is characterized by a decrease in glomerular filtration rate, proteinuria and hyperkalemia. Another adverse effect neurotoxicity manifests as tremors, headache and peripheral neuropathy, and occasionally as seizures. Other major toxicities include hypertension and hyperlipidemia (which are less frequently seen during tacrolimus treatment). New-onset diabetes at the first year is present at as many as 10% of the patients [70].

Hypertrichosis and hirsutism (in at least 50% of patients) and gingival hyperplasia are adverse effects specific for cyclosporine [70]. The patients experiencing these side effects may be put on tacrolimus therapy. Other adverse effects include nausea, vomiting, cholestasis, cholelithiasis and osteoporosis. Immunosuppression with cyclosporine may increase susceptibility to infections and the risk of lymphomas and other malignancies, especially those of the skin.

Tacrolimus

Tacrolimus (TAC) (FK506) is again a prodrug that binds to another immunophilin which is FK506-binding protein 12 (FKBP-12), forming a complex that inhibits the phosphatase activity of the calcineurin and therefore, activation of the T-cells. Tacrolimus is indicated for the prophylaxis of organ rejection in adults receiving allogeneic heart transplants. Concomitant administration with adrenal corticosteroids and azathioprine or mycophenolate mofetil is recommended [71].

In case of persistent or recurrent acute cellular rejection in spite of adequate cyclosporin levels, change from cyclosporin to tacrolimus is a common practice [3]. As hirsutism is a common side effect of cyclosporin, some centers prefer using tacrolimus for all female patients [3].

Tacrolimus is initiated postoperatively once the patient is hemodynamically and renally stable, at least 6 hours after transplantation [3]. IV tacrolimus should be used only when patients are unable to take the oral form. The initial dose of IV tacrolimus is 0.01 mg/kg/day as a continuous infusion [3, 71]. Intravenous dosage in pediatric cardiac transplantation may be raised up to 0.03-0.05 mg/kg/day [3]. As intravenous tacrolimus seems more nephrotoxic than cyclosporine, it should be switched to oral therapy as soon as tolerated (usually 2 to 3 days). The first oral dose should be given 8 to 12 hours after infusion discontinuation [71]. The initial oral tacrolimus dose is 0.075 mg/kg/day in 2 divided doses (given every 12 hours). Dose should be titrated based on clinical assessment of rejection, blood levels, and tolerability [71]. Monitoring of whole blood trough concentrations is considered essential for evaluation of rejection, toxicity, dose adjustments and compliance. Recommended whole blood trough concentration is 10 to 20 nanograms/mL (ng/mL) at 1 to 3 months and 5 to 15 ng/mL at >3 months [71]. Lower doses (0.5 to 2 mg twice daily) may be used for maintenance [3].

While preparing the IV infusion, tacrolimus should be diluted in NS or D5W to a concentration between 0.004 and 0.02 mg/mL in glass or polyethylene containers avoiding polyvinylchloride containers. The diluted solution must be used within 24 hours and must be administered only as continuous IV infusion. Also, polyvinylchloride-free tubing should be used with more diluted solutions (e.g., pediatric dosing) to minimize adsorption. Signs and symptoms of anaphylactic reactions should be monitored during the infusion. Patients should be monitored during the first 30 minutes of infusion and then frequently.

Conventional tacrolimus capsules may be taken with or without food but should be taken the same way to maintain consistency. Administration with food significantly decreases the rate and extent of absorption [71]. On the other hand tacrolimus extended-release capsules should be taken consistently in the morning, preferably on an empty stomach (*i.e.* at least 1 hour before or 2 hours after a meal). Extended-release capsules should not be chewed, divided or crushed. A missed dose may be taken within 14 hours of the scheduled administration time. Beyond the 14-hour window, the missed dose should be skipped and the next regular daily dose should be taken on the usual scheduled time (without duplication) [72].

Major adverse effects of tacrolimus are nephrotoxicity and neurotoxicity, which may commonly manifest as tremors, and is less common with cyclosporine. Insulin-dependent post-transplant diabetes mellitus has been reported for up to 20% of patients receiving tacrolimus. This may be more common when tacrolimus is given with azathioprine than with mycophenolate mofetil [73]. Hypertension and hyperlipidemia are less frequently seen with tacrolimus therapy when compared with cyclosporine. Anemia and alopecia may be other side effects of tacrolimus. Alopecia is usually self-limiting and reversible. Immuno-suppression with tacrolimus may cause increased susceptibility to infections and development of lymphomas. When changing cyclosporine to tacrolimus, a 24-hour period should elapse between cyclosporine discontinuation and commencement of tacrolimus.

Monitoring of serum concentrations (trough for oral therapy) is crucial for prevention of rejection and decreasing drug-related toxicity. Typical whole blood trough concentrations: One week – 3 months: 8-20 ng/mL; 3-18 months: 6-18 ng/mL.

Antiproliferative Agents (Antimetabolites)

Antiproliferative agents interfere with the nucleic acid synthesis and show immunosuppressive effects by the inhibition of T and B lymphocyte proliferation.

Among the antiproliferative agents, mycophenolate mofetil (MMF) exerts a small benefit over azathioprine (AZA) in preventing CAV; and the cyclosporine plus MMF combination presents with a significantly higher survival benefit when compared with cyclosporine plus AZA [74].

Azathioprine

Azathioprine is an imidazolyl derivative of 6-mercaptopurine and acts as an immunosuppressive antimetabolite. The exact mechanism of action is not known, but it is likely that azathioprine antagonises purine nucleotide synthesis and metabolism, and inhibits the synthesis and function of RNA and DNA [75, 76]. As a result of this reduction in intracellular purine synthesis, the numbers of circulating B and T lymphocytes [77, 78], as well as immunoglobulin synthesis and IL-2 secretion [79] decreases. Azathioprine does not reduce serum levels of IL-6 or soluble IL-2R [80]. The mechanism of action of the antineoplastic and immune modulating effects of AZA depends upon intracellular metabolites [81]; therefore, serum drug levels have a little value in monitoring. In order to be effective the drug should be given before antigen exposure or during the early stages. It has little effect on established graft rejection [76]. Currently, azathioprine has been replaced by the other antiproliferative agent, mycophenolate mofetil.

Intravenous dose is equivalent to oral dose. Intravenous dosing should be converted to oral as soon as tolerated. It is recommended that the starting dose for azathioprine is 3-5 mg/kg once daily oral or IV. It may be reduced to 1 and 2 mg/kg/day as maintenance therapy. There is no available drug level assay for

AZA. Daily dosage is adjusted depending on the toxic effects, trying to keep the white blood cell count between 4000/mm^3 and 6000/mm^3.

Major adverse effects of azathioprine are dose-dependent myelosuppression (commonly as leucopenia). If the white blood cell count is <3000/mm^3 or if there is a 50% decrease from the last value, azathioprine treatment should be withheld temporarily. Leucopenia, anemia and thrombocytopenia can occur during the first weeks of therapy and generally resolves in 7-10 days with dose reduction.

Azathioprine can cause life-threatening myelosuppression and should be avoided in patients homozygous for variant TPMT alleles. Heterozygotes have one dysfunctional TPMT allele and below-normal TPMT activity. These patients may need lower azathioprine dosage to achieve similar active metabolite levels as compared to wild-type patients [82]. Chronic immunosuppression with azathioprine increases the risk of neoplasia and serious infections. Other common side effects include nausea and vomiting, and the less common ones are alopecia, hepatotoxicity and pancreatitis, which are reversible on drug discontinuation or dose reduction.

In a double-blind, active-controlled trial, 28 centers randomized 650 patients undergoing their first heart transplant to receive MMF or azathioprine, in addition to cyclosporine and corticosteroids. When compared with the AZA-treated patients, MMF-treated patients had significant reduction in mortality and requirement for rejection treatment at 1 year after cardiac transplantation. However, opportunistic infections, mostly herpes simplex, were more common in the MMF group [83].

Mycophenolate Mofetil

Mycophenolate mofetil (MMF) is a prodrug that is rapidly metabolized to mycophenolic acid (MPA), which is the active metabolite having pharmacological activity.

MPA is a selective, noncompetitive, reversible and potent inhibitor of inosine monophosphate dehydrogenase (IMPDH). IMPDH is a critical enzyme for the de-novo synthesis of guanine nucleotides. While other cell types can use other pathways, T and B-lymphocytes are dependent on the IMPDH activity (de novo pathway for the production of purines necessary for RNA and DNA synthesis) for their proliferation. Therefore, proliferation is selectively inhibited. MPA has potent cytostatic effects on both T- and B-lymphocytes lymphocytes.

Mycophenolate mofetil is more specific in its effects on lymphocytes and has fewer side effects when compared with azathioprine. Therefore, it has been the antimetabolite of choice for many transplant centers. The major disadvantage is its price, which is 6 to 10 times the price of azathioprine.

The initial dose of mycophenolate mofetil is 1-1,5 g twice daily by IV or oral routes. The IV form should be administered as a two-hour infusion every 12 hours. Intravenous solutions should not be given by rapid or bolus injections. First dose should be given within the 12 hours following transplantation. The dose may be subsequently decreased in response to leucopenia or as tolerated. Although therapeutic drug monitoring is not routinely performed, some programs target MPA trough levels between 2-5 ng/mL.

The major adverse effect of mycophenolate mofetil is myelosuppression (risk greater from day 31-180 post-transplant). Clinically significant leucopenia can be reversed by dose reduction or drug discontinuation. Patients receiving higher doses (>3 g/day) experience these adverse effects more frequently. The negative effects of mycophenolate mofetil on bone marrow are caused by the active metabolite, MPA and exert a dose-dependent pattern. Leucopenia associated with mycophenolate mofetil use occurs in up to one-third of patients receiving the treatment [84].

Immunosuppression with mycophenolate mofetil increases the risk for infection and development of lymphoma and skin malignancy. The risk of opportunistic infections is higher with mycophenolate mofetil when compared with azathioprine. Other side effects include nausea, vomiting and diarrhea. While, mycophenolate mofetil may be associated with gastritis, peptic ulcer disease and gastrointestinal bleeding, it is not nephrotoxic.

Summary of Selected Literature

In their 4-year, prospective, multicenter study conducted in nine Spanish heart transplantation centers recruiting 89 patients, Manito *et al.* [85] evaluated the long-term efficacy and safety of the use of mycophenolate mofetil to reduce CNI dose, thus improve renal function. They included patients with chronic renal failure (serum creatinine >1.4 mg/dL) and who were being treated with cyclosporine and prednisone ± azathioprine. They started mycophenolate mofetil and cyclosporine level could be decreased below 100 ng/mL. Survival, acute rejection episodes and creatinine clearance (CrCl) were retrospectively compared with a contemporary cohort of heart transplant recipients who were not treated with mycophenolate mofetil (control group; n=38). After conversion to mycophenolate mofetil, a rapid increase was observed in the CrCl, which was maintained over the follow-up: namely, CrCl at month 6 and at 4 years were 51.0

± 15.6 and 54.1 ± 15.6 mL/min *versus* 41.9 ± 11.1 mL/min at baseline (p<0.0001). No renal function changes were observed among the control group. Acute rejection rates were 5.6% and 2.6% in the mycophenolate mofetil *versus* control groups (p=NS) with 4-year survivals >85%. The authors concluded that the introduction of mycophenolate mofetil allowed a safe reduction of cyclosporine and significantly improved renal function after 4 years [85].

Mycophenolate Sodium (EC-MPS)

Enteric-coated mycophenolate sodium is a delayed release salt of mycophenolic acid developed to avoid gastrointestinal adverse effects of mycophenolate mofetil. 1000 mg mycophenolate mofetil is equivalent to 720 mg mycophenolate sodium.

Proliferation Signal Inhibitors (mTOR Inhibitors)

The mechanistic/mammalian target of rapamycin (mTOR) is a widely expressed serine/threonine kinase of the phosphatidylinositol 3-kinase (PI3K)-like kinase superfamily. It is activated by the IL-2 stimulation of the T-cell IL-2 receptor. It regulates transcription, and hence protein synthesis, cell growth, cell proliferation and cell survival [86]. Unlike tacrolimus and cyclosporine which inhibit the production of cytokines, mTOR inhibitors do not block cytokine production but rather block the response to these cytokines (e.g.IL-2) by causing cell cycle arrest at the G1 to S phase. The result of this is the inhibition of T- and B-cell proliferation. The fact that mTOR inhibitors can reduce the expression of the IL-2 receptor (CD25), independent of their cell cycle progression blocking effect could also contribute to their immunosuppressive effect [87].

The two mTOR inhibitors sirolimus (SIR) and everolimus (EVER), have similar mechanisms of action. They are structurally similar to tacrolimus. The feature of the mTOR inhibitors inhibiting vascular smooth muscle cell growth and proliferation may help reduce the rate of CAV.

In current immunosuppressive protocols mTOR inhibitors can be used in place of MMF or AZA in combination with a CNI and prednisone, or in place of CNIs in combination with MMF or AZA and prednisone especially for those patients with renal issues, as mTOR inhibitors are not nephrotoxic.

Sirolimus

On the first-transplant day a loading dose of 15 mg sirolimus is recommended. This loading dose is followed by a 2-5 mg daily maintenance dose. The maintenance dose is guided by serum trough levels (targeted to 5-10 ng/mL). When used in combination with cyclosporine, sirolimus should be given four hours after the cyclosporine administration.

The whole blood concentrations are measured by HPLC, which is specific for the parent compound. The target concentration range is 10-15 ng/mL when used in combination with a CNI or 15-25 ng/mL without a CNI.

Although sirolimus is not nephrotoxic, it can potentiate the nephrotoxic effects of the CNIs when used together. Therefore, the dose of the CNI should be reduced by 25%.

The most common adverse effects of sirolimus are oral ulcerations, peripheral edema, hypertension, hyperlipidemia, thrombocytopenia, neutropenia and anemia. Hyperlipidemia with peak levels seen within 3 months of therapy usually decreases after 1 year of therapy and is partially responsive to dose reduction. On the other hand myelosuppression seems to be dose dependent and reversible. Thrombocytopenia is seen within the first 2 weeks of therapy.

Delayed would healing and dehiscence are thought to be due to the inhibition of smooth muscle proliferation and intimal thickening. Patients with a body mass index >30 kg/m^2 are at increased risk for impaired wound healing. Other reported adverse effects of sirolimus include pleural and pericardial effusions and pulmonary toxicity. Immunosuppression with sirolimus increases the risk of infection and may be associated with lymphoma development.

Summary of Selected Literature

Yin *et al.* [88] aimed to investigate the effect of sirolimus-based immuno-suppression on heart transplant recipients with chronic renal dysfunction. At their clinic, standard CNI-based immunosuppressive regimen was changed to reduced-dose CNI plus sirolimus due to CNI-related chronic renal dysfunction in 20 out of 138 cardiac transplant recipients. The standard immunosuppressive regimen included steroid, CNI and MMF or AZA. Sirolimus was started at 0.75 - 1.50 mg/d with titration to achieve levels of 5 - 15 µg/L, and CNI dose was reduced gradually to 1/2-2/3 of the baseline level. Cyclosporine dose was reduced from (191.7 ± 60.0) mg/d to (123.6 ± 34.8) mg/d, with blood drug concentration reduced from (175.5 ± 58.0) µg/L to (111.9 ± 56.0) µg/L in 18 patients (p<0.01). Mean tacrolimus dose was reduced from 4.25 mg/d to 3.00 mg/d, with blood drug concentration reduced from 13.5 µg/L to 10.5 µg/L in 2 patients. The authors concluded that change from CNI-based immunosuppressive regimen to reduced-dose CNI plus sirolimus was an effective and safe approach for the management of patients with CNI-related chronic renal dysfunction, leading to an improvement in renal function without compromise in anti-rejection efficacy and with tolerable side effects [88].

The results of non-randomized studies by Raichlin *et al.* [89] and Groetzner *et al.* [60] suggested that switching from CNI- to sirolimus-based immunosuppression improved renal function. Another multicenter randomized trial by Groetzner *et al.* [90] on late heart transplant recipients with renal insufficiency demonstrated that switching to CNI-free immunosuppression (MMF, sirolimus) resulted in improved renal function when compared with CNI-reduced immunosuppression.

Their beneficial effects on CAV assessed by intravascular ultrasound support the inclusion of everolimus and sirolimus in contemporary immunosuppressive regimens [91, 92]. However, the renal dysfunction associated with everolimus/sirolimus - standard-dose CYC combination makes this drug regimen less favorable.

Everolimus

The use of everolimus early after heart transplantation is not recommended because of the increased risk of mortality observed within the first three months following transplantation among patients receiving higher doses (3,0 mg/day) of everolimus.

The initial everolimus dose is 0,75 mg twice daily. This dose is adjusted to reach a target blood trough level of 3-8 ng/mL. It is recommended that everolimus is taken consistently either with or without food.

Coronary intimal thickening and CAV is reduced by everolimus. While the adverse effects of everolimus are mainly similar to those of sirolimus, everolimus use has been associated with reduced rates of CMV infections.

Summary of Selected Literature

In their review, Zuckermann *et al.* [93] concludes that according to the current evidence, the most convincing reasons for using everolimus from the time of heart transplantation are slowing the progression of CAV and lowering the risk of CMV infection [93].

Rosing *et al.* [94] systematically evaluated cardiovascular risk factors in heart transplantation patients whose immunosuppressive therapy was converted to everolimus or was maintained on conventional therapy with CNIs. Among the included patients, 50 were receiving everolimus and 91 were receiving CNI in addition to MMF and low-dose steroids. As a conclusion of the study they stated that everolimus specifically lowered plasma activity and cellular production of lipoprotein-associated phospholipase A2 (Lp-PLA2) and thereby dampened oxidative stress. They suggested that these effects might additionally contribute to the reduced CAV incidence observed in heart transplant recipients receiving everolimus therapy [94].

With the aim of characterization of the action of everolimus on CMV Kobashigawa *et al.* [95] analyzed data from 3 large randomized studies including 1009 de novo cardiac transplant recipients, comparing various everolimus regimens with AZA-based and MMF-based regimens. They concluded that everolimus was associated with a lower incidence of CMV infection compared with AZA and MMF in cardiac transplant recipients, mentioning that this beneficial effect was not dose dependent, was apparent regardless of the type of prophylaxis used and was maintained under concentration-controlled everolimus dosing in combination with reduced dose cyclosporine [95].

Arora *et al.* [96] investigating the effect of everolimus on established CAV in the Nordic Certican Trial in Heart and lung Transplantation sub-study concluded that conversion to everolimus and reduced CNI did not influence CAV progression among maintenance heart transplantation recipients. However, background immunosuppressive therapy was important as AZA + everolimus patients demonstrated attenuated CAV progression and a decline in inflammatory markers, whereas the opposite pattern was seen with everolimus + MMF [96].

The results of a 12-month, multicenter, open-label study where cardiac transplant patients received everolimus with reduced CYC or MMF with standard dose CYC, demonstrated that everolimus with reduced CYC resulted in similar renal failure and equivalent efficacy at 12 months after cardiac transplantation [97].

Table 2. Summary of recommendations on the principles of immunosuppressive regimens in heart transplant recipients [44].

Class I
1. Maintenance therapy should include a CNI in all pediatric HT recipients (*Level: C*).
Class IIa
1. It is reasonable to use CNI-based therapies as the standard immunosuppressive therapy after HT (*Level: B*).
2. MMF, everolimus or sirolimus as tolerated should be included in contemporary immunosuppressive regimens because therapies including these drugs have been shown to reduce onset and progression of CAV (*Level: B*).
3. Immunosuppressive induction with polyclonal antibody preparations may be beneficial in patients at high risk of renal dysfunction when used with the intent to delay or avoid the use of a CNI (*Level: B*).
4. CS avoidance, early CS weaning, or very low-dose maintenance CS therapy are all acceptable therapeutic approaches (*Level: B*). If used, CS weaning should be attempted if there are significant CS side effects and no recent rejection episodes (e.g., within 6 months) (*Level: C*).
5. TAC is the preferred CNI for pediatric HT recipients considered at high immunologic risk (*Level: C*).

(Table 2) cont.....

6. In pediatric HT recipients, routine use of induction therapy with a polyclonal preparation is indicated when complete CS avoidance is planned after HT (*Level: C*).
7. Pediatric recipients with pre-formed alloantibodies and a positive donor-specific cross-match should receive induction therapy, and TAC-based "triple therapy" with CSs and either MMF or an mTOR inhibitor (*Level: C*).
Class IIb
1. It might be reasonable to prefer TAC-based regimens over CYC-based regimens, as the former may be associated with lower rejection rates after HT, although the survival is comparable *(Level: B)*.
2. Routine use of immunosuppressive induction in all patients has not been shown to be superior to immunosuppressive regimens that do not use such therapy *(Level: B)*. Immunosuppressive induction with anti-thymocyte globulin may be beneficial in patients at high risk for acute rejection *(Level: C)*.
3. Adjunctive therapy with an anti-metabolite or a PSI might be considered in most children *(Level: C)*. If a child is intolerant of adjunctive therapy, the decision of replacing it with another agent or not should be made after review of the patient's rejection history and immunologic risk. TAC monotherapy may be considered in patients with a benign rejection history *(Level: C)*. For children diagnosed with CAV, the addition of an mTOR inhibitor should be strongly considered *(Level: C)*.
Classification of Recommendations: **Class I:** Procedure/treatment should be performed/administered (Benefit >>> Risk). **Class II a:** Additional studies with focused objectives needed. It is reasonable to perform procedure/administer treatment (Benefit >> Risk). **Class II b:** Additional studies with broad objectives needed; additional registry data would be helpful. Procedure/treatment may be considered (Benefit ≥ Risk).
Level of Evidence: **Level A**: Multiple populations evaluated; data derived from multiple randomized clinical trials or meta-analyses. **Level B**: Limited populations evaluated; data derived from a single randomized clinical trials or nonrandomized studies. **Level C**: Very limited populations evaluated; only consensus opinion of experts, case studies or standard of care.

CAV: cardiac allograft vasculopathy; CNI: calcineurin inhibitor; CS: corticosteroid; CYC: cyclosporine; HT: heart transplant; MMF: mycophenolate mofetil; mTOR: mammalian target of rapamycin; PSI: proliferation signal inhibitor; TAC: tacrolimus.

COMMON COMPLICATIONS AFTER HEART TRANSPLANTATION

As the long-term survival of heart transplant recipients improved so much, patients today are being exposed to immunosuppressive drugs for long periods. This prolonged exposure resulted in an increased prevalence of immunosuppressive-related complications or comorbidities.

Infection

Immunosuppression with any immunosuppressive agent increases the risk of opportunistic infections in the heart transplant recipient. Infection risk is related to the overall immunosuppression level of the patients and is highest during the postoperative first three months and following the treatment of an acute rejection [98].

Bacterial infections most commonly occur during the postoperative first month and generally manifest as urinary tract infections, infections of the vascular access sites or wounds. Herpes simplex is most commonly responsible for the viral infections of the early postoperative period, while Herpes zoster accounts for many of the late viral infections.

The pathogens of particular concern are cytomegalovirus (CMV) and pneumocystis carinii.

Cytomegalovirus

The incidence of post-transplant CMV infections is between 25-50% [99]. CMV infections develop as primary- or secondary-CMV infections. Primary CMV infection occurs when a CMV-negative recipient receives a CMV-positive donor heart. In secondary CMV infection, the CMV-positive recipient experiences the reactivation of the disease as a result of immunosuppression.

Manifestations of CMV disease are flu-like symptoms (such as fever, myalgia), gastritis, gastric ulcers, colitis, pneumonitis, retinitis, hepatitis, leucopenia and thrombocytopenia. Patients with primary infections usually suffer more from the symptoms than those with secondary infections.

The most sensitive and specific test for diagnosing CMV is quantitative polymerase chain reaction (PCR). Although PCR detects CMV DNA in plasma and measures the quantity of CMV viral load, it is still controversial if the detectable CMV viral load will cause the clinical syndrome and whether to treat those patients without symptoms.

The risk factors for the development and severity of CMV disease include: overall level of immunosuppression, multiple use of high-dose corticosteroids, use of antilymphocyte antibodies or OKT3, serology mismatch (donor CMV-positive and recipient CMV-negative), poor HLA mismatching. Prophylaxis against CMV disease is routinely recommended for all CMV-positive recipients with a CMV-positive donor.

Patients are initially treated with intravenous ganciclovir; then the treatment may be continued with oral valganciclovir or acyclovir. The duration of prophylactic treatment with ganciclovir can vary from center to center. Duration of the therapy may depend on the CMV viral load; therefore, periodic monitoring can be helpful.

Patients at high risk of CMV disease, particularly those with low levels of serum immunoglobulins (<500 mg/dL) may benefit from passive immunization with CMV immunoglobulin. Active CMV disease is treated with intravenous ganciclovir and valganciclovir in non-severe cases for 3-6 weeks. Before discontinuation of the antiviral therapy, an undetectable CMV viral load must be confirmed. For life-long protection against CMV disease, the patient must develop a specific anti-CMV immune response [100].

Cardiac Allograft Vasculopathy

Cardiac allograft vasculopathy (CAV), which is defined as the development of new coronary artery stenoses, is the unique form of post-transplant atherosclerosis which progresses very quickly. At the fifth year of transplantation, angiographically detectable CAV is present in 40–50% of patients. About 5% to 10% of patients develop severe CAV that will lead to heart failure requiring retransplantation or resulting in death [101].

CAV is a leading cause of death in the first year following transplantation [102]. CAV accounts for more than 20% of all deaths after the first post-transplantation year [103, 104]; while it accounts for 17% of all deaths after the third post-transplantation year.

Cardiac allograft vasculopathy has distinct morphological features different from those of atherosclerosis. While focal atherosclerotic plaques characterize the typical CAD lesion, CAV lesions resemble those observed in restenosis after balloon angioplasty and coronary stenting. It is seen that smooth-muscle cell proliferation contributes to the narrowing of the lumen of coronary arteries. Cardiac allograft vasculopathy first develops in the distal vessels and then progress to the proximal sites in a short time. This type of stenosis is characterized by intimal proliferation in early stages and by luminal stenosis of epicardial branches, occlusion of smaller arteries, and myocardial infarction in the later stages [105].

Unlike atherosclerosis, CAV has a unique pathogenesis involving both immunologic and non-immunologic processes. These processes include humoral and cellular rejection, HLA mismatching, invasive CMV infection, ischemia-reperfusion injury, hyperlipidemia, homocysteinemia, diabetes and hypertension. The major issue in CAV is a repeating injury to the vessels and continuous inflammatory response. The initiating event of CAV is thought to be subclinical endothelial cell injury in the allograft coronary artery. This injury may be a consequence of ischemia–reperfusion damage or the host-*vs.*-graft immune response. CAV starts a group of immunologic processes, which result in inflammation and ultimately lead to thrombosis, smooth muscle cell proliferation and vessel constriction [106, 107].

Cardiac allograft vasculopathy presents as ventricular arrhythmias, congestive heart failure and sudden death. Routine performance of a yearly coronary angiogram is recommended for the timely diagnosis of CAV. Other diagnostic tools such as intravascular ultrasound (IVUS), thallium scintigraphy and dobutamine stress echocardiography, pulse-wave tissue Doppler imaging, fast computed tomography (CT) scanning, electron beam CT and MRI may also be used.

The diffuse and distal coronary artery involvement of CAV decreases the effectiveness of percutaneous coronary interventions or bypass surgery [108]; therefore, the prognosis seems to be poor [109]. Today, the only treatment for advanced CAV is retransplantation [110]. Therefore, prophylactic therapy is crucial. Before transplantation, endothelial injury at brain death should be prevented. Reducing cold ischemia time and improving myocardial preservation during storage and transportation can help manage this. After transplantation, measures like cholesterol-lowering dietary restrictions and pharmacotherapeutic management of hyperlipidemia, hypertension control and smoking cessation should be taken.

While, there is still no proven effective prevention strategy for the development of CAV, the mTOR inhibitors (*i.e.* everolimus and sirolimus) may be beneficial in reducing the development as well as severity of CAV and may help to slow disease progression [111, 112]. On the other hand, CAV is reported to happen less frequently in patients treated with statins, angiotensin-converting enzyme inhibitors and calcium-channel blockers [113, 114].

Increased platelet activity may also contribute to CAV development [115]. Therefore, antiplatelet agents, particularly aspirin are routinely used in heart transplant patients. On the other hand, when compared with non-transplant patients, heart transplant recipients seem to be aspirin resistant even at doses as high as 500 mg/day.

Malignancies

The risk of malignancies increases with long-term suppression of the immune system. The incidence, which is between 4 - 18% [116], has been reported to be 3- to 5-fold higher in transplant recipients than in the general population [117] and 10 to 100-fold higher than age-matched non-transplant patients [118]. The risk of malignancy increases, as the duration of immunosuppression gets longer. Nearly half of the patients are reported to be at risk of tumor development after receiving immunosuppressive agents for 25 years [119].

The most common malignancies experienced by the immunosuppressive therapy recipients are skin carcinomas and post-transplant lymphoproliferative disorder (PTLD), which is a type of non-Hodgkin lymphoma; though, any solid-organ tumor can also develop.

The most common of the newly developed malignancies in the post-transplant patients are squamous and basal cell carcinomas of the skin. They both account for almost half of the cancers. In patients receiving immunosuppressant therapy, squamous cell carcinoma happens at a four-fold rate when compared to basal cell carcinoma; while, it is just the opposite for the patients with immunocompetency. The squamous cell carcinoma seen in transplant recipients has a recurrent and metastatic nature [120].

As the risk factors for post-transplant skin cancer include prolonged immunosuppression, increased age and ultraviolet radiation exposure, efforts should be made to decrease skin exposure to ultraviolet rays and lights, decrease the immunosuppressant dose (after the diagnosis of skin cancer) and to arrange dermatology appointments at least once a year [117].

Posttransplant lymphoproliferative disorder, which is the second most common group of malignancies occurring after transplantation is generally associated with prior Epstein-Barr virus infection and may be either B- or T-cell originated [121]. This disorder can present with a wide range of clinical features extending to severe monoclonal lymphoma. The complexity of the therapy increases with the severity of the disorder. Severe disease is usually treated with chemotherapy, radiation and/or surgical resection; also, it would be beneficial to reduce the dose of immunosuppressive therapy and administer high-dose acyclovir to attenuate EBV replication. The most effective therapy is determined depending on the tissue diagnosis. The addition of rituximab may be effective in treating PTLD [118].

The incidence of new malignancies other than skin cancer and PTLD is reported to be between 0.7% and 5.6% at 5 years [122].

In general it is recommended for those taking immunosuppressive to have yearly dermatologic controls besides the usual cancer screening programs such as cervical smears, mammography and faecal occult blood for those over 50. Also it is recommended for the physicians to consider the use of mTOR inhibitor sirolimus as the immunosuppressant drug in preventing cancer development, as clinical data have shown that sirolimus have antitumor and antiangiogenic properties [123].

Renal Dysfunction

Chronic kidney disease or any kind of renal dysfunction is a common complication encountered following heart transplantation. Up to 40% of heart transplant recipients experience a decreased (<60 mL/minute) estimated glomerular filtration rate [124]. In other studies, it is demonstrated that at post-transplantation 4th – 5th years, in 24% to 33% of patients serum creatinine levels were equal to or higher than 2 mg/dL; while, 3% to 8% of the patients developed end-stage renal disease at some time during their lives [125 - 127]. According to the 2005 ISHLT registry report at 9.5 years only 60% of heart transplant recipients are found to be free of severe renal dysfunction (>2.5mg/dL) [102]. The mortality risk is 4-fold increased in those with post-transplantation renal failure [124].

Development of chronic kidney disease is considered mainly due to the long-term use of CNIs. Therefore, the incidence of renal dysfunction depends on the duration and intensity of CNIs used as a component of immunosuppression regimen. Calcineurin inhibitors cause both acute and chronic nephrotoxicity. Acute nephrotoxicity which involves afferent arteriolar vasoconstriction and reduced renal plasma flow is associated with high trough levels and can be predictable [128]; whereas chronic nephrotoxicity involves irreversible structural changes including glomerulosclerosis, tubulointerstitial fibrosis and arteriolopathy, and cannot be predicted by trough level measurements.

Other contributing factors to chronic kidney disease development besides the use of CNIs are pre-transplant renal function impairment, preoperative hypotension, ischemic injury from aortic cross-clamping, intraoperative thrombotic emboli, hypertension, diabetes, and post-transplant acute kidney injury [129]. High venous filling pressures, chronic low-output states and up-regulation of the renin angiotensin aldosterone system may cause renal impairment in patients with preexisting heart failure [118]. Pre-transplant renal function impairment with a serum creatinine level >2.5 mg/dL is associated with extended intensive care unit and hospital stays, long mechanical ventilatory times and impaired wound healing [118].

Although there is no definite effective therapy, several strategies have been proposed to prevent post-transplant chronic kidney disease. These include dose reduction or avoidance of CNI doses and converting to or combining with sirolimus or MMF. Immunosuppression regimens should be individualized according to characteristics of the patient.

On the other hand, it is not known whether angiotensin converting enzyme inhibitors or angiotensin receptor blockers are effective in slowing the progression of CNI-induced renal disease. It should be kept in mind that decreased glomerular filtration rate after transplantation would result in an increased potential for drug-drug interactions.

Cardiovascular Disease

Cardiovascular disease is the most common cause of death in heart transplant patients. Risk of cardiovascular mortality is 2.5-fold and risk of ischemic events is 3-fold greater for the heart transplant recipients when compared with the general population. This increased risk is attributable to the metabolic adverse effects of immunosuppressive therapy consisting of agents such as corticosteroids, cyclosporine and tacrolimus. On the other hand, preexisting risk factors such as hyperglycemia, hyperlipidemia and hypertension may exacerbate in the post-transplantation period and this may result in atherosclerosis which leads to the development of post-transplant cardiovascular diseases, such as ischemic heart disease, congestive heart failure, cerebrovascular accidents and peripheral vascular disease.

For the post-transplant patients risk factor reduction attempts should be more aggressive. Efforts that should be made for prevention of cardiovascular diseases after transplantation include lifestyle modifications (*i.e.* smoking cessation, weight monitoring, healthy eating, *etc.*), management of associated risk factors such as hypertension, dyslipidemia and diabetes (through routine monitoring of blood pressure, serum fasting lipid and glucose levels) and adjusting immunosuppression regimens [130].

Hypertension

In heart transplant recipients the circadian rhythm regulating blood pressure is disturbed in a way avoiding the usual nocturnal blood pressure fall; therefore, the body is affected by a 24-hour hypertensive burden [131].

Systemic hypertension (>140/90 mmHg) is prevalent after heart transplantation affecting 50% to 95% of heart recipients [102, 131, 132]. Newly developed post-transplant hypertension or worsening of preexisting hypertension after transplantation affects 50% to 75% of patients during the first months following transplantation [133]. Hypertension in either form can present hazard for the transplant recipient at short and long term.

The CNIs have been associated with development or worsening of hypertension following transplantation [134]. Majority of the maintenance immunosuppression programs involve the use of CNIs; therefore, hypertension becomes an important cardiovascular issue in heart transplant recipients. Calcineurin inhibitors increase sympathetic tone and endothelin-mediated vasoconstriction, decrease nitric oxide-induced compensatory vasodilation, activate the renin-angiotensin-aldosterone and cause sodium dependent volume expansion [135]. On the other hand, they can also cause hypertension *via* CNI-induced renal dysfunction. Although, both CNIs are associated with hypertension, the incidence is lower in patients treated with tacrolimus when compared with cyclosporine [64].

Blood pressure lowering in the post-operative period is associated with improved graft and patient survival [136]. Effective blood-pressure control is generally difficult and achieved by use of at least one antihypertensive medicine, together with a low sodium diet. The most frequently preferred agents are calcium channel blockers, angiotensin converting enzyme inhibitors and angiotensin receptor blockers. Renal function should be monitored while using ACE inhibitors or angiotensin receptor blockers [118]. While beta-blockers are effective in reducing blood pressure, any potential excessive bradycardia should be avoided in the setting of a denervated heart and it should be considered that beta-blockers blunt the heart-rate response to exercise [118]. Likewise, caution should be exercised with diuretics as they may cause volume depletion and hypotension.

Diabetes Mellitus

New-onset diabetes after transplantation (NODAT) is the development of diabetes following transplantation in patients who were previously non-diabetic. NODAT has been reported in 4% to 40% of heart transplant recipients [104, 137]. The reported incidence seemed to vary likely due to the duration of follow-up and the presence of both modifiable and non-modifiable risks factors [138].

NODAT is particularly associated with the use of corticosteroids, CNIs and sirolimus. Risk factors of NODAT other than the immunosuppressive agents include family history of diabetes, the need for insulin beyond the first 24 hours following transplantation and pre-existing obesity [118]. Among CNIs, tacrolimus is associated with a higher incidence of NODAT than that observed with cyclosporine, particularly when used in high doses and in blacks [139]. Calcineurin inhibitors damaging the pancreatic beta cells, decrease insulin sensitivity and reduce insulin release.

Like NODAT, preexisting diabetes is a risk factor for negative post-transplant outcomes. While, diabetic transplant recipients with no complications have comparable survival rates at 1-year and 3-years, when compared with those without diabetes, diabetic patients with at least one complication have worse mid- and long-term survival rates. On the other hand, patients with multiple diabetic complications are not considered suitable for heart transplantation [118].

In order to do monitoring with HbA1C measurements, it is recommended to wait for three months following transplantation. This is the time period needed for new hemoglobin to be synthesized and glycated; earlier tests may not be valid [140].

Diabetes in the transplant recipient is generally treated the same way it is treated in the non-transplant populations. Besides the usual diabetes treatment, immunosuppression treatment regimens are to be adjusted weighing the risk of allograft rejection against diabetes management. Corticosteroid weaning or dose reduction and prescribing maintenance immunosuppression using agents with less diabetogenic potential are strategies to be followed.

In order to slow the development or progression of the diabetic complications tight glycemic control is recommended. As heart transplant recipients have increased prevalence of renal dysfunction, metformin may be relatively contraindicated in post-transplant diabetic patients. In the case of renal insufficiency short-acting sulfonylureas are preferred over longer-acting ones. On the other hand, it should be kept in mind that thiazolinediones might cause fluid retention and weight gain.

Dyslipidemia

Hyperlipidemia eventually develops in 60% to 81% of patients following heart transplantation [141]. Total cholesterol, LDL cholesterol and triglyceride levels, which increase in three months following transplantation generally, decrease to pre-transplant levels after the first year [142]. Presence of hyperlipidemia increases the prevalence of CAV, cerebrovascular disease and peripheral vascular disease [143]; therefore, cholesterol levels should be kept in the recommended range mentioned in guidelines.

Immunosuppressive drugs (particularly mTOR inhibitors sirolimus and everolimus, calcineurin inhibitors and prednisone), loop diuretics and renal insufficiency may cause dyslipidemia [144]. The hypercholesterolemic effects of tacrolimus are similar, although less marked to those of cyclosporine [145].

Hyperlipidemia in the heart transplant recipients should be managed the same way as in the non-transplant population with the employment of life-style interventions and lipid-lowering pharmacotherapy.

The HMG-CoA reductase inhibitors (statins) are effective in reducing LDL cholesterol level in the transplant patients. Benefits of statins on mortality, CAV and rejection associated with hemodynamic compromise have been demonstrated in heart transplant recipients [146]. This augmented benefit may arise from the immune modulating effects of statins as well as their lipid-lowering effects.

Statins are generally prescribed to heart transplant recipients in a routine manner. The major concern regarding the use of statins is the risk of rhabdomyolysis, particularly for those using CNIs. As pravastatin is not metabolized by cytochrome enzymes, it may have a lower incidence of rhabdomyolysis [147] and generally used at doses of 20 - 40 mg. Statins other than pravastatin are used at doses lower than the maximally approved dose for the non-transplant population. Rhabdomyolysis risk increases when statins are used in higher doses or when combined with niacin or fibrates; and these combinations are contraindicated in patients receiving CNIs [148]. Fibrates may be used for elevated triglyceride levels but they may decrease cyclosporine levels.

Neurologic Complications

Post-transplantation neurologic complications frequently present as encephalopathy, seizures, strokes, peripheral neuropathies and central nervous system infections. Stroke occurs in about 9% of the transplant recipients; while seizures occur in about 15%. Increased age is a risk factor for neurologic complications. Besides, the use of pre-transplant left ventricular assist devices is an additional risk factor for strokes. Seizures due to CNI use or infections usually occur during the post-transplant first month. Tacrolimus and cyclosporine use may lead to an encephalopathy syndrome characterized with seizures, vision changes and headache. Calcineurin inhibitor dose reduction or withdrawal may reverse the syndrome [118].

Gout

Pre-existing gout, obesity, renal insufficiency, use of calcineurin inhibitors and loop diuretics are main causes of gout after heart transplantation [149]. As non-steroidal anti-inflammatory drug and colchicine use are problematic due to drug-drug interaction issues, glucocorticoids are often the preferred agents for the treatment of acute gout. Non-steroidal anti-inflammatory drugs may also worsen renal insufficiency and cause hyperkalemia, particularly in patients taking CNIs. While, prophylactic allopurinol use is effective, doses of both allopurinol and azathioprine must be reduced when used concomitantly. However, this is not a recommended combination as it may cause fatal neutropenia [150]. On the other hand, allopurinol does not interact with mycophenolate mofetil.

Osteoporosis

Osteoporosis is a common problem after heart transplantation; it may result in vertebral fractures. About 50% of the transplant patients have osteopenia and osteoporosis before transplantation as a consequence of advanced heart failure [151]. While corticosteroid use is the major issue contributing to bone loss after transplantation, renal dysfunction and CNIs also have a negative impact on the situation. While, 28% of the heart transplant recipients have osteoporosis by the second post-transplant year, vertebral fractures are reported in about 30% [152]. Most bone loss occurs in the first 6 to 12 months after transplantation when steroid doses are highest [153].

Majority of the bone loss occurs at the lumbar spine and femoral neck at post-transplant first year. Although patient's age and lumbar bone-mineral density are independent predictors of fractures, some patients may have fractures with normal bone-mineral densities [118]. Prevention is first-line therapy. Monitoring should be done by bone mineral densitometry and measurement of creatinine, blood urea nitrogen, calcium, vitamin D metabolite levels and phosphate levels. In non-transplant patients bisphosphonates have been used to prevent glucocorticoid-induced osteoporosis and fractures. Bisphosphonates can also be suggested for those receiving transplantation [154]. Patients receiving >5 mg/day prednisone for at least 3 months are suggested to receive calcium (1500 mg/day) and vitamin D (800 IU/day), as well as a bisphosphonate and regular weight-bearing exercise.

Depression

Depression is reported in about one forth of heart transplant recipients at post-transplant 1 to 3 years [155]. As there is an 18% prevalence of depression at 5 and 10 years after transplantation [156] a large number of heart transplant recipients seem to be taking antidepressant drugs. Therefore, potential interactions between selective serotonin reuptake inhibitors and cyclosporine should be considered when prescribing for depression.

COMMON DRUG INTERACTIONS WITH IMMUNOSUPPRESSIVE AGENTS

Today, the number of medical problems in heart transplant recipients has increased due to aging and complications common to immunosuppressive drugs. The co-existence or emergence of other disease states such as renal dysfunction, infection, diabetes, obesity, hypertension, hyperlipidemia, malignancies, and osteoporosis necessitates the use of other medications. The use of these medications in combination with immunosuppressive agents increases the risk of drug-drug interactions.

Drug–drug interaction risk increases with polypharmacy, advanced age, drugs with narrow therapeutic index or drugs that require intensive monitoring. All these risk factors excluding advanced age are present in heart transplant recipients.

Commonly used immunosuppressive agents are substrates of the cytochrome P450 system; therefore they are more susceptible to interactions with drugs that are substrates or induce or inhibit these series of enzymes, particularly CYP3A4. Cyclosporine, tacrolimus, sirolimus, and everolimus are bio-transformed by CYP3A4. Some medications like cyclosporine, tacrolimus and sirolimus use both the CYP450 enzyme system and P-gp, making them specifically vulnerable to drug interactions.

Calcineurin Inhibitors

Hepatic and intestinal CYP3A are the significant metabolic enzymes for both cyclosporine and tacrolimus. These two drugs are also both inhibitors and substrates of P-gp. So drug interactions reported for cyclosporine are possibly present with tacrolimus as well.

Antihypertensives

Many calcium channel blockers from the dihydropyridine class, diltiazem and verapamil are substrates of both CYP3A4 and P-gp. Diltiazem and verapamil increases serum concentrations of cyclosporine and tacrolimus by 1.5- to 6-fold; therefore, a reduction of 20% to 75% in cyclosporine and tacrolimus doses is required [157]. Amlodipine, nicardipine and felodipine may increase serum concentrations of cyclosporine between 23% and 350% [157]. Concomitant felodipine and nifedipine use caused a 50% rise in tacrolimus serum levels [158, 159]. On the other hand, while nifedipine and isradipine do not seem to have an impact on cyclosporine pharmacokinetics, tacrolimus or cyclosporine are still needed to be initiated or discontinued cautiously while the patient is using dihydropyridines.

Lipid-Lowering Agents

Lipid lowering agents are administered following heart transplant to prevent coronary artery diseases. Taking into consideration the affinity of cyclosporine to plasma lipids, it is assumed that alteration of plasma lipids may result in changes in the disposition and pharmacokinetics of cyclosporine. Akhlaghi *et al.* [160] reported a moderate increase in the apparent oral clearance of cyclosporine when used with lipid lowering agents.

Some of the most commonly prescribed statins (lovastatin, simvastatin and atorvastatin) are substrates of the CYP3A4 system. Pharmacokinetic interactions with cyclosporine and tacrolimus are most likely and potentially lead to myopathy and/or rhabdomyolysis [148]. All the statins other than fluvastatin have a high potential to cause rhabdomyolysis when used together with cyclosporine.

Fluvastatin is metabolized mainly by CYP2C9. Likewise, rosuvastatin is metabolized minimally through the CYP enzyme system [161]. Pravastatin is a substrate of P-gp and metabolized through numerous paths not merely including the CYP enzyme system. Lovastatin and atorvastatin are also substrates of the P-gp. The incidence of myotoxicity escalates with escalating statin dose [147, 148].

When cyclosporine was used in combination with atorvastatin, simvastatin, fluvastatin, lovastatin or rosuvastatin after transplantation, cyclosporine increased the AUC of statins by 3- to 20-fold from the baseline values [157]. Only pravastatin when combined with cyclosporine seems to accumulate minimally after multiple dosages [162, 163]. A potential interaction exists between tacrolimus and lovastatin and simvastatin because they all show comparable affinity for CYP3A in both liver and small intestine. It is recommended to use the lowest therapeutic dose of a lipid-lowering agent, when they are used in combination with cyclosporine. There are no formal dosing recommendations with tacrolimus; however, recommendations made for cyclosporine seem to be applicable for tacrolimus. Pravastatin and fluvastatin seem to be the safest statins in transplant recipients. In case of myopathy or rhabdomyolysis, it is recommended to immediately discontinue cyclosporine, tacrolimus, statins and any other myotoxic agents.

Cyclosporine was reported to increase ezetimibe concentrations by 12-fold but before any recommendations can be made, further evaluation of possible interactions is necessary [157].

The fibric acid derivatives fenofibrate and gemfibrozil are metabolized by CYP3A4 enzyme system. Concomitant fibric acid use causes an 18% to 27% decrease in CYC trough levels [164, 165]. On the other hand, while statin and fibrate combination may lead to myotoxicity, this risk increases with the addition of cyclosporine or tacrolimus.

Antiplatelet Agents

Ticlopidine (250 to 500 mg) may induce CYP3A; thus, decrease cyclosporine serum concentrations by 1.4- to 2.0-fold in a time period ranging from days to months [166, 167]. Therefore, close monitoring of cyclosporine and tacrolimus serum concentrations for several months is recommended at times of ticlopidine initiation or discontinuation. Clopidogrel's active metabolite level may decrease when administered together with cyclosporine or tacrolimus, which theoretically reduces antiplatelet effect of clopidogrel.

Antifungal Agents

Antifungal use is usually common in transplant recipients especially in those receiving heart-lung transplants. All azole derivative antifungals increase the CNI levels to varying extents by reducing their metabolism. Itraconazole and posaconazole were reported to be more potent CYP3A4 inhibitors than voriconazole or fluconazole [168]. Ketoconazole, which is the most potent CYP3A4 inhibitor is intentionally used concomitantly with CNIs to reduce CNI dose and cost for patients [169]. This must be performed along with efficient monitoring to avoid inadvertent withdrawal of ketoconazole, which will lead to therapeutic failure. The interaction between fluconazole and CNI was found to be dose dependent and drug-dependent [170]. With moderate doses of fluconazole (100-200 mg/day), effects on cyclosporine are minor while effects on tacrolimus are moderate to significant. Immunosuppressant dose should be significantly reduced when a fluconazole dose of 400 mg is needed to treat systemic fungal infections [169].

When voriconazole is initiated, an empiric dose reduction is recommended for tacrolimus and cyclosporine; this is reduction by two-thirds of the original maintenance dose of tacrolimus and by half of the original maintenance dose of cyclosporine [170]. Similarly, in the case of posaconazole initiation, an empiric two-thirds dose reduction for tacrolimus and one-fourth dose reduction for cyclosporine in their original maintenance dose is suggested [169].

Oral clotrimazole troches used for the prophylaxis or treatment of oral mucocutaneous candidiasis, were shown to significantly raise tacrolimus serum concentrations. The tacrolimus blood concentrations were doubled in some studies; therefore, CNI drug concentrations should be measured at the time of clotrimazole initiation and discontinuation [169].

Ketoconazole and itraconazole inhibits both CYP3A and P-gp while itraconazole, fluconazole and voriconazole only inhibit CYP3A. *In vitro*, the most potent inhibitor of cyclosporine metabolism is ketoconazole; this is followed by itraconazole and fluconazole. Cyclosporine and tacrolimus trough concentrations increase by 2-folds when used together with ketoconazole, fluconazole, itraconazole and voriconazole [157].

In a research conducted in heart transplant recipients taking cyclosporine, concomitant use of itraconazole, ketoconazole and diltiazem resulted in 75%, 40% and 23% reduction in cyclosporine clearance. The reduction was up to 82% in patients taking both ketoconazole and diltiazem. As a consequence, cyclosporine doses are reduced by 75% in patients taking ketoconazole and by 23% for those on diltizem [171].

In a research involving 40 lung transplant recipients who used tacrolimus and prophylactic itraconazole for more than a year, the required tacrolimus dose increased by 76% with itraconazole discontinuation. (3.26 – 2.1 mg/day during the first 6 months compared with 5.74 – 2.9 mg/day during the following 6 months) [172]. Similar to cyclosporine, tacrolimus as a substrate for CYP3A and P-gp is vulnerable to interactions with any drugs that affect these systems such as calcium-channel blockers, imidazole antifungal agents, erythromycin).

Initially, cyclosporine and tacrolimus doses should be decreased by 50% with ketoconazole, itraconazole and voriconazole. Tacrolimus doses may be decreased by 33% with voriconazole [157].

None of the echinochandin antifungals are significantly metabolized by CYP3A and they are only administered intravenously. Thus they may be convenient alternatives to azole antifungals [169]. Cyclosporine may cause a 35% increase in caspofungin AUC and this results in clinically significant transient rises in liver transaminases [157]. Subsequent studies found neither significant changes in cyclosporine or tacrolimus pharmacokinetics nor any significant increase in hepatotoxicity with caspofungin use [169]. Caspofungin package labeling recommends standard tacrolimus dosing and serum level monitoring. No interaction between micafungin and tacrolimus has been shown [169]. Conversely, in one study cyclosporine concentrations were decreased by 16% by micafungin use, thus monitoring of cyclosporine levels was recommended [173]. Concomitant use with cyclosporine caused a 22% rise in anidulafungin concentrations, but as this was not considered clinically significant, dose modifications were not recommended for both agent [174]. No interaction has been seen with anidulafungin and tacrolimus [175].

Antiretroviral Agents

Many of the antiretroviral medications are substrates of CYP3A4; therefore, severe interactions between antiretroviral medications, particularly protease inhibitors and calcineurin inhibitors are expected, exposing patients to toxicity or under-immunosuppression [169].

HCV Protease Inhibitors

Use of the HCV treatment agents boceprevir and telaprevir has been increasing in liver transplant patients. Both drugs are substrates and inhibitors of CYP3A4. In three liver transplant patients co-administration of cyclosporine and boceprevir resulted in small rise in cyclosporine blood concentrations [169]. In a study involving six liver transplant patients taking telepravir, tacrolimus dosing was adjusted to be once a week or every three days with concomitant drug level monitoring. Based on several small case reports in liver transplant recipients some authors recommend holding calcineurin inhibitors or empirically reducing cyclosporine dose by 75% when combined with boceprevir or telaprevir with appropriate drug level monitoring [169]. But concomitant use of boceprevir and telaprevir with calcineurin inhibitors seems to be safe with effective drug level monitoring [169].

Macrolide Antibiotics

These agents all inhibit CYP3A4 to a moderate to high intensity, with the exception of azithromycin. CYP3A4 inhibition leads to decreased metabolism of cyclosporine and tacrolimus. Erythromycin and clarithromycin have the greatest effect on CNI metabolism compared to other macrolides. This interaction results to 3- to 10-fold increase in CNI concentrations and AUC. The combination of CNIs and macrolides should be avoided; if concomitant use is essential, a 50% decrease in CNI dose may be considered and daily blood levels of CNI should be monitored. Many *in vitro* and *in vivo* reports have showed no interaction with azithromycin but in two case reports elevated cyclosporine concentrations were reported with combination with azithromycin [169]. Tacrolimus levels are also reported to be elevated when used in combination with azithromycin [169]. Drug level monitoring is always advisable with these combinations.

Rifamycins

The plasma levels of CNIs are dramatically reduced when used with rifampin and rifabutin due to the strong CYP3A4 induction effects of rifamycins [169], which persists even in the presence of other CYP3A4 inhibitors. Their combinations should be avoided. When use is inevitable CNI dose should be increased by two-fold at the beginning of rifamycin therapy and subsequently increased rapidly (up to 10-fold); while, regular drug level monitoring is necessary pending dose stabilization. CNI doses must also be monitored and reduced accordingly when rifamycin is stopped [169].

Antidepressants

Most antidepressants are substrates and inhibitors of the CYP enzymes. Fluoxetine, fluvoxamine and nefazodone are all potent inhibitors of CYP3A4; while paroxetine, sertraline and mirtazapine are weak inhibitors of CYP3A4, citalopram is a substrate of CYP3A4, and venlafaxine is both a substrate and inhibitor of CYP2D6. Concomitant use of fluoxetine, fluvoxamine and nefazodone resulted in 2- and 10-fold [157] increase in cyclosporine concentrations; while, a 2- to 5-fold increase in tacrolimus concentrations was reported with concomitant nefazodone use [176, 177]. It is best to avoid nefazodone in patients receiving cyclosporine and tacrolimus; whereas fluvoxamine and fluoxetine may be used with caution, when necessary. Citalopram and venlafaxine may be suitable alternatives in patients taking cyclosporine and tacrolimus. There are reported cases of a 2- to 6- fold decrease in cyclosporine and tacrolimus serum levels in patients concomitantly taking St. John's Wort [157]; therefore, due to the risk of organ rejection, St. John's Wort should not be used in these patients.

Other Agents

When used together, both CNIs and amiodarone can accumulate and cause related toxicities. A 1.8-fold increase in cyclosporine trough concentrations arising from a 50% decrease in its clearance was reported for a heart transplant patient. A different paper reported a 2-fold increase in cyclosporine concentration 3 days after amiodarone was started [157]. The pharmacokinetic effects of amiodarone on cyclosporine may precede for 4 weeks following amiodarone discontinuation. A similar interaction may also be possible between tacrolimus and amiodarone. When starting amiodarone in patients on CNI, the possible lowest dose should be started and the level of CNI must be monitored for a minimum of 4 weeks [157].

Oral phenytoin may decrease the bioavailability and mean half-life of cyclosporine. A similar effect may also be anticipated with tacrolimus. This interaction is thought to be relative to CYP3A induction by phenytoin or potential reduction in cyclosporine absorption. Concomitant use of tacrolimus is reported to elevate phenytoin concentrations [157]. The same effect is expected to occur with cyclosporine. Tacrolimus or cyclosporine serum levels should be monitored regularly for the first 2 weeks on initiation and discontinuation of phenytoin. Before starting phenytoin therapy the cyclosporine dose should be doubled [157].

Carbamazepine and oxcarbazepine may reduce cyclosporine levels by 4-fold due to enzyme induction. It may take up to 4 months for cyclosporine levels to normalize after carbamazepine is discontinued. Similarly, reductions in tacrolimus concentrations are also expected. Other antiepileptics that are not inhibitors of CYP3A such as valproic acid, gabapentin, lamotrigine, tiagabine and vigabatrin may be suitable alternatives [157].

Antigout Agents

Combining colchicine with cyclosporine will results in increased levels of colchicine; thus increasing its toxic effects. This may result in a combination of side effects involving gastrointestinal dysfunction, hepatonephropathy, and neuromyopathy. This syndrome emerges within 1 to 2 weeks following colchicine (0.6 to 3.6 mg/day) initiation and it resolves 3 to 4 weeks after colchicine is stopped and/or cyclosporine dose is reduced. Patients with kidney dysfunction are more vulnerable to this syndrome [178]. Colchicine should be given in the lowest possible dose and for a limited time in patients taking CNIs. Colchicine should be stopped immediately when patients show signs of nausea, vomiting, jaundice, muscle weakness, muscle wasting, myalgias, and distal paresthesias [178].

Target of Rapamycin Inhibitors

Sirolimus and everolimus are absorbed readily after oral administration. Sirolimus has a 14% bioavailability due to extensive metabolization in the entero-hepatic circle by CYP3A4 and counter-transport by intestinal P-gp. There are few interaction reports on these drugs.

Antihypertensives

No effects of CYP3A4 inhibiting agents like dihydropyridines, diltiazem or verapamil on everolimus serum levels were reported from multicenter efficacy trials. In renal transplant recipients, the AUC of sirolimus rose by 60% when used with diltiazem [179].

Macrolide Antibiotics

CYP3A4 inhibition leads to decreased metabolism of mTOR inhibitors [169]. Erythromycin and clarithromycin inhibit this enzyme more strongly than other macrolides. The combination of macrolides with mTOR inhibitors leads to very significant (3- to 10-fold) escalations in immunosuppressant blood levels; therefore mTOR inhibitors should not be used with erythromycin/clarithromycin. When the concomitant use of these agents are unavoidable, mTOR inhibitor blood levels should be monitored every three days. Many *in vitro* and *in vivo* reports have showed no interaction between azithromycin and mTOR inhibitors [169].

Antifungal Agents

In a cadaveric renal transplant patient, it was reported that oral fluconazole raised sirolimus trough levels 3.5-fold. Package labeling does not recommend combining sirolimus with ketoconazole or voriconazole. Itraconazole may diminish everolimus clearance by 71% [180]. Combinations of commonly used azole antifungal agents and sirolimus/everolimus should be used cautiously.

Azole derivative antifungal agents (itraconazole, posaconazole, fluconazole, voriconazole, ketoconazole) decrease the metabolism of mTOR inhibitors leading to great rises in serum levels and AUC. Ketoconazole has been revealed to be the most potent CYP3A4 inhibitor and has been used with mTOR inhibitor-based immunosuppression in order to reduce immunosuppressive dose requirements and cost for transplant patients [169]. When used with voriconazole and posaconazole, sirolimus blood concentrations may promptly rise by 10-fold and 9-fold, respectively; therefore these combinations are contraindicated [169]. If inevitable, voriconazole and sirolimus can be used only with low doses of sirolimus (0.5–1.0 mg/day) as reported in a small case series. The same situation is also valid for everolimus. Everolimus prescribing information discourages its concomitant administration with voriconazole. But case reports show their possible use with lower doses of everolimus [181, 182]. A 3.8-fold rise in everolimus blood levels with concomitant posaconazole use was reported in a renal transplant recipient [181]. Drug level monitoring is always recommended at initiation, during and after discontinuation of voriconazole or posaconazole. In renal transplant recipients, the AUC of sirolimus rose by 990% when used with ketoconazole [179].

Itraconazole caused a 74% decrease while fluconazole had no influence on everolimus clearance [180]. In 13 lung and heart-lung transplant patients, a 2.3-fold higher everolimus trough concentration was reported in patients receiving concomitant azole antifungals when compared to others [183]. Itraconazole and ketoconazole had a stronger effect while fluconazole appeared to have the least influence [184]. Micafungin product information notes a 21% increase in sirolimus AUC at sirolimus steady-state and recommends sirolimus serum level monitoring with appropriate dose adjustments.

Antiretroviral Agents

Many antiretroviral agents are CYP3A4 substrates; therefore, interactions of mTOR inhibitors with protease inhibitors can be dangerous [185]. Regular monitoring is needed in these patients.

Rifamycins

Rifamycins (rifampin, rifabutin, rifapentine) are all strong inducers of CYP3A4. Combination of these agents with mTOR inhibitors should not be used. In situations where combination is a must, like in tuberculosis patients, doses of mTOR inhibitors should be increased at the beginning of combined therapy. This should be followed by subsequent increases (up to 10-fold reported) and frequent drug serum concentration monitoring is recommended until dosing is stabilized. Rifamycin therapy should cautiously be discontinued [169]. In renal transplant recipients, the AUC of sirolimus is reduced by 82% with rifampicin [179]. Rifampin was reported to enhance everolimus clearance by 172% and shorten the t1/2 from 32 to 24 hours, resulting in a 63% decrease in AUC [184].

Other Agents

When cyclosporine is used with sirolimus, the time of administration affects sirolimus pharmacokinetics. In the package labeling it is reported that sirolimus should be given 4 hours after cyclosporine [157].

The combination of everolimus and cyclosporine resulted in increase in everolimus Cmax and AUC. Therefore, close monitoring of everolimus serum levels is required for 1 to 2 weeks after cyclosporine is initiated or discontinued.

When administered with cyclosporine microemulsion (not the oil-based formulation), the AUC of sirolimus increases by 50-80% as a result of inhibition of CYP3A and P-gp by cyclosporine, but there is no change in cyclosporine AUC [186]. Synergistic pharmacodynamic interactions have been reported with sirolimus and cyclosporine [186], being the reason why sirolimus is used as a cyclosporine-sparing agent.

Antiproliferative Agents

Lipid-Lowering Agents

Co-administration of mycophenolate mofetil and cholestyramine causes a 40% decrease in MPA AUC and is not recommended in the package labeling [157].

Other Immunosuppresives

A randomized study carried out on 60 heart transplant patients revealed that patients on tacrolimus (n=30) required lower mycophenolate mofetil doses to reach mycophenolate mofetil trough concentrations of 0.45–4.0 mg/L (1.6–0.8 *vs* 2.8–1.0 g/day at 1 year post-transplantation, p=0.00004), than those on cyclosporine (n=30) [184]. Another prospective, randomized controlled study involving 50 heart transplant recipients compared the mycophenolate mofetil/tacrolimus (n=25) and the mycophenolate mofetil/cyclosporine (n=25) combinations in terms of efficacy, toxicity and pharmacokinetics. The patients on cyclosporine required higher mycophenolate mofetil dose to reach similar trough concentrations [184]. In 30 adult stable lung transplant patients mycophenolate mofetil trough concentrations were 50% lower in recipients taking cyclosporine even with higher doses of mycophenolate mofetil [187].

In summary, when determining the mycophenolate mofetil dose, the accompanying immunosuppressant (cyclosporine, tacrolimus, sirolimus) must be considered, as the clinical outcome may be strongly affected by under-immunosuppression [187].

Antigout Agents

Both allopurinol and oxypurinol; the active metabolite of allopurinol, increase the myelosuppressive side effects of 6-mercaptopurine. Reversible anemia, leukopenia and thrombocytopenia have been reported in patients who used oral azathioprine and allopurinol simultaneously. There may be no possible interaction with intravenous azathioprine. 75% to 80% reductions should be made in the oral doses of both allopurinol and azathioprine when they are co-administered. Complete blood count ought to be performed regularly [157].

Other Agents

Mycophenolate mofetil can form chelates with antacids and iron. Therefore, mycophenolate mofetil and iron/antacids should be administered 2 to 4 hours apart [188].

Resistance to warfarin anticoagulation may be induced by Azathioprine (100 mg). In some patients 1.5- to 2.5-fold increase in initial weekly warfarin dose was required to maintain adequate anticoagulation. Close monitoring of the prothrombin time is recommended when these agents are used together [188].

CONCLUSION

Successful surgery is the first step in the survival of transplant recipients. After surgery, survival depends on successful postoperative care and the use of relevant immunosuppressive regimens. While immunosuppressive therapy increases the survival rate of the heart transplant recipient, this complex therapy requires constant need for patient monitoring. It may be harmful or inefficient if immunosuppressants are not selected and organized properly. The choice of the immunosuppressive regimen should first depend on the patient characteristics. Other factors such as drug adverse effects, interactions and accessibility also affect the choice of immunosuppressants. Some studies have shown the importance of induction immunosuppression, but the risk of malignancy and their inability to reduce late rejection rates have made their use controversial. Induction immunosuppression may be initiated in patients with predisposing kidney disease thereby avoiding early introduction of calcineurin inhibitors. The choice of drugs in the maintenance immunosuppressive regimens must be done to achieve maximum benefit with minimum adverse effects. Dosing must be done effectively and patients must be monitored continuously. Drugs must be selected based on the comorbid disease states and the drugs used by the patients. Drug interactions are usually common with immunosuppressants. These drug interactions may reduce the effectiveness of immunosuppressants thereby, increasing rejection risk. Therefore, as pharmacists are experts in drug therapy with their comprehensive knowledge of medications, it would be wise to have a pharmacist in the multidisciplinary transplant team.

CONFLICT OF INTEREST

The authors confirm that they have no conflict of interest to declare for this publication.

ACKNOWLEDGEMENTS

Declared none.

REFERENCES

[1]   Roger VL, Go AS, Lloyd-Jones DM, *et al.* Heart disease and stroke statistics2011 update: a report from the American Heart Association. Circulation 2011; 123(4): e18-e209.
[http://dx.doi.org/10.1161/CIR.0b013e3182009701] [PMID: 21160056]

[2]   Lund LH, Edwards LB, Kucheryavaya AY, *et al.* The Registry of the International Society for Heart and Lung Transplantation: Thirty-second Official Adult Heart Transplantation Report2015; Focus Theme: Early Graft Failure. J Heart Lung Transplant 2015; 34(10): 1244-54.
[http://dx.doi.org/10.1016/j.healun.2015.08.003] [PMID: 26454738]

[3]   Abrahams Z, Mullens W, Boyle A. Cardiac transplantation. In: Griffin BP, Topol EJ, Eds. Manual of cardiovascular medicine. 3rd ed. PA, USA: Lippincott Williams & Wilkins Philadelphia 2009; pp. 171-90.

[4]   2009 annual report of the U.S. Organ Procurement and Transplantation Network and the Scientific Registry of Transplant Recipients: Transplant Data 1999-2008. U.S. Department of Health and Human services, Health Resources and Services Administration, Healthcare Systems Bureau, Division of Transplantation, Rockville, MD. Available from: http://www.ustransplant.org/annual_reports/current. [accessed 1st Feb 2014].

[5]   Stehlik J, Edwards LB, Kucheryavaya AY, *et al.* The Registry of the International Society for Heart and Lung Transplantation: twenty-seventh official adult heart transplant report2010. J Heart Lung Transplant 2010; 29(10): 1089-103.
[http://dx.doi.org/10.1016/j.healun.2010.08.007] [PMID: 20870164]

[6]   Stehlik J, Edwards LB, Kucheryavaya AY, *et al.* Registry of the International Society for Heart and Lung Transplantation: twenty-eighth adult heart transplant report-2011. J Heart Lung Transplant 2011; 30(10): 1078-94.
[http://dx.doi.org/10.1016/j.healun.2011.08.003] [PMID: 21962016]

[7]   Johnson MR, Mullen GM, OSullivan EJ, *et al.* Risk/benefit ratio of perioperative OKT3 in cardiac transplantation. Am J Cardiol 1994; 74(3): 261-6.
[http://dx.doi.org/10.1016/0002-9149(94)90368-9] [PMID: 8037132]

[8]   Opelz G, Döhler B. Lymphomas after solid organ transplantation: a collaborative transplant study report. Am J Transplant 2004; 4(2): 222-30.
[http://dx.doi.org/10.1046/j.1600-6143.2003.00325.x] [PMID: 14974943]

[9]   Rinaldi M, Pellegrini C, DArmini AM, *et al.* Neoplastic disease after heart transplantation: single center experience. Eur J Cardiothorac Surg 2001; 19(5): 696-701.
[http://dx.doi.org/10.1016/S1010-7940(01)00674-1] [PMID: 11343955]

[10]   Aliabadi A, Grömmer M, Cochrane A, Salameh O, Zuckermann A. Induction therapy in heart transplantation: where are we now? Transpl Int 2013; 26(7): 684-95.
[http://dx.doi.org/10.1111/tri.12107] [PMID: 23656308]

[11]   Higgins R, Kirklin JK, Brown RN, *et al.* To induce or not to induce: do patients at greatest risk for fatal rejection benefit from cytolytic induction therapy? J Heart Lung Transplant 2005; 24(4): 392-400.
        [http://dx.doi.org/10.1016/j.healun.2004.01.002] [PMID: 15797738]

[12]   Whitson BA, Kilic A, Lehman A, *et al.* Impact of induction immunosuppression on survival in heart transplant recipients: a contemporary analysis of agents. Clin Transplant 2015; 29(1): 9-17.
        [http://dx.doi.org/10.1111/ctr.12469] [PMID: 25284138]

[13]   Mazimba S, Tallaj JA, George JF, Kirklin JK, Brown RN, Pamboukian SV. Infection and rejection risk after cardiac transplantation with induction *vs.* no induction: a multi-institutional study. Clin Transplant 2014; 28(9): 946-52.
        [http://dx.doi.org/10.1111/ctr.12395] [PMID: 24930563]

[14]   Penninga L, Møller CH, Gustafsson F, Gluud C, Steinbrüchel DA. Immunosuppressive T-cell antibody induction for heart transplant recipients. Cochrane Database Syst Rev 2013; 12(12): CD008842.
        [PMID: 24297433]

[15]   Caillat-Zucman S, Blumenfeld N, Legendre C, *et al.* The OKT3 immunosuppressive effect. *In situ* antigenic modulation of human graft-infiltrating T cells. Transplantation 1990; 49(1): 156-60.
        [http://dx.doi.org/10.1097/00007890-199001000-00035] [PMID: 2137271]

[16]   Norman DJ. Mechanisms of action and overview of OKT3. Ther Drug Monit 1995; 17(6): 615-20.
        [http://dx.doi.org/10.1097/00007691-199512000-00012] [PMID: 8588230]

[17]   Jensen PB, Birkeland SA, Rohrp N, Elbirk A, Jørgensen KA. Development of anti-OKT3 antibodies after OKT3 treatment. Scand J Urol Nephrol 1996; 30(3): 227-30.
        [http://dx.doi.org/10.3109/00365599609181304] [PMID: 8837256]

[18]   Hammond EH, Wittwer CT, Greenwood J, *et al.* Relationship of OKT3 sensitization and vascular rejection in cardiac transplant patients receiving OKT3 rejection prophylaxis. Transplantation 1990; 50(5): 776-82.
        [http://dx.doi.org/10.1097/00007890-199011000-00008] [PMID: 2122559]

[19]   Wilde MI, Goa KL. Muromonab CD3: a reappraisal of its pharmacology and use as prophylaxis of solid organ transplant rejection. Drugs 1996; 51(5): 865-94.
        [http://dx.doi.org/10.2165/00003495-199651050-00010] [PMID: 8861551]

[20]   Delgado JF, Vaqueriza D, Sánchez V, *et al.* Induction treatment with monoclonal antibodies for heart transplantation. Transplant Rev (Orlando) 2011; 25(1): 21-6.
        [http://dx.doi.org/10.1016/j.trre.2010.10.002] [PMID: 21126660]

[21]   Almenar L, García-Palomar C, Martínez-Dolz L, *et al.* Influence of induction therapy on rejection and survival in heart transplantation. Transplant Proc 2005; 37(9): 4024-7.
        [http://dx.doi.org/10.1016/j.transproceed.2005.09.154] [PMID: 16386616]

[22]   Cuppoletti A, Perez-Villa F, Vallejos I, Roig E. Experience with single-dose daclizumab in the prevention of acute rejection in heart transplantation Transplant Proc 2005; 37(9): 4036 8.
        [http://dx.doi.org/10.1016/j.transproceed.2005.10.086] [PMID: 16386620]

[23]   Chin C, Pittson S, Luikart H, *et al.* Induction therapy for pediatric and adult heart transplantation: comparison between OKT3 and daclizumab. Transplantation 2005; 80(4): 477-81.
        [http://dx.doi.org/10.1097/01.tp.0000168153.50774.30] [PMID: 16123721]

[24]   Segovia J, Rodríguez-Lambert JL, Crespo-Leiro MG, *et al.* A randomized multicenter comparison of basiliximab and muromonab (OKT3) in heart transplantation: SIMCOR study. Transplantation 2006; 81(11): 1542-8.
        [http://dx.doi.org/10.1097/01.tp.0000209924.00229.e5] [PMID: 16770243]

[25]   Product Information: ATGAM(R) IV injection, lymphocyte immune globulin, anti-thymocyte globulin [equine] sterile IV injection. Pharmacia & Upjohn Company, Kalamazoo, MI, 2005.

[26] Schonder KS, Johnson HJ. Solid organ transplantation. In: DiPiro JT, Talbert RL, Yee GC, Eds. Pharmacotherapy: A pathophysiologic approach. 7th ed. New York: McGraw-Hill 2008; pp. 1459-82.

[27] Thrush PT, Gossett JG, Costello JM, *et al.* Role for immune monitoring to tailor induction prophylaxis in pediatric heart recipients. Pediatr Transplant 2014; 18(1): 79-86.
[http://dx.doi.org/10.1111/petr.12193] [PMID: 24283506]

[28] Czer LS, Phan A, Ruzza A, *et al.* Antithymocyte globulin induction therapy adjusted for immunologic risk after heart transplantation. Transplant Proc 2013; 45(6): 2393-8.
[http://dx.doi.org/10.1016/j.transproceed.2013.02.114] [PMID: 23953554]

[29] Rafiei M, Kittleson M, Patel J, *et al.* Anti-thymocyte gamma-globulin may prevent antibody production after heart transplantation. Transplant Proc 2014; 46(10): 3570-4.
[http://dx.doi.org/10.1016/j.transproceed.2014.08.042] [PMID: 25498091]

[30] Ansari D, Lund LH, Stehlik J, *et al.* Induction with anti-thymocyte globulin in heart transplantation is associated with better long-term survival compared with basiliximab. J Heart Lung Transplant 2015; 34(10): 1283-91.
[http://dx.doi.org/10.1016/j.healun.2015.04.001] [PMID: 26087667]

[31] Goland S, Czer LS, Coleman B, *et al.* Induction therapy with thymoglobulin after heart transplantation: impact of therapy duration on lymphocyte depletion and recovery, rejection, and cytomegalovirus infection rates. J Heart Lung Transplant 2008; 27(10): 1115-21.
[http://dx.doi.org/10.1016/j.healun.2008.07.002] [PMID: 18926403]

[32] Koch A, Daniel V, Dengler TJ, Schnabel PA, Hagl S, Sack FU. Effectivity of a T-cell-adapted induction therapy with anti-thymocyte globulin (Sangstat). J Heart Lung Transplant 2005; 24(6): 708-13.
[http://dx.doi.org/10.1016/j.healun.2004.04.014] [PMID: 15949731]

[33] Cantarovich M, Giannetti N, Barkun J, Cecere R. Antithymocyte globulin induction allows a prolonged delay in the initiation of cyclosporine in heart transplant patients with postoperative renal dysfunction. Transplantation 2004; 78(5): 779-81.
[http://dx.doi.org/10.1097/01.TP.0000130179.18176.3D] [PMID: 15371689]

[34] Delgado DH, Miriuka SG, Cusimano RJ, Feindel C, Rao V, Ross HJ. Use of basiliximab and cyclosporine in heart transplant patients with pre-operative renal dysfunction. J Heart Lung Transplant 2005; 24(2): 166-9.
[http://dx.doi.org/10.1016/j.healun.2003.09.043] [PMID: 15701432]

[35] Carlsen J, Johansen M, Boesgaard S, *et al.* Induction therapy after cardiac transplantation: a comparison of anti-thymocyte globulin and daclizumab in the prevention of acute rejection. J Heart Lung Transplant 2005; 24(3): 296-302.
[http://dx.doi.org/10.1016/j.healun.2003.12.014] [PMID: 15737756]

[36] Carrier M, Leblanc MH, Perrault LP, *et al.* Basiliximab and rabbit anti-thymocyte globulin for prophylaxis of acute rejection after heart transplantation: a non-inferiority trial. J Heart Lung Transplant 2007; 26(3): 258-63.
[http://dx.doi.org/10.1016/j.healun.2007.01.006] [PMID: 17346628]

[37] Mattei MF, Redonnet M, Gandjbakhch I, *et al.* Lower risk of infectious deaths in cardiac transplant patients receiving basiliximab *versus* anti-thymocyte globulin as induction therapy. J Heart Lung Transplant 2007; 26(7): 693-9.
[http://dx.doi.org/10.1016/j.healun.2007.05.002] [PMID: 17613399]

[38] Flaman F, Zieroth S, Rao V, Ross H, Delgado DH. Basiliximab *versus* rabbit anti-thymocyte globulin for induction therapy in patients after heart transplantation. J Heart Lung Transplant 2006; 25(11): 1358-62.
[http://dx.doi.org/10.1016/j.healun.2006.09.002] [PMID: 17097501]

[39] Mullen JC, Kuurstra EJ, Oreopoulos A, Bentley MJ, Wang S. A randomized controlled trial of

daclizumab *versus* anti-thymocyte globulin induction for heart transplantation. Transplant Res 2014; 3: 14.
[http://dx.doi.org/10.1186/2047-1440-3-14] [PMID: 25093077]

[40]   Beniaminovitz A, Itescu S, Lietz K, *et al.* Prevention of rejection in cardiac transplantation by blockade of the interleukin-2 receptor with a monoclonal antibody. N Engl J Med 2000; 342(9): 613-9.
[http://dx.doi.org/10.1056/NEJM200003023420902] [PMID: 10699160]

[41]   Hershberger RE, Starling RC, Eisen HJ, *et al.* Daclizumab to prevent rejection after cardiac transplantation. N Engl J Med 2005; 352(26): 2705-13.
[http://dx.doi.org/10.1056/NEJMoa032953] [PMID: 15987919]

[42]   Mehra MR, Zucker MJ, Wagoner L, *et al.* A multicenter, prospective, randomized, double-blind trial of basiliximab in heart transplantation. J Heart Lung Transplant 2005; 24(9): 1297-304.
[http://dx.doi.org/10.1016/j.healun.2004.09.010] [PMID: 16143248]

[43]   Lund LH, Edwards LB, Kucheryavaya AY, *et al.* The registry of the International Society for Heart and Lung Transplantation: thirty-first official adult heart transplant report2014; focus theme: retransplantation. J Heart Lung Transplant 2014; 33(10): 996-1008.
[http://dx.doi.org/10.1016/j.healun.2014.08.003] [PMID: 25242124]

[44]   Costanzo MR, Dipchand A, Starling R. International Society of Heart and Lung Transplantation Guidelines. The International Society of Heart and Lung Transplantation Guidelines for the care of heart transplant recipients. J Heart Lung Transplant 2010; 29(8): 914-56.

[45]   Auphan N, DiDonato JA, Rosette C, Helmberg A, Karin M. Immunosuppression by glucocorticoids: inhibition of NF-kappa B activity through induction of I kappa B synthesis. Science 1995; 270(5234): 286-90.
[http://dx.doi.org/10.1126/science.270.5234.286] [PMID: 7569976]

[46]   Scheinman RI, Cogswell PC, Lofquist AK, Baldwin AS Jr. Role of transcriptional activation of I kappa B alpha in mediation of immunosuppression by glucocorticoids. Science 1995; 270(5234): 283-6.
[http://dx.doi.org/10.1126/science.270.5234.283] [PMID: 7569975]

[47]   Schweiger M. Immunosuppressive therapy after cardiac transplantation. Cardiac transplantation, InTech 2012. Available from: http://www.intechopen.com/books/cardiac-transplantation/ immunosupp-ressive-is-therapy-after-cardiac-transplantation. [cited 27th Nov 2015].
[http://dx.doi.org/10.5772/26031]

[48]   Kobashigawa JA, Stevenson LW, Brownfield ED, *et al.* Corticosteroid weaning late after heart transplantation: relation to HLA-DR mismatching and long-term metabolic benefits. J Heart Lung Transplant 1995; 14(5): 963-7.
[PMID: 8800734]

[49]   Kirk R, Edwards LB, Kucheryavaya AY, *et al.* The Registry of the International Society for Heart and Lung Transplantation: thirteenth official pediatric heart transplantation report2010. J Heart Lung Transplant 2010; 29(10): 1119-28.
[http://dx.doi.org/10.1016/j.healun.2010.08.009] [PMID: 20870166]

[50]   Ajmal M, Matas AJ, Kuskowski M, Cheng EY. Does statin usage reduce the risk of corticosteroid-related osteonecrosis in renal transplant population? Orthop Clin North Am 2009; 40(2): 235-9.
[http://dx.doi.org/10.1016/j.ocl.2009.01.004] [PMID: 19358908]

[51]   Baraldo M, Gregoraci G, Livi U. Steroid-free and steroid withdrawal protocols in heart transplantation: the review of literature. Transpl Int 2014; 27(6): 515-29.
[http://dx.doi.org/10.1111/tri.12309] [PMID: 24617420]

[52]   Faulhaber M, Mäding I, Malehsa D, Raggi MC, Haverich A, Bara CL. Steroid withdrawal and reduction of cyclosporine A under mycophenolate mofetil after heart transplantation. Int Immunopharmacol 2013; 15(4): 712-7.
[http://dx.doi.org/10.1016/j.intimp.2013.02.012] [PMID: 23454241]

[53]   Crespo-Leiro MG. Calcineurin inhibitors in heart transplantation. Transplant Proc 2005; 37(9): 4018-20.
[http://dx.doi.org/10.1016/j.transproceed.2005.09.155] [PMID: 16386614]

[54]   Morioka M, Hamada J, Ushio Y, Miyamoto E. Potential role of calcineurin for brain ischemia and traumatic injury. Prog Neurobiol 1999; 58(1): 1-30.
[http://dx.doi.org/10.1016/S0301-0082(98)00073-2] [PMID: 10321795]

[55]   Rao A, Luo C, Hogan PG. Transcription factors of the NFAT family: regulation and function. Annu Rev Immunol 1997; 15: 707-47.
[http://dx.doi.org/10.1146/annurev.immunol.15.1.707] [PMID: 9143705]

[56]   Serfling E, Berberich-Siebelt F, Chuvpilo S, *et al.* The role of NF-AT transcription factors in T cell activation and differentiation. Biochim Biophys Acta 2000; 1498(1): 1-18.
[http://dx.doi.org/10.1016/S0167-4889(00)00082-3] [PMID: 11042346]

[57]   Hogan PG, Chen L, Nardone J, Rao A. Transcriptional regulation by calcium, calcineurin, and NFAT. Genes Dev 2003; 17(18): 2205-32.
[http://dx.doi.org/10.1101/gad.1102703] [PMID: 12975316]

[58]   Macian F. NFAT proteins: key regulators of T-cell development and function. Nat Rev Immunol 2005; 5(6): 472-84.
[http://dx.doi.org/10.1038/nri1632] [PMID: 15928679]

[59]   Hertz MI, Aurora P, Christie JD, *et al.* Registry of the International Society for Heart and Lung Transplantation: a quarter century of thoracic transplantation. J Heart Lung Transplant 2008; 27(9): 937-42.
[http://dx.doi.org/10.1016/j.healun.2008.07.019] [PMID: 18765185]

[60]   Groetzner J, Kaczmarek I, Schulz U, *et al.* Mycophenolate and sirolimus as calcineurin inhibitor-free immunosuppression improves renal function better than calcineurin inhibitor-reduction in late cardiac transplant recipients with chronic renal failure. Transplantation 2009; 87(5): 726-33.
[http://dx.doi.org/10.1097/TP.0b013e3181963371] [PMID: 19295318]

[61]   Cornu C, Dufays C, Gaillard S, *et al.* Impact of the reduction of calcineurin inhibitors on renal function in heart transplant patients: a systematic review and meta-analysis. Br J Clin Pharmacol 2014; 78(1): 24-32.
[http://dx.doi.org/10.1111/bcp.12289] [PMID: 24251918]

[62]   Kobashigawa JA, Miller LW, Russell SD, *et al.* Tacrolimus with mycophenolate mofetil (MMF) or sirolimus *vs.* cyclosporine with MMF in cardiac transplant patients: 1-year report. Am J Transplant 2006; 6(6): 1377-86.
[http://dx.doi.org/10.1111/j.1600-6143.2006.01290.x] [PMID: 16686761]

[63]   Baran DA, Zucker MJ, Arroyo LH, *et al.* Randomized trial of tacrolimus monotherapy: tacrolimus in combination, tacrolimus alone compared (the TICTAC trial). J Heart Lung Transplant 2007; 26(10): 992-7.
[http://dx.doi.org/10.1016/j.healun.2007.07.022] [PMID: 17919618]

[64]   Taylor DO, Barr ML, Radovancevic B, *et al.* A randomized, multicenter comparison of tacrolimus and cyclosporine immunosuppressive regimens in cardiac transplantation: decreased hyperlipidemia and hypertension with tacrolimus. J Heart Lung Transplant 1999; 18(4): 336-45.
[http://dx.doi.org/10.1016/S1053-2498(98)00060-6] [PMID: 10226898]

[65]   Grimm M, Rinaldi M, Yonan NA, *et al.* Superior prevention of acute rejection by tacrolimus vs. cyclosporine in heart transplant recipientsa large European trial. Am J Transplant 2006; 6(6): 1387-97.
[http://dx.doi.org/10.1111/j.1600-6143.2006.01300.x] [PMID: 16686762]

[66]   Reichart B, Meiser B, Viganò M, *et al.* European Multicenter Tacrolimus (FK506) Heart Pilot Study: one-year resultsEuropean Tacrolimus Multicenter Heart Study Group. J Heart Lung Transplant 1998; 17(8): 775-81.

[PMID: 9730426]

[67]   Eisen HJ, Hobbs RE, Davis SF, *et al.* Safety, tolerability, and efficacy of cyclosporine microemulsion
        in heart transplant recipients: a randomized, multicenter, double-blind comparison with the oil-based
        formulation of cyclosporineresults at 24 months after transplantation. Transplantation 2001; 71(1): 70-
        8.
        [http://dx.doi.org/10.1097/00007890-200101150-00012] [PMID: 11211198]

[68]   NEORAL(R) oral soft gelatin capsules, oral solution, cyclosporine oral soft gelatin capsules, oral
        solution Novartis Pharmaceuticals Corporation (per FDA). NJ: East Hanover 2013.

[69]   Sandimmune(R) oral soft gelatin capsules, oral solution, intravenous injection, cyclosporine oral soft
        gelatin capsules, oral solution, intravenous injection Novartis Pharmaceuticals Corporation (per FDA).
        NJ: East Hanover 2013.

[70]   Lindenfeld J, Miller GG, Shakar SF, *et al.* Drug therapy in the heart transplant recipient: part II:
        immunosuppressive drugs. Circulation 2004; 110(25): 3858-65.
        [http://dx.doi.org/10.1161/01.CIR.0000150332.42276.69] [PMID: 15611389]

[71]   Product Information: PROGRAF(R) oral capsules, IV injection, tacrolimus oral capsules, IV injection.
        Astellas Pharma US, Inc. (per manufacturer), Deerfield, IL, 2011.

[72]   Product Information: ASTAGRAF XL(TM) oral extended-release capsules, tacrolimus oral extended-
        release capsules. Astellas Pharma US, Inc. (per manufacturer), Northbrook, Il, 2013.

[73]   Montori VM, Basu A, Erwin PJ, Velosa JA, Gabriel SE, Kudva YC. Posttransplantation diabetes: a
        systematic review of the literature. Diabetes Care 2002; 25(3): 583-92.
        [http://dx.doi.org/10.2337/diacare.25.3.583] [PMID: 11874952]

[74]   Keogh A. Calcineurin inhibitors in heart transplantation. J Heart Lung Transplant 2004; 23(5)
        (Suppl.): S202-6.
        [http://dx.doi.org/10.1016/j.healun.2004.03.008] [PMID: 15093806]

[75]   Carrico CK, Sartorelli AC. Effects of 6-thioguanine on macromolecular events in regenerating rat
        liver. Cancer Res 1977; 37(6): 1868-75.
        [PMID: 870191]

[76]   AMA drug evaluation. 5th ed., Chicago: American Medical Association 1983.

[77]   McKendry RJ. Purine analogues. Second line agents in the treatment of rheumatic diseases. New
        York: Marcel Decker 1991.

[78]   Trotter JL, Rodey GE, Gebel HM. Azathioprine decreases suppressor T cells in patients with multiple
        sclerosis. N Engl J Med 1982; 306(6): 365-6.
        [http://dx.doi.org/10.1056/NEJM198202113060615] [PMID: 6459531]

[79]   Bacon PA, Salmon M. Modes of action of second-line agents. Scand J Rheumatol Suppl 1987; 64: 17-
        24.
        [http://dx.doi.org/10.3109/03009748709096717] [PMID: 3124265]

[80]   Crilly A, McInnes IB, Capell HA, Madhok R. The effect of azathioprine on serum levels of interleukin
        6 and soluble interleukin 2 receptor. Scand J Rheumatol 1994; 23(2): 87-91.
        [http://dx.doi.org/10.3109/03009749409103034] [PMID: 8165444]

[81]   Nyhan WL, Sweetman L, Carpenter DG, Carter CH, Hoefnagel D. Effects of azathiprine in a disorder
        of uric acid metabolism and cerebral function. J Pediatr 1968; 72(1): 111-8.
        [http://dx.doi.org/10.1016/S0022-3476(68)80413-5] [PMID: 5634933]

[82]   Liang JJ, Geske JR, Boilson BA, *et al.* TPMT genetic variants are associated with increased rejection
        with azathioprine use in heart transplantation. Pharmacogenet Genomics 2013; 23(12): 658-65.
        [http://dx.doi.org/10.1097/FPC.0000000000000005] [PMID: 24121523]

[83]   Kobashigawa J, Miller L, Renlund D, *et al.* A randomized active-controlled trial of mycophenolate

mofetil in heart transplant recipients. Transplantation 1998; 66(4): 507-15.
[http://dx.doi.org/10.1097/00007890-199808270-00016] [PMID: 9734496]

[84] Urbanowicz T, Straburzyńska-Migaj E, Klotzka A, *et al.* Induction therapy, tacrolimus plasma concentration, and duration if intensive care unit stay are risk factors for peripheral leucopenia following heart transplantation. Ann Transplant 2014; 19: 494-8.
[http://dx.doi.org/10.12659/AOT.890816] [PMID: 25274118]

[85] Manito N, Rábago G, Palomo J, *et al.* Improvement in chronic renal failure after mycophenolate mofetil introduction and cyclosporine dose reduction: four-year results from a cohort of heart transplant recipients. Transplant Proc 2011; 43(7): 2699-706.
[http://dx.doi.org/10.1016/j.transproceed.2011.04.017] [PMID: 21911149]

[86] Hay N, Sonenberg N. Upstream and downstream of mTOR. Genes Dev 2004; 18(16): 1926-45.
[http://dx.doi.org/10.1101/gad.1212704] [PMID: 15314020]

[87] Woerly G, Brooks N, Ryffel B. Effect of rapamycin on the expression of the IL-2 receptor (CD25). Clin Exp Immunol 1996; 103(2): 322-7.
[http://dx.doi.org/10.1046/j.1365-2249.1996.d01-616.x] [PMID: 8565319]

[88] Yin D, Huang J, Feng L, *et al.* [Sirolimus use in heart transplantation recipients with chronic renal dysfunction]. Zhonghua Xin Xue Guan Bing Za Zhi 2012; 40(2): 136-40.
[PMID: 22490714]

[89] Raichlin E, Khalpey Z, Kremers W, *et al.* Replacement of calcineurin-inhibitors with sirolimus as primary immunosuppression in stable cardiac transplant recipients. Transplantation 2007; 84(4): 467-74.
[http://dx.doi.org/10.1097/01.tp.0000276959.56959.69] [PMID: 17713429]

[90] Groetzner J, Kaczmarek I, Schulz U, *et al.* Mycophenolate and sirolimus as calcineurin inhibitor-free immunosuppression improves renal function better than calcineurin inhibitor-reduction in late cardiac transplant recipients with chronic renal failure. Transplantation 2009; 87(5): 726-33.
[http://dx.doi.org/10.1097/TP.0b013e3181963371] [PMID: 19295318]

[91] Eisen HJ, Tuzcu EM, Dorent R, *et al.* Everolimus for the prevention of allograft rejection and vasculopathy in cardiac-transplant recipients. N Engl J Med 2003; 349(9): 847-58.
[http://dx.doi.org/10.1056/NEJMoa022171] [PMID: 12944570]

[92] Keogh A, Richardson M, Ruygrok P, *et al.* Sirolimus in de novo heart transplant recipients reduces acute rejection and prevents coronary artery disease at 2 years: a randomized clinical trial. Circulation 2004; 110(17): 2694-700.
[http://dx.doi.org/10.1161/01.CIR.0000136812.90177.94] [PMID: 15262845]

[93] Zuckermann A, Wang SS, Epailly E, *et al.* Everolimus immunosuppression in de novo heart transplant recipients: what does the evidence tell us now? Transplant Rev (Orlando) 2013; 27(3): 76-84.
[http://dx.doi.org/10.1016/j.trre.2013.03.002] [PMID: 23643624]

[94] Rosing K, Fobker M, Kannenberg F, *et al.* Everolimus therapy is associated with reduced lipoprotein-associated phospholipase A2 (Lp-Pla2) activity and oxidative stress in heart transplant recipients. Atherosclerosis 2013; 230(1): 164-70.
[http://dx.doi.org/10.1016/j.atherosclerosis.2013.07.007] [PMID: 23958269]

[95] Kobashigawa J, Ross H, Bara C, *et al.* Everolimus is associated with a reduced incidence of cytomegalovirus infection following de novo cardiac transplantation. Transpl Infect Dis 2013; 15(2): 150-62.
[http://dx.doi.org/10.1111/tid.12007] [PMID: 23013440]

[96] Arora S, Ueland T, Wennerblom B, *et al.* Effect of everolimus introduction on cardiac allograft vasculopathyresults of a randomized, multicenter trial. Transplantation 2011; 92(2): 235-43.
[http://dx.doi.org/10.1097/TP.0b013e31822057f1] [PMID: 21677600]

[97] Lehmkuhl HB, Arizon J, Viganò M, *et al.* Everolimus with reduced cyclosporine *versus* MMF with

standard cyclosporine in de novo heart transplant recipients. Transplantation 2009; 88(1): 115-22.
[http://dx.doi.org/10.1097/TP.0b013e3181aacd22] [PMID: 19584690]

[98]   Thaler SJ, Rubin RH. Opportunistic infections in the cardiac transplant patient. Curr Opin Cardiol
         1996; 11(2): 191-203.
         [http://dx.doi.org/10.1097/00001573-199603000-00013] [PMID: 8736691]

[99]   da Cunha-Bang C, Sørensen SS, Iversen M, *et al.* Factors associated with the development of
         cytomegalovirus infection following solid organ transplantation. Scand J Infect Dis 2011; 43(5): 360-
         5.
         [http://dx.doi.org/10.3109/00365548.2010.549836] [PMID: 21306196]

[100]   Legendre C, Pascual M. Improving outcomes for solid-organ transplant recipients at risk from
         cytomegalovirus infection: late-onset disease and indirect consequences. Clin Infect Dis 2008; 46(5):
         732-40.
         [http://dx.doi.org/10.1086/527397] [PMID: 18220478]

[101]   Costanzo MR, Naftel DC, Pritzker MR, *et al.* Heart transplant coronary artery disease detected by
         coronary angiography: a multiinstitutional study of preoperative donor and recipient risk factors.
         Cardiac Transplant Research Database. J Heart Lung Transplant 1998; 17(8): 744-53.
         [PMID: 9730422]

[102]   Taylor DO, Edwards LB, Boucek MM, *et al.* Registry of the International Society for Heart and Lung
         Transplantation: twenty-second official adult heart transplant report2005. J Heart Lung Transplant
         2005; 24(8): 945-55.
         [http://dx.doi.org/10.1016/j.healun.2005.05.018] [PMID: 16102427]

[103]   Taylor DO, Edwards LB, Mohacsi PJ, *et al.* The registry of the International Society for Heart and
         Lung Transplantation: twentieth official adult heart transplant report2003. J Heart Lung Transplant
         2003; 22(6): 616-24.
         [http://dx.doi.org/10.1016/S1053-2498(03)00186-4] [PMID: 12821159]

[104]   Hertz MI, Taylor DO, Trulock EP, *et al.* The registry of the international society for heart and lung
         transplantation: nineteenth official report-2002. J Heart Lung Transplant 2002; 21(9): 950-70.
         [http://dx.doi.org/10.1016/S1053-2498(02)00498-9] [PMID: 12231366]

[105]   Billingham ME. Histopathology of graft coronary disease. J Heart Lung Transplant 1992; 11(3 Pt 2):
         S38-44.
         [PMID: 1622997]

[106]   Day JD, Rayburn BK, Gaudin PB, *et al.* Cardiac allograft vasculopathy: the central pathogenetic role
         of ischemia-induced endothelial cell injury. J Heart Lung Transplant 1995; 14(6 Pt 2): S142-9.
         [PMID: 8719476]

[107]   Hollenberg SM, Klein LW, Parrillo JE, *et al.* Coronary endothelial dysfunction after heart
         transplantation predicts allograft vasculopathy and cardiac death. Circulation 2001; 104(25): 3091-6.
         [http://dx.doi.org/10.1161/hc5001.100796] [PMID: 11748106]

[108]   Redonnet M, Tron C, Koning R, *et al.* Coronary angioplasty and stenting in cardiac allograft
         vasculopathy following heart transplantation. Transplant Proc 2000; 32(2): 463-5.
         [http://dx.doi.org/10.1016/S0041-1345(00)00818-6] [PMID: 10715480]

[109]   Benza RL, Zoghbi GJ, Tallaj J, *et al.* Palliation of allograft vasculopathy with transluminal
         angioplasty: a decade of experience. J Am Coll Cardiol 2004; 43(11): 1973-81.
         [http://dx.doi.org/10.1016/j.jacc.2004.02.045] [PMID: 15172400]

[110]   Kass M, Haddad H. Cardiac allograft vasculopathy: pathology, prevention and treatment. Curr Opin
         Cardiol 2006; 21(2): 132-7.
         [http://dx.doi.org/10.1097/01.hco.0000203184.89158.16] [PMID: 16470150]

[111]   Mancini D, Pinney S, Burkhoff D, *et al.* Use of rapamycin slows progression of cardiac transplantation
         vasculopathy. Circulation 2003; 108(1): 48-53.

[http://dx.doi.org/10.1161/01.CIR.0000070421.38604.2B] [PMID: 12742978]

[112] Eisen H, Kobashigawa J, Starling RC, Valantine H, Mancini D. Improving outcomes in heart transplantation: the potential of proliferation signal inhibitors. Transplant Proc 2005; 37(4) (Suppl.): 4S-17S.
[http://dx.doi.org/10.1016/j.transproceed.2005.02.118] [PMID: 15809102]

[113] Wenke K, Meiser B, Thiery J, *et al.* Simvastatin initiated early after heart transplantation: 8-year prospective experience. Circulation 2003; 107(1): 93-7.
[http://dx.doi.org/10.1161/01.CIR.0000043241.32523.EE] [PMID: 12515749]

[114] Mehra MR, Ventura HO, Smart FW, Stapleton DD. Impact of converting enzyme inhibitors and calcium entry blockers on cardiac allograft vasculopathy: from bench to bedside. J Heart Lung Transplant 1995; 14(6 Pt 2): S246-9.
[PMID: 8719495]

[115] Shaddy RE, Hammond EH, Yowell RL. Immunohistochemical analysis of platelet-derived growth factor and basic fibroblast growth factor in cardiac biopsy and autopsy specimens of heart transplant patients. Am J Cardiol 1996; 77(14): 1210-5.
[http://dx.doi.org/10.1016/S0002-9149(96)00164-6] [PMID: 8651097]

[116] Toyoda Y, Guy TS, Kashem A. Present status and future perspectives of heart transplantation. Circ J 2013; 77(5): 1097-110.
[http://dx.doi.org/10.1253/circj.CJ-13-0296] [PMID: 23614963]

[117] Girlanda R. Complications of post-transplant immunosuppression. Regenerative medicine and tissue engineering InTech 2013. Available from: http://www.intechopen.com/books/regenerative-medicine-and-tissue-engineering/complications-of-post-transplant-immunosuppression. [cited 27th Nov 2015].
[http://dx.doi.org/10.5772/55614]

[118] Murphy L, Pinney SP. Clinical outcomes following heart transplantation. Mt Sinai J Med 2012; 79(3): 317-29.
[http://dx.doi.org/10.1002/msj.21311] [PMID: 22678856]

[119] Wimmer CD, Rentsch M, Crispin A, *et al.* The janus face of immunosuppression - de novo malignancy after renal transplantation: the experience of the Transplantation Center Munich. Kidney Int 2007; 71(12): 1271-8.
[http://dx.doi.org/10.1038/sj.ki.5002154] [PMID: 17332737]

[120] Euvrard S, Kanitakis J, Pouteil-Noble C, Claudy A, Touraine JL. Skin cancers in organ transplant recipients. Ann Transplant 1997; 2(4): 28-32.
[PMID: 9869876]

[121] Blaes AH, Morrison VA. Post-transplant lymphoproliferative disorders following solid-organ transplantation. Expert Rev Hematol 2010; 3(1): 35-44.
[http://dx.doi.org/10.1586/ehm.09.76] [PMID: 21082932]

[122] Torbenson M. Emerging causes of morbidity and mortality in organ transplant patients. Curr Opin Organ Transplant 2006; 11: 304-10.
[http://dx.doi.org/10.1097/01.mot.0000227850.44699.8d]

[123] Leblanc KG Jr, Hughes MP, Sheehan DJ. The role of sirolimus in the prevention of cutaneous squamous cell carcinoma in organ transplant recipients. Dermatol Surg 2011; 37(6): 744-9.
[PMID: 21605234]

[124] Ojo AO, Held PJ, Port FK, *et al.* Chronic renal failure after transplantation of a nonrenal organ. N Engl J Med 2003; 349(10): 931-40.
[http://dx.doi.org/10.1056/NEJMoa021744] [PMID: 12954741]

[125] van Gelder T, Balk AH, Zietse R, Hesse C, Mochtar B, Weimer W. Survival of heart transplant recipients with cyclosporine-induced renal insufficiency. Transplant Proc 1998; 30(4): 1122-3.
[http://dx.doi.org/10.1016/S0041-1345(98)00177-8] [PMID: 9636455]

[126] Zietse R, Balk AH, vd Dorpel MA, Meeter K, Bos E, Weimar W. Time course of the decline in renal function in cyclosporine-treated heart transplant recipients. Am J Nephrol 1994; 14(1): 1-5.
[http://dx.doi.org/10.1159/000168677] [PMID: 8017475]

[127] Goldstein DJ, Zuech N, Sehgal V, Weinberg AD, Drusin R, Cohen D. Cyclosporine-associated end-stage nephropathy after cardiac transplantation: incidence and progression. Transplantation 1997; 63(5): 664-8.
[http://dx.doi.org/10.1097/00007890-199703150-00009] [PMID: 9075835]

[128] Van Buren DH, Burke JF, Lewis RM. Renal function in patients receiving long-term cyclosporine therapy. J Am Soc Nephrol 1994; 4(8) (Suppl.): S17-22.
[PMID: 8193290]

[129] Bahirwani R, Campbell MS, Siropaides T, *et al.* Transplantation: impact of pretransplant renal insufficiency. Liver Transpl 2008; 14(5): 665-71.
[http://dx.doi.org/10.1002/lt.21367] [PMID: 18433034]

[130] Svensson M, Jardine A, Fellström B, Holdaas H. Prevention of cardiovascular disease after renal transplantation. Curr Opin Organ Transplant 2012; 17(4): 393-400.
[PMID: 22790074]

[131] Starling RC, Cody RJ. Cardiac transplant hypertension. Am J Cardiol 1990; 65(1): 106-11.
[http://dx.doi.org/10.1016/0002-9149(90)90035-Y] [PMID: 2403729]

[132] Frohlich ED, Ventura HO, Ochsner JL. Arterial hypertension after orthotopic cardiac transplantation. J Am Coll Cardiol 1990; 15(5): 1102-3.
[http://dx.doi.org/10.1016/0735-1097(90)90248-N] [PMID: 2312965]

[133] Zbroch E, Małyszko J, Myśliwiec M, Przybyłowski P, Durlik M. Hypertension in solid organ transplant recipients. Ann Transplant 2012; 17(1): 100-7.
[http://dx.doi.org/10.12659/AOT.882641] [PMID: 22466914]

[134] Krämer BK, Zülke C, Kammerl MC, *et al.* Cardiovascular risk factors and estimated risk for CAD in a randomized trial comparing calcineurin inhibitors in renal transplantation. Am J Transplant 2003; 3(8): 982-7.
[http://dx.doi.org/10.1034/j.1600-6143.2003.00156.x] [PMID: 12859533]

[135] Curtis JJ. Hypertensinogenic mechanism of the calcineurin inhibitors. Curr Hypertens Rep 2002; 4(5): 377-80.
[http://dx.doi.org/10.1007/s11906-002-0067-5] [PMID: 12217256]

[136] Opelz G, Döhler B. Improved long-term outcomes after renal transplantation associated with blood pressure control. Am J Transplant 2005; 5(11): 2725-31.
[http://dx.doi.org/10.1111/j.1600-6143.2005.01093.x] [PMID: 16212633]

[137] Davidson J, Wilkinson A, Dantal J, *et al.* New-onset diabetes after transplantation: 2003 International consensus guidelines. Proceedings of an international expert panel meeting. Barcelona, Spain, 19 February 2003. Transplantation 2003; 75(10) (Suppl.): SS3-SS24.
[PMID: 12775942]

[138] Pham P-T, Pham P-M, Pham SV, Pham P-A, Pham P-C. New onset diabetes after transplantation (NODAT): an overview. Diabetes Metab Syndr Obes 2011; 4: 175-86.
[http://dx.doi.org/10.2147/DMSO.S19027] [PMID: 21760734]

[139] Heisel O, Heisel R, Balshaw R, Keown P. New onset diabetes mellitus in patients receiving calcineurin inhibitors: a systematic review and meta-analysis. Am J Transplant 2004; 4(4): 583-95.
[http://dx.doi.org/10.1046/j.1600-6143.2003.00372.x] [PMID: 15023151]

[140] Wilkinson A, Davidson J, Dotta F, *et al.* Guidelines for the treatment and management of new-onset diabetes after transplantation. Clin Transplant 2005; 19(3): 291-8.
[http://dx.doi.org/10.1111/j.1399-0012.2005.00359.x] [PMID: 15877787]

[141] Lindenfeld J, Page RL II, Zolty R, *et al.* Drug therapy in the heart transplant recipient: Part III: common medical problems. Circulation 2005; 111(1): 113-7.
[http://dx.doi.org/10.1161/01.CIR.0000151609.60618.3C] [PMID: 15630040]

[142] Akhlaghi F, Jackson CH, Parameshwar J, Sharples LD, Trull AK. Risk factors for the development and progression of dyslipidemia after heart transplantation. Transplantation 2002; 73(8): 1258-64.
[http://dx.doi.org/10.1097/00007890-200204270-00012] [PMID: 11981418]

[143] Johnson MR. Transplant coronary disease: nonimmunologic risk factors. J Heart Lung Transplant 1992; 11(3 Pt 2): S124-32.
[PMID: 1622991]

[144] Webster AC, Lee VW, Chapman JR, Craig JC. Target of rapamycin inhibitors (sirolimus and everolimus) for primary immunosuppression of kidney transplant recipients: a systematic review and meta-analysis of randomized trials. Transplantation 2006; 81(9): 1234-48.
[http://dx.doi.org/10.1097/01.tp.0000219703.39149.85] [PMID: 16699448]

[145] Taylor DO, Barr ML, Meiser BM, Pham SM, Mentzer RM, Gass AL. Suggested guidelines for the use of tacrolimus in cardiac transplant recipients. J Heart Lung Transplant 2001; 20(7): 734-8.
[http://dx.doi.org/10.1016/S1053-2498(00)00222-9] [PMID: 11448799]

[146] Wenke K, Meiser B, Thiery J, *et al.* Simvastatin reduces graft vessel disease and mortality after heart transplantation: a four-year randomized trial. Circulation 1997; 96(5): 1398-402.
[http://dx.doi.org/10.1161/01.CIR.96.5.1398] [PMID: 9315523]

[147] Jamal SM, Eisenberg MJ, Christopoulos S. Rhabdomyolysis associated with hydroxymethylglutaryl-coenzyme A reductase inhibitors. Am Heart J 2004; 147(6): 956-65.
[http://dx.doi.org/10.1016/j.ahj.2003.12.037] [PMID: 15199341]

[148] Ballantyne CM, Corsini A, Davidson MH, *et al.* Risk for myopathy with statin therapy in high-risk patients. Arch Intern Med 2003; 163(5): 553-64.
[http://dx.doi.org/10.1001/archinte.163.5.553] [PMID: 12622602]

[149] Clive DM. Renal transplant-associated hyperuricemia and gout. J Am Soc Nephrol 2000; 11(5): 974-9.
[PMID: 10770978]

[150] Cummins D, Sekar M, Halil O, Banner N. Myelosuppression associated with azathioprine-allopurinol interaction after heart and lung transplantation. Transplantation 1996; 61(11): 1661-2.
[http://dx.doi.org/10.1097/00007890-199606150-00023] [PMID: 8669118]

[151] Shane E, Mancini D, Aaronson K, *et al.* Bone mass, vitamin D deficiency, and hyperparathyroidism in congestive heart failure. Am J Med 1997; 103(3): 197-207.
[http://dx.doi.org/10.1016/S0002-9343(97)00142-3] [PMID: 9316552]

[152] Shane E, Rivas MC, Silverberg SJ, Kim TS, Staron RB, Bilezikian JP. Osteoporosis after cardiac transplantation. Am J Med 1993; 94(3): 257-64.
[http://dx.doi.org/10.1016/0002-9343(93)90057-V] [PMID: 8452149]

[153] Berguer DG, Krieg MA, Thiébaud D, *et al.* Osteoporosis in heart transplant recipients: a longitudinal study. Transplant Proc 1994; 26(5): 2649-51.
[PMID: 7940827]

[154] Shane E, Addesso V, Namerow PB, *et al.* Alendronate *versus* calcitriol for the prevention of bone loss after cardiac transplantation. N Engl J Med 2004; 350(8): 767-76.
[http://dx.doi.org/10.1056/NEJMoa035617] [PMID: 14973216]

[155] Dew MA, Kormos RL, DiMartini AF, *et al.* Prevalence and risk of depression and anxiety-related disorders during the first three years after heart transplantation. Psychosomatics 2001; 42(4): 300-13.
[http://dx.doi.org/10.1176/appi.psy.42.4.300] [PMID: 11496019]

[156] Dobbels F, De Geest S, Martin S, Van Cleemput J, Droogne W, Vanhaecke J. Prevalence and correlates of depression symptoms at 10 years after heart transplantation: continuous attention

required. Transpl Int 2004; 17(8): 424-31.
[http://dx.doi.org/10.1111/j.1432-2277.2004.tb00465.x] [PMID: 15338116]

[157] Page RL II, Miller GG, Lindenfeld J. Drug therapy in the heart transplant recipient: part IV: drug-drug interactions. Circulation 2005; 111(2): 230-9.
[http://dx.doi.org/10.1161/01.CIR.0000151805.86933.35] [PMID: 15657387]

[158] Butani L, Berg G, Makker SP. Effect of felodipine on tacrolimus pharmacokinetics in a renal transplant recipient. Transplantation 2002; 73(1): 159-60.
[http://dx.doi.org/10.1097/00007890-200201150-00033] [PMID: 11793001]

[159] Seifeldin RA, Marcos-Alvarez A, Gordon FD, Lewis WD, Jenkins RL. Nifedipine interaction with tacrolimus in liver transplant recipients. Ann Pharmacother 1997; 31(5): 571-5.
[PMID: 9161650]

[160] Akhlaghi F, McLachlan AJ, Keogh AM, Brown KF. Effect of simvastatin on cyclosporine unbound fraction and apparent blood clearance in heart transplant recipients. Br J Clin Pharmacol 1997; 44(6): 537-42.
[http://dx.doi.org/10.1046/j.1365-2125.1997.t01-1-00625.x] [PMID: 9431828]

[161] Cheng-Lai A. Rosuvastatin: a new HMG-CoA reductase inhibitor for the treatment of hypercholesterolemia. Heart Dis 2003; 5(1): 72-8.
[http://dx.doi.org/10.1097/01.HDX.0000050417.89309.F8] [PMID: 12549990]

[162] Kliem V, Wanner C, Eisenhauer T, *et al.* Comparison of pravastatin and lovastatin in renal transplant patients receiving cyclosporine. Transplant Proc 1996; 28(6): 3126-8.
[PMID: 8962211]

[163] Olbricht C, Wanner C, Eisenhauer T, *et al.* Accumulation of lovastatin, but not pravastatin, in the blood of cyclosporine-treated kidney graft patients after multiple doses. Clin Pharmacol Ther 1997; 62(3): 311-21.
[http://dx.doi.org/10.1016/S0009-9236(97)90034-5] [PMID: 9333107]

[164] Fehrman-Ekholm I, Jogestrand T, Angelin B. Decreased cyclosporine levels during gemfibrozil treatment of hyperlipidemia after kidney transplantation. Nephron 1996; 72(3): 483.
[http://dx.doi.org/10.1159/000188918] [PMID: 8852502]

[165] Boissonnat P, Salen P, Guidollet J, *et al.* The long-term effects of the lipid-lowering agent fenofibrate in hyperlipidemic heart transplant recipients. Transplantation 1994; 58(2): 245-7.
[http://dx.doi.org/10.1097/00007890-199407270-00018] [PMID: 7726891]

[166] Birmelé B, Lebranchu Y, Bagros P, Nivet H, Furet Y, Pengloan J. Interaction of cyclosporin and ticlopidine. Nephrol Dial Transplant 1991; 6(2): 150-1.
[http://dx.doi.org/10.1093/ndt/6.2.150-a] [PMID: 1857531]

[167] Feriozzi S, Massimetti C, Ancarani E. Treatment with ticlopidine is associated with reduction of cyclosporin a blood levels. Nephron 2002; 92(1): 249-50.
[http://dx.doi.org/10.1159/000064474] [PMID: 12187118]

[168] Brüggemann RJ, Alffenaar JW, Blijlevens NM, *et al.* Clinical relevance of the pharmacokinetic interactions of azole antifungal drugs with other coadministered agents. Clin Infect Dis 2009; 48(10): 1441-58.
[http://dx.doi.org/10.1086/598327] [PMID: 19361301]

[169] Trofe-Clark J, Lemonovich TL. Interactions between anti-infective agents and immunosuppressants in solid organ transplantation. Am J Transplant 2013; 13 (Suppl. 4): 318-26.
[http://dx.doi.org/10.1111/ajt.12123] [PMID: 23465024]

[170] Page RL II, Mueller SW, Levi ME, Lindenfeld J. Pharmacokinetic drug-drug interactions between calcineurin inhibitors and proliferation signal inhibitors with anti-microbial agents: implications for therapeutic drug monitoring. J Heart Lung Transplant 2011; 30(2): 124-35.

[http://dx.doi.org/10.1016/j.healun.2010.09.001] [PMID: 21115368]

[171] Monchaud C, Marquet P. Pharmacokinetic optimization of immunosuppressive therapy in thoracic transplantation: part I. Clin Pharmacokinet 2009; 48(7): 419-62.
[http://dx.doi.org/10.2165/11317230-000000000-00000] [PMID: 19691367]

[172] Shitrit D, Ollech JE, Ollech A, *et al.* Itraconazole prophylaxis in lung transplant recipients receiving tacrolimus (FK 506): efficacy and drug interaction. J Heart Lung Transplant 2005; 24(12): 2148-52.
[http://dx.doi.org/10.1016/j.healun.2005.05.003] [PMID: 16364864]

[173] Hebert MF, Townsend RW, Austin S, *et al.* Concomitant cyclosporine and micafungin pharmacokinetics in healthy volunteers. J Clin Pharmacol 2005; 45(8): 954-60.
[http://dx.doi.org/10.1177/0091270005278601] [PMID: 16027407]

[174] Dowell JA, Stogniew M, Krause D, Henkel T, Weston IE. Assessment of the safety and pharmacokinetics of anidulafungin when administered with cyclosporine. J Clin Pharmacol 2005; 45(2): 227-33.
[http://dx.doi.org/10.1177/0091270004270146] [PMID: 15647416]

[175] Dowell JA, Stogniew M, Krause D, Henkel T, Damle B. Lack of pharmacokinetic interaction between anidulafungin and tacrolimus. J Clin Pharmacol 2007; 47(3): 305-14.
[http://dx.doi.org/10.1177/0091270006296764] [PMID: 17322142]

[176] Garton T. Nefazodone and cyp450 3a4 interactions with cyclosporine and tacrolimus1. Transplantation 2002; 74(5): 745.
[http://dx.doi.org/10.1097/00007890-200209150-00028] [PMID: 12352898]

[177] Olyaei AJ, deMattos AM, Norman DJ, Bennett WM. Interaction between tacrolimus and nefazodone in a stable renal transplant recipient. Pharmacotherapy 1998; 18(6): 1356-9.
[PMID: 9855339]

[178] Simkin PA, Gardner GC. Colchicine use in cyclosporine treated transplant recipients: how little is too much? J Rheumatol 2000; 27(6): 1334-7.
[PMID: 10852250]

[179] Stenton SB, Partovi N, Ensom MH. Sirolimus: the evidence for clinical pharmacokinetic monitoring. Clin Pharmacokinet 2005; 44(8): 769-86.
[http://dx.doi.org/10.2165/00003088-200544080-00001] [PMID: 16029064]

[180] Kovarik JM, Hsu CH, McMahon L, Berthier S, Rordorf C. Population pharmacokinetics of everolimus in de novo renal transplant patients: impact of ethnicity and comedications. Clin Pharmacol Ther 2001; 70(3): 247-54.
[http://dx.doi.org/10.1067/mcp.2001.118022] [PMID: 11557912]

[181] Billaud EM, Antoine C, Berge M, *et al.* Management of metabolic cytochrome P450 3A4 drug-drug interaction between everolimus and azole antifungals in a renal transplant patient. Clin Drug Investig 2009; 29(7): 481-6.
[http://dx.doi.org/10.2165/00044011-200929070-00006] [PMID: 19499965]

[182] Pea F, Baccarani U, Tavio M, *et al.* Pharmacokinetic interaction between everolimus and antifungal triazoles in a liver transplant patient. Ann Pharmacother 2008; 42(11): 1711-6.
[http://dx.doi.org/10.1345/aph.1L330] [PMID: 18812562]

[183] Kovarik JM, Snell GI, Valentine V, *et al.* Everolimus in pulmonary transplantation: pharmacokinetics and exposure-response relationships. J Heart Lung Transplant 2006; 25(4): 440-6.
[http://dx.doi.org/10.1016/j.healun.2005.12.001] [PMID: 16563975]

[184] Monchaud C, Marquet P. Pharmacokinetic optimization of immunosuppressive therapy in thoracic transplantation: part II. Clin Pharmacokinet 2009; 48(8): 489-516.
[http://dx.doi.org/10.2165/11317240-000000000-00000] [PMID: 19705921]

[185] Frassetto LA, Browne M, Cheng A, *et al.* Immunosuppressant pharmacokinetics and dosing modifications in HIV-1 infected liver and kidney transplant recipients. Am J Transplant 2007; 7(12):

2816-20.
[http://dx.doi.org/10.1111/j.1600-6143.2007.02007.x] [PMID: 17949460]

[186] Kahan BD, Keown P, Levy GA, Johnston A. Therapeutic drug monitoring of immunosuppressant drugs in clinical practice. Clin Ther 2002; 24(3): 330-50.
[http://dx.doi.org/10.1016/S0149-2918(02)85038-X] [PMID: 11952020]

[187] Gerbase MW, Fathi M, Spiliopoulos A, Rochat T, Nicod LP. Pharmacokinetics of mycophenolic acid associated with calcineurin inhibitors: long-term monitoring in stable lung recipients with and without cystic fibrosis. J Heart Lung Transplant 2003; 22(5): 587-90.
[http://dx.doi.org/10.1016/S1053-2498(02)01159-2] [PMID: 12742423]

[188] Walker J, Mendelson H, McClure A, Smith MD. Warfarin and azathioprine: clinically significant drug interaction. J Rheumatol 2002; 29(2): 398-9.
[PMID: 11838865]

CHAPTER 5

PCSK9 Inhibition with Evolocumab Reaching Physiologic LDL-C Levels for Reducing Atherosclerotic Burden and Cardiovascular Disease-The Full Landscape

Enrique C. Morales-Villegas[1,*] and **Kausik K. Ray[2]**

[1] *Cardiometabolic Research Center, Aguascalientes, Mexico*

[2] *Imperial Centre for Cardiovascular Disease Prevention, London, UK*

Abstract: Physiologically, in the presence of an intracellular deficit of cholesterol, the LDLR synthesis, expression and function increase, thus uptaking and providing cholesterol to the cell. This process is counter-regulated by PCSK9 expression, the protease inducing LDLR proteolysis, thereby limiting its function maintaining a constant cholesterol intracellular concentration. Accordingly, the balance between PCSK9 and LDLR regulates the intracellular concentration of cholesterol and in consequence has impact on circulating LDL-cholesterol.

This chapter reviews the brief and amazing recent history with PCSK9 inhibition from basic science to current clinical recommendations for MAbs-PCSK9. In 2003 and 2005, respectively, the *pcsk9* gene mutations, determinants of the *"gain of function"* of PCSK9 and severe hypercholesterolemia, and the *pcsk9* gene mutations with *"loss of function"* of PCSK9, determinants of hypocholesterolemia were described; subsequently, in 2006, the association between the *pcsk9* gene mutations and the *"loss of function"* of PCSK9 with hypocholesterolemia and reduction of up to 88% for the risk of a coronary event in the "mutant" population versus the control population was published.

Since evolocumab clinical research program has completed and published their phases I, II and III results including its cardiovascular outcomes trial, this chapter is focused in reviewing the results of evolocumab clinical research program. In 2009, the effect of a *"full human"* monoclonal antibody vs PCSK9 in mice and non-human primates was first reported; MAb-PCSK9, AMG-145 (evolocumab) produced in cynomolgus monkeys a doubling in the number of LDLR and an average 75% reduction in circulating LDL-cholesterol. In 2012, the first phase I study with evolocumab versus placebo were reported; this program informed very significant reductions in LDL-cholesterol in healthy subjects and patients with familial and non-familial hyper-

* **Corresponding author Enrique C. Morales-Villegas:** Cardiometabolic Research Center, Aguascalientes, Mexico. Republica del Perú 102-201C. Las Américas, Aguascalientes, Mexico, 20230; Tel: +52-4499782545; Fax: +52-4499715862 ; E-mail: drmorvi@prodigy.net.mx

Atta-ur-Rahman & M. Iqbal Choudhary (Eds.)

cholesterolemia treated without/with statins; tolerability and safety of evolocumab were similar to placebo. With this evidence, the phase II and III investigations with evolocumab initiated; four years later, the OSLER trial allowed us to envisage the following scenario: MAb-PCSK9 evolocumab have a favorable effect on LDL-cholesterol, other apo-B100 lipoproteins and overall mortality and myocardial infarction; all the aforementioned with a very favorable safety and tolerability profile. In the same direction, in 2016 was published the GLAGOV trial, wich demonstrates for the first time that the addition of a non-statin therapy -evolocumab- to the optimal treatment with statins is associated with atheroregression; and finally, in 2017, the FOURIER and the EBBINGHAUS trials were presented, wich confirmed that the addition of evolocumab to the optimal treatment with statins is associated with an additional and significant 20% relative risk reduction -26 months of follow-up- for cardiovascular mortality, myocardial infarction and/or ischemic stroke, all without neurocognitive risk.

Beyond the currently approved indications by regulatory agencies, considering the high cost of PCSK9 inhibitors and financial restraints within healthcare budgets, for now and before definitive and necessary cost-effectiveness analysis and price optimization are in place, evolocumab is recommended in specific clinical scenarios reviewed in this chapter.

Keywords: PCSK9, Mabs-PCSK9, Alirocumab, Bococizumab, Evolocumab, Familial hypercholesterolemia, Non-familial hypercholesterolemia.

BASIC EVIDENCE

Proprotein Convertase Subtilisin Kexin Type 9

Characterized in 2003 as NARC-1 by Nabil Seidah *et al.*, this protein currently called PCSK9 is the ninth member of the proprotein convertase family or subtilases [1]. These proteins are serine proteases that regulate the activation, inactivation and/or intracellular translation of secretory proteins such as transcription or growth factors, prohormones and membrane receptors, some of which are related to cardiovascular health and disease [2]. Nine subtilases have been identified; seven belonging to the kexin subfamily in bacteria and fungi and two belonging to the kexin-like subfamily in mammals; in humans, the SKI-1/S1P subtilase regulates the activity of the transcription factor SREBP and the growth factor BDNF, and the PCSK9 subtilase regulates LDLR activity [3 - 5].

PCSK9 is encoded by the *pcsk9* gene located on the small arm of the chromosome 1p32 and contains 12 exons and 11 introns. The PCSK9 primordium or prepro-PCSK9 is synthesized in the liver, small intestine and kidney as an inactive glycoprotein of 692 amino acids with 4 domains [6]. Amino acids 1-30 constitute the signal peptide domain; amino acids 31-152 constitute the inhibition propeptide domain; amino acids 153-452 constitute the subtilisin-like or catalytic peptide domain; and amino acids 453-692 constitute the cysteine-rich or C-terminal peptide domain. After the synthesis, in the endoplasmic reticulum, through two autocatalytic steps, the prepro-PCSK9 of 692 amino acids is transformed into PCSK9 of 540 amino acids. During the first step, the prepro-PCSK9 loses the 30 amino acids of the signal peptide, and during the second step, the pro-PCSK9 loses the 121 amino acids of the inhibition propeptide; the resulting molecule with 540 amino acids constitutes the secretory PCSK9 with two domains, the subtilisin-like or catalytic domain and the C-terminal domain [1, 6]. The secretory PCSK9 circulates freely in plasma and associated to the LDL, and its mean plasma concentration is 608 ng/ml on average for males and 646 ng/ml on average for females [3, 7]. The first secretory PCSK9 target to be identified was the LDLR at the surface of liver hepatocytes [8].

Low Density Lipoprotein Receptor

The exact dimension of the importance of the secretory PCSK9 in cellular cholesterol metabolism is understood in terms of its interaction with the LDLR. The LDLR was identified by Goldstein and Brown in the 70s [9]. It is encoded on chromosome 19 and is constituted as a glycoprotein structure with five domains; the extracellular ligand-binding, domain 1 (apo-B100 binding site), the extracellular epidermal growth factor-A homology, domain 2 (PCSK9 binding site), the extracellular sugar-rich, domain 3, the transmembrane, domain 4, and the intracytoplasmic, domain 5 [9, 10].

Under physiological conditions, circulating LDLs, each with an average content of 1,500 esterified cholesterol molecules, are identified in the single molecule of apo-B100 by the extracellular ligand-binding domain 1 of the LDLR. The LDL-LDLR binomial is introduced into the cell by receptor-mediated endocytosis. In the endosome, by type-V ATPases-induced acidification, the LDLR is allosterically dissociated from the LDL and is recycled to the cell membrane; by membrane fusion, the LDL is transferred from endosomes to lysosomes where the lipid and protein components are hydrolyzed and incorporated into the cellular metabolism; the half-life of an LDLR is 20 hours and the time of a membrane-endosome-membrane cycle is 10 minutes [9].

In other words, each LDLR is able to uptake 120 LDL molecules, each with 1,500 esterified cholesterol molecules equivalent to 180,000 esterified cholesterol molecules up taken by each LDLR. The aforementioned reflects the high efficiency of the LDLR to fulfill the function of up taking LDL, integrating its esterified cholesterol content to the cellular metabolism and facilitating the hepato-biliary-enteral elimination of the excess of this pro-atherogenic lipid.

PCSK9 and LDLR Reciprocal Regulation

The incorporation of esterified cholesterol into the cell via LDLR is a process finely counter-regulated by the PCSK9. The concentration of intracellular cholesterol, especially in the Golgi apparatus and the endoplasmic reticulum membranes, is the biological constant that regulates the expression of the transcription factor SREBP1-2 [11, 12]. In the presence of an intracellular cholesterol reduction, the SREBP1-2 transcription factor is activated. The activation of this transcription factor determines the following processes: activation of intracellular cholesterol synthesis by activation of the synthesis and expression of HMGCoAR, activation of the uptake and incorporation of LDL-cholesterol by activation of the synthesis and expression of LDLR, and activation of cell autophagy [9]. All the aforementioned with the purpose of correcting intracellular cholesterol depletion.

However, in parallel and paradoxically at first sight, in the presence of intracellular cholesterol reduction, the SREBP1-2 transcription factor also determines the activation of the synthesis and expression of PCSK9 [12]. This counter-regulation aims to maintain the intracellular cholesterol concentration stable, since the absence of the counter-regulation of cholesterol synthesis by HMGCoAR, the uptake of LDL-cholesterol by the LDLR and autophagy, would cause an intracellular cytotoxic cholesterol increase. This phenomenon is prevented by the PCSK9 action that keeps the number of functional LDLR constant [13, 14]. The circulating secretory PCSK9 (extracellular pathway) has as a ligand the domain 2 with homology to the epidermal growth factor of the LDLR and related receptors [10]. Once PCSK9 is bound to LDLR, in the presence or absence of LDL, the PCSK9-LDLR complex (wich includes other associated proteins) is endocytosed and is unable to dissociate at acidic pHs, being transferred from the endosomes to the lysosomes for proteolysis of both molecules [8, 15].

PCSK9 in Transgenic and Knockout Models

Knowing the genome and especially the *pcsk9* gene location was feasible to develop classical experiments aimed to understanding the function of this gene and its consequences; adenoviral-mediated overexpression and deletion of the *pcsk9* gene experiments were crucial for recognizing PCSK9 as a very potential therapeutic target [16].

Adenoviral-mediated overexpression of human PCSK9 results in an intermediate LDLR-knockout phenotype in mice; these mice are viable, fertile, hyper-cholesterolemic with a five-fold increase of LDL-cholesterol and accelerated atherosclerosis [16]. This model has been replicated in minipigs with similar results [17]. Deletion of the *pcsk9* gene results in a *pcsk9* knockout mice; these mice are viable, fertile, hypocholesterolemic with an 80% drop in LDL-cholesterol and atherosclerosis protection [18].

GENETIC EVIDENCE IN HUMANS

Gene pcsk9 Mutations with "Gain of Function"

Marianne Abifadel, Catherine Boileau *et al.*, in 2003 reported in a brief communication, the characterization of a third form of autosomal dominant hypercholesterolemia [19]. In a French population with familial hypercholesterolemia phenotype, the authors described the association with two mutations in the *pcsk9* gene, the S127R (625T → A) mutation in exon 2 and F216L (890T → C) mutation in exon 4. This third form of autosomal dominant hypercholesterolemia was called FH3. Prior to the report of Abifadel/Boileau, the familial hypercholesterolemia phenotype was associated with mutations in the *ldlr* gene and mutations in the *apoB* gene. Hypercholesterolemia associated with mutations in the *ldlr* gene or Familial Hypercholesterolemia, the one associated with mutations in *apoB* gene or Familial Hypercholesterolemia by defective apo-B100 and the one associated with mutations described by Abifadel/Boileau *et al.* determine a phenotype characterized by severe hypercholesterolemia (LDL cholesterol > 500 mg/dL), cholesterol deposits in tissues, tendon and skin xanthomas, corneal arcus and early atherosclerotic cardiovascular disease [19].

Abifadel *et al.*, postulated that given the association between hypercholesterolemia with an autosomal dominant pattern and mutations in the *pcsk9* gene, such mutations in the gene encoding the PCSK9, may constitute a *"gain of function"* of the protease as the determining mechanism of hypercholesterolemia. Based on this observation, even in a lack of awareness of the intrinsic mechanism of action of PCSK9, the authors postulated that research on this topic would be the key to discovering new ways in cholesterol metabolism with therapeutic potential. Clearly, this discovery, in addition to describing a third etiology of autosomal dominant hypercholesterolemia, was the key to start researching a new therapeutic strategy against hypercholesterolemia.

Gene pcsk9 Mutations with "Loss of Function"

Jonathan Cohen, Helen Hobbs *et al.*, in 2005, in a letter, published the characterization of a new form of hypocholesterolemia [20]. In the cohort of the Dallas Heart Study (52% African-American, 29% European-American, 17% Hispanic, and 2% other ethnicities), subjects with hypocholesterolemia (LDL cholesterol <58 mg/dL) were selected. In this subpopulation of 32 subjects, the authors described two *"nonsense"* mutations in the *pcsk9* gene; the Y142X (426C

→ G) mutation in exon 3, which introduces a stop codon at residue 142 and the C679X (20137C → A) mutation in exon 12, which introduces an early termination signal at codon 679. These mutations had a prevalence of 0.4% (Y142X) and 1.4% (C679X) in African Americans and a negligible prevalence in European-Americans (<0.1%) and Hispanics (<0.2%).

Expanding the research to a Cook County population in Illinois and a Nigeria native population, Cohen found that the prevalence of Y142X and C679X mutations was 0.6% and 1.6% in the Cook population and 0% and 1.4% in the Nigeria population (average prevalence of both mutations 2% in African-American subjects) [20]. The phenotype of these subjects was characterized by LDL-cholesterol levels between the 1st percentile and the 50th percentile, with an average LDL-cholesterol level 40% lower than the control population (p <0.001). By measuring latosterol (cholesterol biosynthesis) and camposterol (cholesterol absorption), the authors discarded the inhibition of the synthesis and/or the inhibition of the absorption of cholesterol as determinant factors of hypocholesterolemia.

With these findings, Cohen *et al.*, postulated a *"loss of function"* of the PCSK9 as the determining mechanism of hypocholesterolemia, anticipating the interaction between PCSK9 and LDLR as the mechanism potentially involved.

Genetic-Epidemiological Evidence

Jonathan Cohen, Helen Hobbs *et al.*, in 2006, published as an original article, the association between the *pcsk9* gene mutations with PCSK9 *"loss of function"*, low LDL-cholesterol levels and low prevalence of coronary events [21]. Considering the high frequency of mutations Y142X and C679X in African-Americans [20] and mutation R46L in White subjects [22], Cohen analyzed the prevalence of such mutations and their correlation with LDL-cholesterol level and the incidence of coronary events within a period of 15 years; to that end, Cohen assessed 3,363 African-American subjects and 9,524 Euro-American subjects aged between 45 and 64 years of the study ARIC.

Mutations Y142X and C679X had a prevalence of 0.8 and 1.8% in African-American subjects and <0.01 in White subjects; the average level of LDL-cholesterol was 100 mg/dL in the carrier population and 138 mg/dL in the control population (p <0.001). During a 15-year follow-up period, the incidence of coronary events was 1.2% in the carrier population and 9.7% in the control population, representing an H.R of 0.11 in the carrier population vs. the control population (p 0.003), or a reduction of 89% of the relative risk of coronary events. Mutation R46L had a prevalence of 3.2% in White subjects and 0.7 in African-American subjects; the average level of LDL-cholesterol was 116mg/dL in the carrier population and 137 mg/dL in the control population (p <0.001). During a 15-year follow-up period, the incidence of coronary events was 6.3% in the carrier population and 11.8% in the control population, representing an H.R of 0.53 in the carrier population vs. the control population (p 0.003) or a relative risk reduction of 47% of coronary events. In all three types of mutations, the numbers remained statistically significant after multivariable adjustment for age, sex and non-lipid cardiovascular risk factors (p <0.05).

Based on these findings the following statement was postulated: The reduction of 1mmol equivalent to 40 mg/dL or 0.5 mmol equivalent to 20 mg/dL of LDL-cholesterol throughout the entire life of an individual represents a reduction of up to 89% and 47%, respectively, in the relative risk of coronary events. Such cumulative benefit of low LDL-cholesterol level is much higher than the reported with an equivalent drug reduction of LDL-cholesterol initiated in adulthood and opened the door to the concept of *"starting early and maintaining for a long-term the reduction in LDL-cholesterol"*.

During discussion, while recognizing that the intrinsic mechanism explaining the association between *pcsk*9 gene mutations and LDL-cholesterol reduction was not completely defined, Cohen postulated the inhibition of PCSK9 as a highly attractive therapeutic strategy focused on LDL-cholesterol reduction and the incidence of cardiovascular events associated with atherosclerosis. Additionally, he emphasized that the protection conferred by the low *"for life"* level of LDL-cholesterol was observed in a population such as the African-American ARIC with 50% prevalence of hypertension, 30% prevalence of smoking and 20% prevalence of diabetes mellitus.

EVIDENCE WITH MONOCLONAL ANTIBODIES *VS.* PCSK9

Animal Experimental Evidence in Non-Human Primates

The Joyce Chan *et al.*, -AMGEN- [23] group pioneered the development of *"full human"* MAbs-PCSK9. Briefly, these antibodies are produced in the mouse by removing the genomic sequences encoding immunoglobulin synthesis, followed by replacing the corresponding human genomic sequences; thus, the *"humanized"* mouse produces 100% human immunoglobulins and by being immunized with human PCSK9, *"full human"* MAbs-PCSK9 are synthesized. High quality secretory B lymphocytes of MAbs-PCSK9 are selected and used for creating producer hybridomas of MAbs-PCSK9- [24].

Chan´s group showed that "full human" MAbs-PCSK9, AMG-145, had a high affinity for the catalytic site of secretory PCSK9, inhibiting its binding to the LDLR and increasing recycling and survival of the receptor. In mice analyses and especially in non-human primates *"cynomolgus monkeys"*, AMGEN group reported that the administration of AMG-145 produced an almost total reduction in the level of circulating PCSK9, a doubling of the number of LDLR and a reduction up to 75% in circulating LDL-cholesterol [23].

These experiments expanded the knowledge of the PCSK9 and its inhibition with Mabs-PCSK9 and opened the door for the efficacy, safety and tolerability study of AMG-145 in human phase I studies.

Human Clinical Evidence with AMG-145 (Evolocumab)

Human Phase I Clinical Evidence with Evolocumab

Clampton Dias *et al.*, reported in November 6th, 2012, the results of two studies of their phase I program with AMG-145 (evolocumab) [25]. The first study included seven cohorts of healthy subjects and the second study included 7 cohorts of subjects with hypercholesterolemia treated with statins (6 Non-FH and 1 HeFH). In the first study, five single S.C doses (7 mg, 21 mg, 70 mg, 210 mg and 420 mg) and two single I.V. doses (21 mg and 420 mg) of evolocumab versus placebo were tested; in the second group, five multiple S.C doses (14 mg/week, 35 mg/week, 140 mg/2 weeks, 280 mg/2 weeks and 420 mg/4 weeks) of evolocumab versus placebo were tested.

The TEAE incidence was similar between the active treatment groups and placebo. In the first single dose study, LDL-cholesterol reduction versus placebo was dose-dependent; of up to -64.0% with a maximum S.C dose of 420 mg and of -61% with a maximum I.V. dose of 420 mg. In the second multiple dose study, LDL-cholesterol reduction was also dose dependent; up to -73%, -75% and -66% with doses of 140 mg/2 weeks, 280 mg/2 weeks, and 420 mg/4 weeks, respectively. The type of hypercholesterolemia and the type of the baseline treatment did not determine a difference in the therapeutic response. The levels of non-HDL cholesterol, apolipoprotein-B and lipoprotein (a) had proportional and significant reductions, and the levels of HDL-cholesterol and apolipoprotein-A1 had also significant increases.

The authors highlighted several important aspects, including: the significant and proportional reduction in LDL-cholesterol and other atherogenic lipoproteins with doses of 140 mg S.C/2 weeks and 420 mg S.C/4 weeks; the direct relationship between the reduction of the level of circulating PCSK9 and LDL-cholesterol; and ultimately the safety and tolerability of evolocumab.

Human Phase II and III Clinical Evidence with AMG-145 (Evolocumab)

a) Homozygous Familial Hypercholesterolemia

Evan Stein *et al.*, reported in September 6th, 2013 *"The Trial Evaluating PCSK9 Antibody in Subjects with LDL Receptor Abnormalities"* or TESLA-Pilot study [26]. This open-label, single arm, phase II study with AMG-145 (evolocumab) included a cohort of 8 subjects (12 to 65 years old and bodyweight >40 kg) with receptor defective or negative HoFH either by genetic confirmation or clinical diagnosis, on statin therapy and other lipid lowering drugs (apheresis, lomitapide and mipomersen excluded), at stable doses for a period equal to or greater than 4 weeks, and LDL-cholesterol level >130 mg/dL. The cohort was treated with open-label evolocumab 420 mg S.C/4 weeks for 12 weeks with an extension phase of 12 weeks and then 420 mg S.C/2 weeks for 12 weeks.

All patients had LDL-receptor mutations confirmed in both alleles; the LDL receptor activity was defective in six and negative in two patients. The mean baseline LDL-cholesterol level measured by ultracentrifugation was 441.7 mg/dL and the percentage reduction in LDL-cholesterol after 12 weeks of evolocumab 420 mg S.C/4 weeks was -17% (+5% to -44%), with differences among individual responses (-19% among defective LDLR individuals). Four patients experiencing a reduction in LDL-cholesterol ≥15% and three patients ≥30%, without response in the two patients with negative LDLR activity; after 12 weeks of evolocumab 420 mg S.C/2 weeks the mean percentage reduction in LDL-cholesterol was -26% among defective LDLR individuals. Reduction in other lipid fractions with apolipoprotein B was proportional to the reduction in LDL-cholesterol. Six of the eight patients reported adverse events, all of wich were considered not serious and unrelated to treatment.

TESLA-Pilot, a proof of concept study, demonstrates for the first time that LDL-cholesterol lowering is achievable with a Mab-PCSK9 (evolocumab 420 mg S.C/4 weeks) in individuals with HoFH, specifically in those with LDLR defective mutations.

Frederick Rall *et al.*, reported in October 2nd, 2014 *"The Trial Evaluating PCSK9 Antibody in Subjects with LDL Receptor Abnormalities"* or TESLA-B trial [27]. This randomized, double-blind, placebo-controlled, phase III study with AMG-145 (evolocumab) included a cohort of 50 subjects (12 years and older and bodyweight >40 kg) with receptor defective or negative HoFH either by genetic confirmation or clinical diagnosis, on statin therapy and other lipid lowering drugs (apheresis, lomitapide and mipomersen excluded), at stable doses for a period equal to or greater than 4 weeks, and LDL-cholesterol level >130 mg/dL. The cohort was randomized to evolocumab 420 mg S.C/4 weeks or placebo S.C/4 weeks for 12 weeks.

All patients, except one (genetic heterozygote) had mutations confirmed in both alleles: 22 patients were true homozygous with the same mutation in both LDLR alleles, 23 patients were compound heterozygous with different mutation in both LDLR alleles; one patient had mutations in both apolipoprotein B alleles; one patient was triple heterozygote with mutations in both apolipoprotein B alleles and in one LDLR allele; one patient had autosomal recessive hyper-cholesterolemia. The mean baseline LDL-cholesterol level measured by ultracentrifugation was 350 mg/dL and the percentage reduction in LDL-cholesterol of evolocumab 420 mg S.C/4 weeks versus placebo at week 12 was -30.9% (-43.9% to -18%); the mean absolute reduction in LDL-cholesterol versus placebo at week 12 was -94 mg/dL (-144 mg/dL to -43 mg/dL). According to the LDL receptor function there was a gradient in the therapeutic response: null response for LDLR negative mutations in both alleles and autosomal recessive hypercholesterolemia; non-significant -17.9% reduction in LDLR mutations in both alleles in wich one or both were unclassified; significant -24.5% reduction in LDLR mutations in both alleles in wich one was defective and the other one was negative; and significant -40.8% reduction in LDLR mutations in both alleles in wich one or both were defective; the two patients with apolipoprotein B mutations were assigned to placebo. In general, the reduction in other lipid fractions with apolipoprotein B (excluding lipoprotein "a") was proportional to the reduction in LDL-cholesterol.

In the evolocumab treatment group, the safety, tolerance, treatment discontinuation and reaction in site injection assessment to evolocumab was better or similar to placebo, without detection of binding or neutralizing anti-evolocumab antibodies.

TESLA-B study supports the TESLA-Pilot trial results and demonstrates that in individuals with HoFH, evolocumab 420 mg S.C/4 weeks, significantly reduces LDL-cholesterol levels by 31% compared with placebo, with a surprising LDL-cholesterol reduction of 41% in individuals with LDLR defective activity mutations, all of that with an excellent safety and tolerability profile.

b) Heterozygous Familial Hypercholesterolemia

Frederick Rall *et al.*, reported in November 5th, 2012 *"The Reduction of LDL-C with PCSK9 Inhibition in Heterozygous Familial Hypercholesterolemia Disorder Randomized Trial"* or RUTHERFORD-1 trial [28]. This phase II study with AMG-145 (evolocumab) included a cohort of 167 subjects with HeFH according to the Simon Broome criteria, on statin therapy with/without ezetimibe and other lipid lowering drugs, at stable doses for a period equal to or greater than 4 weeks, and LDL-cholesterol level >100 mg/dL. The cohort was divided into three treatment groups: placebo S.C/4 weeks, evolocumab 350 mg S.C/4 weeks and evolocumab 420 mg S.C/4 weeks (3 doses).

In both active treatment groups, the safety and tolerance assessment to evolocumab was similar to placebo. Baseline LDL-cholesterol level measured by ultracentrifugation, the percentage reduction in LDL-cholesterol versus placebo, and the p value were: evolocumab 350 mg: 163.8 mg/dL, -43.8% and <0.001; evolocumab 420 mg: 152.1 mg/dL, -56.4% and <0.001. These results were similar regardless of baseline therapy. Reduction in other lipid fractions with apolipoprotein B was proportional to the reduction in LDL-cholesterol. The percentage where LDL-cholesterol level was <100 mg/dL and <70 mg/dL where: evolocumab 350 mg: 70% and 44%; evolocumab 420 mg: 89% and 65%, respectively.

RUTHERFORD-1 demonstrates that inhibition of PCSK9 with evolocumab versus placebo, provides significant additional LDL-cholesterol reduction in individuals with HeFH treated with background high intensity statins with or without ezetimibe, reaching LDL-cholesterol levels <100 mg/dL and < 70 mg/dL in 9 and 7 of each 10 individuals, respectively, treated with evolocumab 420 mg S.C/4 weeks.

Frederick Rall *et al.*, reported in October 4th, 2014 *"The Reduction of LDL-C with PCSK9 Inhibition in Heterozygous Familial Hypercholesterolemia Disorder Randomized Trial"* or RUTHERFORD-2 trial [29]. This phase-III study with AMG-145 (evolocumab) included a cohort of 331 subjects with HeFH according to the Simon Broome criteria, on statin therapy with/without ezetimibe and other lipid lowering drugs, at stable doses for a period equal to or greater than 4 weeks, and LDL-cholesterol level >100 mg/dL. The cohort was divided into four treatment groups: evolocumab 140 mg S.C/2 weeks, evolocumab 420 mg S.C/4 weeks, placebo S.C/2 weeks and placebo S.C/4 weeks for 12 weeks.

Mutations associated with HeFH were recorded in 211 of 264 (80%) individuals; in seven individuals (3%) mutations were recorded in both LDLR alleles, consistent with HoFH or compound HeFH, among the other 204 individuals with a single mutation in LDLR alleles, 75 (37%) had defective alleles, 66 (32%) had null or negative alleles and 54 (26%) had non-classified mutations. Nine individuals (4%) has mutations in the apolipoprotein B gene. Baseline calculated LDL-cholesterol level (measured by ultracentrifugation if LDL-cholesterol was <40 mg/dL and/or triglycerides >400 mg/dL), the percentage reduction in LDL-cholesterol versus placebo at week 12, and the p value were: evolocumab 140 mg

S.C/2 weeks: 182.5 mg/dL, -59.2% and <0.0001; evolocumab 420 mg S.C/4 weeks: 154.4 mg/dL, -61.3% and <0.0001. The percentage where LDL-cholesterol level was <70 mg/dL where: evolocumab 140mg S.C/2 weeks: 68%; evolocumab 420 mg S.C/4 weeks: 63%; placebo (both groups): 2%. These results were similar regardless of baseline characteristics, type of mutation or baseline therapy. Reduction in other lipid fractions with apolipoprotein B was proportional to the reduction in LDL-cholesterol without change in hs-CRP level. In both evolocumab treatment groups, the safety and tolerance assessment to evolocumab was similar to placebo.

RUTHERFORD-2 study reinforces the RUTHERFORD-1 trial results and confirms that inhibition of PCSK9 with evolocumab versus placebo, provides with safety and tolerability, significant additional LDL-cholesterol reduction in individuals with HeFH treated with background high intensity statins with or without ezetimibe, achieving LDL-cholesterol levels <70 mg/dL in 6-7 of each 10 individuals treated with evolocumab 140 mg S.C/2 weeks or 420 mg S.C/4 weeks; notably this response is not related to the underlying genetic mutations, that it indicates that genetic analysis may not be helpful in the therapeutic approach to patients with HeFH unlike individuals with HoFH.

c) Predominant Non-Familial Hypercholesterolemia

Robert Giugliano *et al.*, reported in November 6th, 2012 the *"LDL-C Assessment with PCSK9 Monoclonal Antibody Inhibition Combined with Statin Therapy"* or LAPLACE-1-TIMI-57 trial [30]. This phase II study with AMG-145 (evolocumab) included a cohort of 631 subjects with HC, on statin therapy with/without ezetimibe, at stable doses for a period equal to or greater than 4 weeks, and LDL-cholesterol level >85 mg/dL. The cohort was divided into eight treatment groups: placebo, evolocumab 70 mg, 105 mg or 140 mg S.C/2 weeks (6 doses), and placebo, evolocumab 280 mg, 350 mg or 420 mg S.C/ 4 weeks (3 doses).

In all active treatment groups, the safety and tolerance assessment to evolocumab was similar to placebo. The baseline LDL-cholesterol level measured by utracentrifugation, the percentage reduction in LDL-cholesterol versus placebo, and the p value were: evolocumab 70 mg: 120.9 mg/dL, -41.8% and <0.0001; evolocumab 105 mg: 128.7 mg/dL, -60.2% and <0.0001; evolocumab 140 mg: 120.9 mg, -66.1% and <0.0001; evolocumab 280 mg: 124.8 mg/dL, -41.8% and <0.0001; evolocumab 350 mg: 124.8 mg/dL, -50% and <0.0001; evolocumab 420 mg: 120.9 mg, -50.3% and <0.0001. These results were similar regardless of baseline clinical characteristics or therapy. Reduction in other lipid fractions with apolipoprotein B was proportional to the reduction in LDL-cholesterol. The percentage where LDL-cholesterol level was <70 mg/dL, non-HDL-cholesterol level <100 mg/dL and apolipoprotein B <80 g/L (triple goal) where: evolocumab 70 mg: 48.7%, 65.4% and 75.5%; evolocumab 105 mg: 79.5%, 83.3% and 88.5%; evolocumab 140 mg: 93.5%, 96.1% and 96.1%; evolocumab 280 mg: 56.4%, 68% and 73.1%; evolocumab 350 mg: 72.2%, 77.2% and 82.3%; evolocumab 420 mg: 71.8%, 83.3% and 85.9%.

LAPLACE-1 demonstrates that inhibition of PCSK9 with evolocumab versus placebo, provides significant additional LDL-cholesterol reduction in individuals with HC treated with background statins with or without ezetimibe, achieving and ideal triple goal with LDL-C <70 mg/dL, non-HDL-C <100 mg/dL and apolipoprotein-B <80 g/L in 94%, 96% and 96% of individuals treated with evolocumab 140 mg S.C/2 weeks. Evolocumab had an excellent safety and tolerability profile without immunogenicity concerns.

Michael Koren *et al.*, reported in November 6th, 2012 the *"Monoclonal Antibody Against PCSK9 to Reduce Elevated LDL-C in Patients Currently Not Receiving Drug Therapy for Easing Lipid Levels"* or MENDEL-1 trial [31]. This phase II study with AMG-145 (evolocumab) included a cohort of 406 subjects with HC and ASCVD risk <10% calculated with Framingham algorithm, without treatment for lipids, and LDL-cholesterol level from 100 to 180 mg/dL. The cohort was divided into nine treatment groups: placebo, evolocumab 70 mg, 105 mg or 140 mg S.C/2 weeks (6 doses); placebo, evolocumab 280 mg, 350 mg or 420 mg S.C/4 weeks (3 doses); and placebo S.C/4 weeks + ezetimibe 10 mg (3 doses).

In all active treatment groups, the safety and tolerance assessment to evolocumab was similar to placebo. Baseline LDL-cholesterol level (measured by utracentrifugation), the percentage reduction in LDL-cholesterol versus placebo and versus ezetimibe, and the p value for both comparisons were: evolocumab 70 mg: 148.2 mg/dL, -37.3%, -26.7% and <0.0001; evolocumab 105 mg: 144.3 mg/dL, -40.2%, -29.6% and <0.0001; evolocumab 140 mg: 140.4 mg, -42.2%, -36.7% and <0.0001; evolocumab 280 mg: 147.2 mg/dL, -43.6%, -25.2% and <0.0001; evolocumab 350 mg: 136.5 mg/dL, -47.7%, -29.3% and <0.0001; evolocumab 420 mg: 140.4 mg, -50.3%, -34.3% and <0.0001. Reduction in other lipid fractions with apolipoprotein B was proportional to the reduction in LDL-cholesterol.

MENDEL-1 is the first study with an Mab-PCSK9 in patients with HC without pharmacologic treatment, this trial demonstrates that inhibition of PCSK9 with evolocumab versus placebo and ezetimibe, provides significant LDL-cholesterol reduction in individuals with HC drug-naïve; this finding has especial relevance in patients with moderate or severe HC with high cardiovascular risk and statin intolerance.

Michael Koren *et al.*, reported in January 14th[h], 2014 the *"Open-Label Study of Long-term Evaluation Against LDL-C"* or OSLER-LDL-cholesterol trial [32]. This phase III open-label extension (52 weeks) study with AMG-145 (evolocumab) included a cohort of 1,104 participants in four phase-II trials with evolocumab (MENDEL-1, LAPLACE-1-TIMI-57, GAUSS-1 and RUTHERFORD-1 trials). The OSLER-LDL-C trial included subjects who had no adverse events leading to treatment discontinuation during the phase II study, who did not require an urgent modification of their baseline therapy during the first 12 weeks of OSLER participation and who achieved clinical stability. The cohort was divided into two treatment groups: evolocumab 420 mg S.C/4 weeks + standard of care (SOC) and SOC alone (control arm) for 12 weeks, after the first 12 weeks, central laboratory results were unblinded, and investigators could adjust SOC therapies in both treatment groups.

Mean baseline LDL-cholesterol level of the pooled phase II trials was 141.1 mg/dL. Individuals not taking evolocumab in the phase II trials and randomized to evolocumab 420 mg S.C/4 weeks in the open-label extension had a LDL-cholesterol reduction of -51.8% at week 12 and -52.3% at week 52 (p <0.0001 for both comparisons). Individuals taking evolocumab in the phase II trials and randomized to evolocumab 420 mg S.C/4 weeks in the open-label extension had persistent reductions in LDL-cholesterol from -50.4% at the end of phase II trials to -52.1% at week 52 (p <0.31). Individuals who discontinued evolocumab after phase II trials and were randomized to SOC without evolocumab in the open-label extension had a rapid return to baseline LDL-cholesterol level from -53.1% at the end of phase II trials to -17.9% at week 4 and -5.8% at week 12, without rebound effect during follow up. Among the patients who had at least one ultracentrifugation LDL-cholesterol result post-baseline during OSLER, a value of <100 mg/dL, <70 mg/dL, <50 mg/dL or <25 mg/dL of LDL-cholesterol was achieved in 96%, 82.8%, 55.3% and 13.5% in the evolocumab 420 mg S.C/4 weeks group versus 32.4%, 3.6%, 0.5% and 0% in the SOC without evolocumab group (p <0.0001 for all comparisons). Modification in other lipid fractions with apolipoprotein B tracked those observed for LDL-cholesterol.

In all evolocumab treatment group, the safety assessment was similar to SOC regardless of the LDL-cholesterol level achieved (<100, <70, <50 or <25 mg/dL), in the evolocumab 420 mg S.C/4 weeks, treatment discontinuation was reported in 3.7%, reaction in site injection was reported in 5.2%, with two cases report of transient binding anti-evolocumab antibodies without neutralizing anti-evolocumab antibodies.

OSLER-LDL-C study is the first open-label, long-term study evaluating evolocumab efficacy, safety and tolerability in a selected and heterogenous group of patients with HC; in this group SOC + evolocumab versus SOC without evolocumab reduced LDL-cholesterol in average 50% at week 12 without attenuation of its efficacy at week 52, achieving and LDL-C level <100 mg/dL in 72% of participants. In OSLER-LDL-C trial the safety and tolerability of evolocumab was excellent without immunogenicity concerns.

Dirk Blom *et al.*, reported in March 19th, 2014 the *"Durable Effect of PCSK9 Antibody Compared with Placebo Study"* or DESCARTES trial [33]. This phase III study with AMG-145 (evolocumab) included a cohort of 905 subjects with HC and LDL-cholesterol >75 mg/dL. In an initial stabilization open-label-phase, the cohort was divided into four treatment groups according with baseline LDL-cholesterol level, background lipid treatment and ASCVD risk: diet alone, diet + atorvastatin 10 mg, diet + atorvastatin 80 mg and diet + ezetimibe 10mg for four weeks. In a second open-label phase all patients with LDL-cholesterol level ≥75 mg/dL were included; those patients with coronary heart disease or equivalent with LDL-cholesterol level ≥75 and < 100 mg/dL and those patients without coronary heart disease or equivalent with LDL-cholesterol level ≥75 mg/dL and <130 mg/dL were randomized. Among patients in whom lipid-goal had not been reached, therapy was increased to the next level for an additional 4 weeks; patients reaching atorvastatin 80mg + ezetimibe 10 mg with LDL-cholesterol above the therapeutic goal were eligible for randomization. Selected patients were randomized in two treatment groups: evolocumab 420 mg S.C/4 weeks or placebo S.C/4 weeks for 48 weeks (the monthly 6 ml injection could be split in two 3 ml injections or three 2 ml injections).

Of 901 patients randomized who received a study drug, 111 received diet alone, 383 received atorvastatin 10 mg, 218 received atorvastatin 80 mg and 189 received atorvastatin 80 mg + ezetimibe 10 mg as background lipid-lowering therapy. Baseline calculated LDL-cholesterol level (measured by ultracentrifugation), the mean percentage reduction in LDL-cholesterol at week 52, the LDL-cholesterol achieved at week 52 and the percentage with LDL-cholesterol <70 mg/dL at week 52 were: Diet alone + evolocumab 420 mg: 111.6 mg/dL, -51.5%, 53.5 mg/dL and 83.6%; diet + placebo: 112.3 mg/dL, +4.2%, 117.3 mg/dL and 3.2%. Atorvastatin 10 mg + evolocumab 420 mg: 101.3 mg/dL, -54.7%, 44.7 mg/dL and 90.1%; atorvastatin 10 mg + placebo: 98.4 mg/dL, +6.9%, 103.9 mg/dL and 5.3%. Atorvastatin 80mg + evolocumab 420 mg: 94.6 mg/dL, -46.7%, 49.6 mg/dL and 80.8%; atorvastatin 80 mg + placebo: 96.2 mg/dL, +10.1%, 104.6 mg/dL and 6.1%. Atorvastatin 80 mg + ezetimibe 10 mg + evolocumab 420 mg: 116.8 mg/dL, -46.8%, 63.9 mg/dL and 67%; atorvastatin 80mg + ezetimibe 10 mg + placebo: 119.8 mg/dL, +1.7%, 115 mg/dL and 11.1%.

All groups: evolocumab 420 mg: 104.2 mg/dL, -50.1%, 50.9 mg/dL and 83.2%; all placebo groups: 104 mg/dL, +6.8%, 107.9 mg/dL and 6.4%. Reduction in other lipid fractions with apolipoprotein B was proportional to the reduction in LDL-cholesterol.

In the evolocumab treatment groups, the safety, tolerance, treatment discontinuation and reaction in site injection assessment to evolocumab was similar to placebo with 1 case report of transient binding anti-evolocumab antibodies without neutralizing anti-evolocumab antibodies.

DESCARTES study is an interesting forced risk-based lipid lowering trial ranged from diet alone to atorvastatin 80 mg plus ezetimibe 10 mg as background lipid-lowering therapy. In this trial evolocumab versus placebo reduced LDL-cholesterol in average 57% at week 52 (a reduction similar to that reported in OSLER-LDL-C trial), with variation from 48.5% in the group treated with atorvastatin 80 mg plus ezetimibe 10mg to 61.6% in the group treated with atorvastatin 10 mg, achieving with evolocumab 420 mg S.C/4 weeks an LDL-C level <70 mg/dL in 83% of participants. As in other trials, the safety and tolerability of evolocumab 420 mg S.C/4 weeks was excellent without immunogenicity concerns.

Jennifer Robinson *et al.*, reported in May 14th, 2014 the *"LDL-C Assessment with PCSK9 Monoclonal Antibody Inhibition Combined with Statin Therapy"* or LAPLACE-2 trial [34]. This comprehensive but complex phase III study with AMG-145 (evolocumab) included a cohort of 2,067 subjects with HC and LDL-cholesterol >150 mg/dL without lipid-lowering treatment, >100 mg/dL with non-intensive lipid-lowering treatment and >80 mg/dL with intensive lipid-lowering treatment. In a first stabilization open-label-phase, the cohort was divided into five treatment groups: atorvastatin 10 mg, rosuvastatin 5 mg, simvastatin 40mg, atorvastatin 80 mg and rosuvastatin 40 mg for four weeks. In a second phase, patients were randomized in 24 treatment groups as follows:

. Atorvastatin 10 mg (six groups): evolocumab 140 mg S.C/2 weeks + placebo oral daily; evolocumab 420 mg S.C/4 weeks + placebo oral daily; placebo S.C/2 weeks + placebo oral daily; placebo S.C/4 weeks + placebo oral daily; placebo S.C/2 weeks + ezetimibe 10 mg daily; placebo S.C/4 weeks + ezetimibe 10 mg oral daily for 12 weeks.

. Rosuvastatin 5 mg (four groups): evolocumab 140 mg S.C/2 weeks; evolocumab 420 mg S.C/4 weeks; placebo S.C/2 weeks; placebo S.C/4 weeks for 12 weeks.

. Simvastatin 40 mg (four groups): evolocumab 140 mg S.C/2 weeks; evolocumab 420 mg S.C/4 weeks; placebo S.C/2 weeks; placebo S.C/4 weeks for 12 weeks.

. Atorvastatin 80 mg (six groups): evolocumab 140 mg S.C/2 weeks + placebo oral daily; evolocumab 420 mg S.C/4 weeks + placebo oral daily; placebo S.C/2 weeks + placebo oral daily; placebo S.C/4 weeks + placebo oral daily; placebo S.C/2 weeks + ezetimibe 10 mg daily; placebo S.C/4 weeks + ezetimibe 10mg oral daily for 12 weeks.

. Rosuvastatin 40 mg (four groups): evolocumab 140 mg S.C/2 weeks; evolocumab 420 mg S.C/4 weeks; placebo S.C/2 weeks; placebo S.C/4 weeks for 12 weeks.

Baseline calculated LDL-cholesterol level (measured by ultracentrifugation if LDL-cholesterol <40 mg/dL and/or triglycerides >400 mg/dL), the mean LDL-cholesterol achieved at week 10-12, the mean percentage reduction in LDL-cholesterol at week 10-12, and the percentage with LDL-cholesterol <70 mg/dL were as follows:

. Atorvastatin 10 mg (six groups): evolocumab 140 mg S.C/2 weeks + placebo oral daily: 124.2 mg/dL, 47.9 mg/dl, -61.4% and 85.8%; evolocumab 420 mg S.C/4 weeks + placebo oral daily: 126.1 mg/dL, 46.6 mg/dL, -62.5% and 85.8%; placebo S.C/2 weeks + placebo oral daily: 123 mg/dL, 126.2 mg/dL, +8.5% and 5.7%; placebo S.C/4 weeks + placebo oral daily: 123.7 mg/dL, 123.7 mg/dL, +0.4% and 5.6%; placebo S.C/2 weeks + ezetimibe 10 mg daily: 126.8 mg/dL, 95 mg/dL, -23.9% and 20%; placebo S.C/4 weeks + ezetimibe 10mg oral daily: 119.3 mg/dL, 94.2 mg/dL, -19% and 16.7%.

. Rosuvastatin 5 mg (four groups): evolocumab 140 mg S.C/2 weeks: 118.7 mg/dL, 48.9 mg/dL, -59.3% and 88.7%; evolocumab 420 mg S.C/4 weeks: 122.9 mg/dL, 43.3 mg/dL, -63.8% and 89.9%; placebo S.C/2 weeks: 115.6 mg/dL, 121.6 mg/dL, +7.6% and 7%; placebo S.C/4 weeks for 12 weeks: 119.9 mg/dL, 121.5 mg/dL, +2.8% and 5.3%.

. Simvastatin 40 mg (four groups): evolocumab 140 mg S.C/2 weeks: 114.5 mg/dL, 39 mg/dL, -66.2% and 93.6%; evolocumab 420 mg S.C/4 weeks: 123.7 mg/dL, 48.4 mg/dL, -62.4% and 88.5%; placebo S.C/2 weeks: 110.3 mg/dL, 111.8 mg/dL, +3.3% and 1.9%; placebo S.C/4 weeks for 12 weeks: 108.6 mg/dL, 114.4 mg/dL, +6% and 3.9%.

. Atorvastatin 80 mg (six groups): evolocumab 140 mg S.C/2 weeks + placebo oral daily: 94.2 mg/dL, 35.3 mg/dL, -61.8% and 94.4%; evolocumab 420 mg S.C/4 weeks + placebo oral daily: 93.8 mg/dL, 34,8 mg/dL, -65.1% and 92.5%; placebo S.C/2 weeks + placebo oral daily: 100.3 mg/dL, 109.5 mg/dL, +13.1% and 13.7%; placebo S.C/4 weeks + placebo oral daily: 94.7 mg/dL, 100.1 mg/dL, +9.8% and 9.3%; placebo S.C/2 weeks + ezetimibe 10 mg daily: 98.7 mg/dL, 85.6

mg/dL, -16.9% and 50.9%; placebo S.C/4 weeks + ezetimibe 10mg oral daily: 92.3 mg/dL, 72.1 mg/dL, -21.3% and 62.3%.

. Rosuvastatin 40 mg (four groups): evolocumab 140 mg S.C/2 weeks: 88.5 mg/dL, 37.5 mg/dL, -59.1% and 93.5%; evolocumab 420 mg S.C/4 weeks: 88.5 mg/dL, 33 mg/dL, -62.9% and 94.5%; placebo S.C/2 weeks: 77.4 mg/dL, 81.5 mg/dL, +6.6% and 38.9%; placebo S.C/4 weeks: 102.9 mg/dL, 96.6 mg/dL, 0% and 28.8%. Reduction in other lipid fractions with apolipoprotein B was proportional to the reduction in LDL-cholesterol.

In all evolocumab treatment groups, the safety, tolerance, treatment discontinuation and reaction in site injection assessment to evolocumab was similar to placebo with 1 case (0.1%) report of binding anti-evolocumab antibodies without neutralizing anti-evolocumab antibodies.

LAPLACE-2 study is a complex but very comprehensive trial wich explore the efficacy, safety and tolerability of evolocumab versus placebo and ezetimibe in 24 treatment arms including, moderate-intensity doses of simvastatin, rosuvastatin and atorvastatin, and high-intensity doses of rosuvastatin and atorvastatin as background lipid-lowering treatment. In this trial evolocumab versus placebo reduced LDL-cholesterol up to 66%, achieving and LDL-C level <70 mg/dL in 86% of individuals treated with moderate-intensity statins and 94% of individuals treated with high-intensity statins, in comparison, ezetimibe versus placebo reduced LDL-cholesterol up to 24%, achieving an LDL-C level <70 mg/dL in 17% of individuals treated with moderate-intensity statins and 62% of individuals treated with high-intensity statins. Other relevant finding of this trial was to demonstrate for first time that the addition of evolocumab results in similar percent reductions in LDL-cholesterol regardless of statin type, dose or intensity across the 3 statins used. As in other trials, the safety and tolerability of evolocumab was excellent without immunogenicity concerns.

Michael Koren *et al.,* reported in June 17th, 2014 the *"Monoclonal Antibody Against PCSK9 to Reduce Elevated LDL-C in Patients Currently Not Receiving Drug Therapy for Easing Lipid Levels"* or MENDEL-2 trial [35]. This phase III study with AMG-145 (evolocumab) included a cohort of 615 subjects with HC with ASCVD risk <10% calculated with Framingham algorithm, without treatment for lipids, and LDL-cholesterol level 100 to 189 mg/dL. The cohort was divided into six treatment groups: oral daily placebo + placebo S.C/2 weeks; oral daily placebo + placebo S.C/4 weeks; ezetimibe 10 mg + placebo S.C/2 weeks; ezetimibe 10 mg + placebo S.C/4 weeks; oral daily placebo + evolocumab 140 mg S.C/2 weeks and oral daily placebo + evolocumab 420 mg S.C/4 weeks, all for 12 weeks.

Baseline LDL-cholesterol level, the percentage reduction in LDL-cholesterol versus placebo and ezetimibe at week 12, the p value for comparisons and the percentage with LDL-cholesterol <70 mg/dL achievement were: oral daily placebo + placebo S.C/2 weeks: 140 mg/dL, +0.1%, N.A, N.A and 1.4%; oral daily placebo + placebo S.C/4 weeks: 144 mg/dL, -1.3%, N.A, N.A and 0%; ezetimibe 10 mg + placebo S.C/2 weeks: 143 mg/dL, -17.8%, N.A, N.A and 1.4%; ezetimibe 10 mg + placebo S.C/4 weeks: 144 mg/dL, -18.6%, N.A, N.A and 0%; oral daily placebo + evolocumab 140 mg S.C/2 weeks: 142 mg/dL, -57.1%, -39.3%, 0.001 (for both comparisons) and 72.9%; oral daily placebo + evolocumab 420 mg S.C/4 weeks: 144 mg/dL, -54.8%, -37.6%, <0.001 (for both comparisons) and 65.4%. These results were similar regardless of baseline characteristics. Reduction in other lipid fractions with apolipoprotein B was proportional to the reduction in LDL-cholesterol.

In all evolocumab treatment groups, the safety, tolerance, treatment discontinuation and reaction in site injection assessment to evolocumab was similar to placebo/ezetimibe groups without detection of binding or neutralizing anti-evolocumab antibodies.

MENDEL-2 study amplifies the MENDEL-1 trial results in patients with HC without pharmacologic treatment, this trial corroborates that inhibition of PCSK9 with evolocumab versus placebo and ezetimibe, provides significant LDL-cholesterol reduction in individuals with HC drug-naïve; this finding as was mentioned before, has especial relevance for patients with moderate or severe HC with high cardiovascular risk and statin intolerance or contraindication.

d) Long-term Trials

Marc Sabatine *et al.*, reported in March 15th, 2015 the *"Open-Label Study of Long-term Evaluation Against LDL-C 1-2"* or OSLER-1-2 trial [36]. This trial was planned with the aim of evaluating the medium-term safety, tolerance and efficacy in reducing LDL-cholesterol of evolocumab; this analysis also included an exploratory analysis of the blindly adjudicated incidence of cardiovascular events: death, myocardial infarction, angina pectoris requiring hospitalization, coronary revascularization, stroke, transient ischemic attack, and heart failure requiring hospitalization. The OSLER-1 study included subjects who had completed any of the 5 *"parent"* phase II studies (MENDEL-1, LAPLACE--TIMI-57, GAUSS-1, RUTHERFORD-1 and YUKAWA trials), and the OSLER-2 study included subjects who had completed any of the 7 *"parent"* phase III studies (MENDEL-2, LAPLACE-2, GAUSS-2, RUTHERFORD-2, DESCARTES, THOMAS-1 and THOMAS-2 trials). Of the 12 *"parent"* studies, those subjects who had no adverse events leading to treatment discontinuation during the study, who did not require an urgent modification of their baseline therapy and who achieved clinical stability, were randomly assigned in a 2:1 ratio to receive open-label evolocumab 420 mg S.C/4 weeks (OSLER-1) versus SOC therapy without evolocumab for 56 weeks, or evolocumab 140 mg S.C/2 weeks or 420 mg S.C/4 weeks (patient's choice in OSLER- 2) versus SOC therapy without evolocumab for 48 weeks.

The study included 74.1% of the *"parent study cohort"*, totaling 4,465 subjects (1,324 in OSLER-1 and 3,141 in OSLER-2); 2,976 were assigned to evolocumab and 1,489 continued their SOC therapy without evolocumab. The mean follow-up was 11.1 months. With a baseline, LDL-cholesterol level of 120 mg/dL, at week 12 the LDL-cholesterol reduction was -61% in the evolocumab group (-59% to - 63% with a p value of <0.001); the mean absolute reduction of LDL-cholesterol was 73 mg/dL with a mean circulating LDL-cholesterol value of 48 mg/ dL; 90.2% and 73.6% of subjects in the evolocumab group had an LDL-cholesterol level of <100 mg/dL and <70 mg/dL, respectively, against 26% and 3.8% in the control group. These figures remained stable throughout the follow-up. The figures for non-HDL cholesterol, apolipoprotein B, total cholesterol and triglycerides had a reduction of -52%, -47.3%, -36.1% and -12.6%, respectively. The HDL-cholesterol and apolipoprotein-A figures increased 7% and 4.2%, respectively.

The incidence of adverse events, serious adverse events and hepatic and muscle enzyme elevations were similar between the evolocumab group and the control group, with no difference related to LDL cholesterol levels during treatment (<40 mg/dL or <25 mg/dL); in the evolocumab group there was a low (<1%) although a higher incidence of neurocognitive adverse events, with no association to LDL-cholesterol level. Injection site reactions with evolocumab were reported in 4.3%, leading to discontinuation in 0.2%; binding anti-evolocumab antibodies were reported in 0.3% in both evolocumab groups and anti-evolocumab neutralizing antibodies were reported in 0%.

In this exploratory study, the estimated incidence of cardiovascular events at 12 months was 0.95% in the evolocumab group versus 2.18% in the control group, representing an H.R of 0.47 (0.28 to 0.78 with a p value of 0.003); this trend was progressive throughout the follow-up.

OSLER-1-2 has concordant results with OSLER-LDL-C [32] trial and confirms the medium-term efficacy, safety and tolerability of evolocumab, providing for first time a positive signal regarding the reduction of cardiovascular events with evolocumab compared to that achieved with statins and other non-statin therapies being worth to mention the methodological limitations of this study, specifically the selected population included (subjects who had no adverse events leading to treatment discontinuation during the *"parent"* study, who did not require an urgent modification of their baseline therapy and who achieved clinical stability) and the open-label design of the trial.

Michael Koren *et al.*, reported in March 14th, 2017 the *"Open-Label Study of Long-term Evaluation Against LDL-C 1-2, 4 years extension study"* or OSLER---2 trial, 4 years extension [36]. As we reviewed previously, the OSLER-1-2 Long-Term Study [37] was planned with the aim of evaluating the long-term lipid lowering efficacy, persistence, and safety of evolocumab. This four-year extension study reports data from the first enrollment in October 2011 to August 2016.

The OSLER-1-2 included 1,324 of the 1,650 eligible *"parent trials"* patients (80.2%), of those, 882 patients received evolocumab plus SOC and 442 received SOC without evolocumab; after one year, 1,255 of the 1,324 OSLER-1 eligible patients (94.7%) received at least one evolocumab open-label dose; 886 were taking statins (28% high-intensity, 47% intermediate-intensity and 25% low-intensity) and 369 (29%) were not taking HMGCoAR inhibitors.

As of August 2016, 1,215 (96.8%), 1,122 (85%), 1,057 (80%), and 812 (61%) of patients had lipid measurements available at 1, 2, 3, and 4 years of follow-up, respectively. With a baseline *"parent trials"* LDL-cholesterol level of 133 mg/dL, at week 12 in the OSLER-1-2 trial the LDL-cholesterol reduction was -61% in the evolocumab group (-63% to -60%) versus -2% in the control group (-5% to -0.2%) with a mean circulating LDL-cholesterol value of 53 mg/dL in the evolocumab group versus 133 mg/dL in the control group (p <0.001). At weeks 64, 100, 160, and 208 of OSLER-1-2 follow-up the LDL-cholesterol reductions compared with baseline *"parent trials"* were 60% (61% to 59%), 59% (-60% to -57%), 59% (-61% to -58%), and 57% (-59% to -55%), respectively.

The annualized incidence of new-onset diabetes was 2.8% in the evolocumab group versus 4% in the control group; neurocognitive event rates were 0.4% in the evolocumab group versus 0% in the control group, and no neutralizing anti-evolocumab antibodies were detected.

OSLER 1-2 four-year extension study, despite inherent selected population included and open-label design limitations reaffirms the OSLER-1-2 [36] trial results and confirms the long-term (4 years follow-up) efficacy, safety and tolerability of evolocumab with an excellent persistence treatment rate of 79% for 44 months without evidence of immunogenicity.

e) Cardiovascular Outcomes Trial

Marc Sabatine *et al.*, reported in March 17th, 2015 the "*Further Cardiovascular Outcomes Research with PCSK9 Inhibition in Subjects with Elevated Risk*" or FOURIER trial [38], this, is the first randomized, placebo controlled trial published to determine the efficacy, safety and tolerability of one MAb-PCSK9 (evolocumab) in patients with ASCVD optimally treated. Based on the evidence of phase II and III trials with the use of evolocumab, the study FOURIER was planned with the aim of defining at what extent the incidence of new ASCVD events is reduced by the use of evolocumab in patients with chronic ASCVD optimally treated with the SOC for ASCVD, including statins/ezetimibe.

The FOURIER study is a multinational RCT (49 countries and 1,242 sites) which included adult subjects with clinical ASCVD. Subjects included were required to have 40 to 85 years of age, clinically evident ASCVD (history of myocardial infarction, non-hemorrhagic stroke or symptomatic peripheral artery disease with ABI <0.85 or revascularization/amputation history) with ≥ 1 additional major cardiovascular risk factor (diabetes mellitus, age ≥ 65 years, myocardial infarction or non-hemorrhagic stroke in the previous 6 months, additional myocardial infarction or non-hemorrhagic stroke, current daily cigarette smoking or additional symptomatic peripheral artery disease) or ≥ 2 additional minor cardiovascular risk factor (history of non-myocardial infarction-related coronary revascularization, residual coronary stenosis $\geq 40\%$ in ≥ 2 coronary arteries, HDL-cholesterol <40/<50 mg/dL in men/women, respectively, hsCRP >2 mg/L, LDL-cholesterol or non-HDL-cholesterol ≥ 130 or ≥ 160 mg/dL, respectively, or metabolic syndrome) to be treated with a high/moderate intensity statin therapy (with or without ezetimibe) and to have an LDL-cholesterol level ≥ 70mg/dL and/or non-HDL-cholesterol level ≥ 100 mg/dL with triglycerides levels ≤ 400 mg/dL.

The selected subjects were randomly assigned in a 1:1 ratio to receive, evolocumab 140 mg S.C/2 weeks or 420 mg S.C/4 weeks or placebo S.C/2 weeks or placebo S.C/4 weeks according to patient preference. The primary efficacy end-point of the study was the composite of cardiovascular death, myocardial infarction, stroke, hospitalization for unstable angina, or coronary revascularization. The secondary efficacy end-point of the study was the composite of cardiovascular death, myocardial infarction, or stroke. Safety was assessed through collection of data on adverse events and central laboratory results. A central-blinded clinical-events committee (TIMI Study Group) adjudicated all potential efficacy and safety end-points.

The study included 27,564 individuals, 13,784 in the evolocumab group and 13,780 in the placebo group; the baseline characteristics of the patients in the two groups were well matched; the mean age was 63 years, 24.6% were women, 81.1%, 19.4% and 13.2% had a history of myocardial infarction, non-hemorrhagic stroke and symptomatic peripheral artery disease, respectively; 69.3%, 30.4% and 5.2% were on high-intensity statin, medium intensity statin and ezetimibe, respectively. The median duration of follow-up was 26 months (22 to 30 months) and ascertainment of the primary efficacy end-point was complete in 99.5% of potential patients-years of follow-up.

Lipids results: With a baseline LDL-cholesterol of 92 mg/dL in both groups, at 48 weeks, in the evolocumab group versus placebo group, the mean LDL-cholesterol percentage reduction was -59% (-58% to -60% with a p value of <0.001) equivalent to a mean absolute reduction of 56 mg/dL (55 to 57 mg/dl) with a median of 30 mg/dL (19-46 mg/dL) of LDL-cholesterol in the evolocumab group. At 48 weeks, in the evolocumab group, 87%, 67% and 42% of the patients reduced the LDL-colesterol level to ≤70 mg/dL, ≤40 mg/dL and ≤25 mg/dL, versus 18%, 0.5 and less than 0.1%, respectively, in the placebo group (p <0.001 for all comparisons). In the evolocumab group, non-HDL-cholesterol and apolipoprotein-B levels were reduced -52% and -49%, respectively (p <0.001 for both).

Primary efficacy end-point: The primary efficacy endpoint occurred in 1,344 of 13,784 patients in the evolocumab group (9.8%) and in 1,563 of 13,780 patients in the placebo group (11.3%) (H.R 0.85: 0.79 to 0.92 with a p value of <0.001). The magnitude of the primary endpoint of risk reduction tended to increase over time (12% in the first year and 19% afterwards).

Secondary efficacy end-point: The secondary efficacy endpoint occurred in 816 of 13,784 patients in the evolocumab group (5.9%) and in 1,013 of 13,780 patients in the placebo group (7.4%) (H.R 0.80: 0.73 to 0.88 with a p value of <0.001). As with, the primary efficacy endpoint, the magnitude of the secondary endpoint of risk reduction tended to increase over time (16% in the first year and 25% afterwards). The primary and secondary endpoint benefit with evolocumab was consistent across key subgroups, across all LDL-cholesterol quartiles, across both statin intensity treatments with or without ezetimibe, and irrespective of the evolocumab treatment regimen (140 mg S.C/2 weeks or 420 mg S.C/4 weeks).

Safety and tolerability: The safety, including cataract, neurocognitive abnormalities or diabetes mellitus de-novo, and the tolerability profiles of the evolocumab group did not show significant differences compared to those observed in the placebo group. Injection site reactions were reported in 2.1% in the evolocumab group vs 1.6% in the placebo group, with no differences in treatment interruption between groups (0.1% for both groups). Allergic reactions were similar between groups, 3.1% for evolocumab and 2.9% for placebo, with new anti-evolocumab binding antibodies detected in 0.3% of patients and no anti-evolocumab neutralizing antibodies detected (0%).

FOURIER trial demonstrates for the first time that the addition of Mab-PCSK9, in this case evolocumab, to the optimal treatment with statins with or without ezetimibe in a median period of 26 months is associated with a significant 15% reduction in the risk of cardiovascular death, myocardial infarction, stroke, hospitalization for unstable angina, or coronary revascularization, and a significant 20% reduction in the risk of cardiovascular death, myocardial infarction, or stroke, both with an excellent safety and tolerability profile. These results are aligned with the findings of PROVE-IT, TNT trial IMPROVE-IT and GLAGOV trials and show that continued cardiovascular benefit can be accrued even when LDL-cholesterol levels are reduced to 20 to 25 mg/dL, a level that is well below of the current therapeutic targets or under a personal perspective, a level that is well close to the biologically active LDL-cholesterol level postulated for Myant, Reich, Goldstein and Brown in 1978.

f) Statin Intolerance Trials

David Sullivan *et al.,* reported in November 5th, 2012 the *"Goal Achievement After Utilizing an Anti PCSK9 antibody in Statin Intolerant Subjects"* or GAUSS-1 trial [39]. This phase II study with AMG-145 (evolocumab) included a cohort of 160 subjects with statin muscle intolerance, defined as the inability to tolerate at least one statin at any dose or an increase in the dose above weekly doses of rosuvastatin 35 mg, atorvastatin 70 mg, simvastatin 140 mg, pravastatin 140 mg, lovastatin 140 mg or fluvastatin 240 mg with symptoms improvement or resolution with statin discontinuation, and LDL-cholesterol level >100 mg/dL, >130 mg/dL or >160 mg/dl according to ATP-III NCEP. The cohort was divided into five treatment groups: evolocumab 280 mg, evolocumab 350 mg and evolocumab 420 mg S.C/4 weeks (3 doses); evolocumab 420 mg S.C/4 weeks + open-label ezetimibe 10mg daily, and placebo S.C/4weeks + open-label ezetimibe 10mg daily (3 doses).

The cohort included 50% of patients with intermediate or high and 50% with low ASCVD risk; 100% of patients were unable to tolerate at least 1 statin, 77% could not tolerate 2 or more statins, 32%, could not tolerate 3 or more, and 11%, could not tolerate 4 or more statins; baseline muscle-related statin side effects reported were myalgia 90%, myositis 9% and rhabdomyolysis 1%.

Baseline LDL-cholesterol level measured by ultracentrifugation, the mean percentage reduction in LDL-cholesterol, the absolute change in LDL-cholesterol and the LDL-cholesterol level achievement <100 mg/dl and < 70 mg/dL were: evolocumab 280 mg: 194.8 mg/dl, -40.8%, -66.8 mg/dL, 47% and 9% ; evolocumab 350 mg: 190.3 mg/dL, -42.6%, -69.7 mg/dL, 51% and 16%; evolocumab 420 mg S.C/4 weeks: 203.5 mg/dL, -50.7%, -90.8 mg/dL, 61% and 28%; evolocumab 420 mg S.C/4 weeks + ezetimibe 10mg daily: 194.4 mg/dL, -63%%, -109.8 mg/dL, 99.1% and 63%; placebo S.C/4weeks + ezetimibe 10mg daily 182.9 mg/dL, -14.8%, -14.2 mg/dL, 7% and 0% (p<0.001 for all comparisons with placebo and ezetimibe). Reduction in other lipid fractions with apolipoprotein B was proportional to the reduction in LDL-cholesterol.

Overall 58% of patients in the evolocumab treatment groups, 67% in the evolocumab/ezetimibe group and 59% in the placebo/ezetimibe group reported TEAEs; myalgia was reported in 7.4%, 20% and 3.1% in the evolocumab, evolocumab + ezetimibe and placebo + ezetimibe groups, respectively; two patient in the evolocumab groups had CK elevations greater >10xULN, both events associated with unusually physical activity, one resolved spontaneously, the other resolved after rosuvastatin and evolocumab interruption; one patient in placebo/ezetimibe group has CK elevation >5xULN. No binding or neutralizing anti-evolocumab antibodies were detected.

GAUSS-1 study shows and excellent muscle tolerability profile of AMG-145 (evolocumab) in a short-term trial of a cohort of patients with history of statin intolerance, and opened the door to long-term trials oriented to demonstrate long-term muscle tolerability to Mabs-PCSK9 in patients with statin intolerance, a real unmet therapeutic challenge.

Erik Stroes *et al.,* reported in June 17th, 2014 the *"Goal Achievement After Utilizing an Anti PCSK9 antibody in Statin Intolerant Subjects"* or GAUSS-2 trial [40]. This phase III study with AMG-145 (evolocumab) included a cohort of 307 subjects with statin muscle intolerance, defined as the inability to tolerate at least two statins at any dose or an increase in the dose above the smallest tablet strength because intolerable muscle-related side effects, and LDL-cholesterol level >100 mg/dL, >130 mg/dL or >160 mg/dl according to ATP-III NCEP. The cohort was divided into four treatment groups: ezetimibe 10 mg daily + placebo S.C/2 weeks, placebo oral daily + evolocumab 140 mg S.C/2 weeks, ezetimibe 10 mg daily + placebo S.C/4 weeks and placebo oral daily + evolocumab 420 mg S.C/4 weeks.

The cohort included 56% of patients with high ASCVD risk. Overall 44% of patients were intolerant to 2 statins, 34% were intolerant to 3 statins, and 22% were intolerant to 4 statins; baseline muscle-related statin side effects reported were myalgia 80.75%, myositis 17% and rhabdomyolysis 2%.

Baseline LDL-cholesterol level measured by ultracentrifugation, the mean percentage reduction in LDL-cholesterol, the absolute change in LDL-cholesterol and LDL-cholesterol level achievement < 70 mg/dL at week 12 were: ezetimibe 10 mg daily + placebo S.C/2 weeks: 195 mg/dL, -18.1%, -36.2 mg/dL and 2%; placebo oral daily + evolocumab 140 mg S.C/2 weeks: 192 mg/dL, -56.1%, -106 mg/dL and 45.5%; ezetimibe 10 mg daily + placebo S.C/4 weeks: 195 mg/dL, -15.1%- -30.2 mg/dL and 0%; placebo oral daily + evolocumab 420 mg S.C/4 weeks: 192 mg/dL, -52.6%, -99 mg/dL and 42% (p<0.001 for all comparisons with placebo and ezetimibe). Reduction in other lipid fractions with apolipoprotein B was proportional to the reduction in LDL-cholesterol.

Overall 66% of patients in the evolocumab treatment groups and 73% in the ezetimibe treatment groups reported TEAEs; myalgia and myositis were reported in 8% and <1% in the evolocumab treatment groups, and 18% and 0% in the ezetimibe treatment groups, respectively; CK elevations >5 and >10xULN were reported in 1% and 0% in the evolocumab treatment groups, and 3% and 1% in the ezetimibe groups, respectively. No binding or neutralizing anti-evolocumab antibodies were detected.

GAUSS-2 study confirms the GAUSS-1 trial results [39] showing and excellent muscle tolerability profile of AMG-145 (evolocumab) in a medium-term trial of a cohort of individuals with history of statin intolerance, and supported the need of one trial with blinded rechallenge to statins in order to include patients with real statin (intolerance to statins without intolerance to placebo).

Steven Nissen *et al.*, reported in April 5th, 2015 the *"Goal Achievement After Utilizing an Anti PCSK9 antibody in Statin Intolerant Subjects"* or GAUSS-3 trial [41]. This comprehensive phase III study with AMG-145 (evolocumab) was designed as a two-stage randomized trial to first identify patients with statin-induced muscle symptoms and subsequently to compare the effectiveness and tolerability of ezetimibe and evolocumab. The trial included a cohort of 511 patients with history of statin muscle intolerance, defined as the inability to tolerate atorvastatin 10 mg or any other statin at any dose, or 3 or more statins with one at the lowest average daily starting dose and 2 other at any dose because muscle-related side effects, and LDL-cholesterol level above the goal according the ASCVD risk (>100 mg/dL for patients with ASCVD, >130 mg/dL for patients without ASCVD with ≥2 risk factors, >160 mg/dL with 1 risk factor and >190 mg/dL without additional risk factors). After inclusion, all patients were included in a washout phase for 4 weeks in wich all statins and lipid-lowering drugs were discontinued. Phase A included 492 patients, was a double-blind, placebo-controlled crossover procedure to rechallenge with atorvastatin; patients were randomly assigned to atorvastatin 20 mg or matching placebo for 10 weeks, then underwent a 2 weeks washout period, followed by crossover to the alternate therapy for 10 weeks. Phase B included 218 patients who experienced muscle-related adverse events with atorvastatin 20 mg but not with placebo (real intolerance) or patients with documented CK increase >10xULN and muscle symptoms while receiving statin therapy and resolution at discontinuation; patients included in phase B were randomized into two treatment groups: ezetimibe 10 mg daily + placebo S.C/4 weeks and placebo oral daily + evolocumab 420 mg S.C/4 weeks (three 140 mg doses).

The phase A cohort included 62.5% of patients with high ASCVD risk, 11%, 14.9% and 11.6% with moderately-high, moderate and low ASCVD risk, respectively; 18.5% with intolerance to one statin and 81.5% with intolerance to ≥ 3 statins; 83.5%, 15.1% and 0.4% with myalgia, myositis or rhabdomyolysis history, respectively. The phase B cohort included 56% of patients with high ASCVD risk, 13.3%, 17.4% and 13.3% with moderately-high, moderate and low ASCVD risk, respectively; 3.4% with intolerance to 1 statin, 14.5% with intolerance to two statins and 82.1% with intolerance to ≥ 3 statins; 77.2%, 16.6% and 6.2% with myalgia, myositis or rhabdomyolysis history, respectively.

Overall 42.6% of patients with a history of muscle-related adverse events reported intolerable symptoms in phase A with atorvastatin but no with placebo (199 entered in phase B together with 19 patients with myalgia and CK increase >10xULN during statin administration); conversely 26.5% reported intolerable symptoms with placebo but no with atorvastatin.

Baseline LDL-cholesterol level measured by ultracentrifugation, the mean percentage reduction in LDL-cholesterol, absolute change in LDL-cholesterol and LDL-cholesterol level achievement < 70 mg/dL at week 24 of the phase B were: ezetimibe 10 mg daily + placebo S.C/4 weeks: 221.9 mg/dL, -16.7%, -31.2 mg/dL and 0%; placebo oral daily + evolocumab 420 mg S.C/4 weeks: 218.8 mg/dL, -52.8%, -102.9 mg/dL and 27.4% (p<0.001 for all comparisons with ezetimibe). Reduction in other lipid fractions with apolipoprotein B was proportional to the reduction in LDL-cholesterol.

Overall 20.7% of patients in the evolocumab treatment groups and 28.8% in the ezetimibe treatment groups reported muscle-related events; treatment (oral and S.C) discontinuation percentage was low and similar in both groups as were other adverse events reported. One patient (0.7%) developed binding anti-evolocumab antibodies and 0% developed anti-evolocumab neutralizing antibodies.

GAUSS-3 study demonstrates for the first time that among individuals with history of statin intolerance, using a blinded rechallenge design with atorvastatin 20mg and placebo, 42.5% of patients with history of statin intolerance have intolerance to the statin but not to the placebo (real intolerance) and 26.5% have intolerance to the placebo but not to the statin (nocebo effect), suggesting that reported muscle symptoms are not always related to statin use. Among patients with real statin tolerance, evolocumab reduced LDL-cholesterol by 50% versus ezetimibe that reduced LDL-cholesterol by 16.7%, achievement of a LDL-C level <70 mg/dL was 0% for ezetimibe versus 27.4% for evolocumab. The muscle-tolerability for evolocumab was excellent with 0.7% of discontinuation because muscle-related events versus 6.8% for ezetimibe. This trial demonstrates the efficacy and excellent muscle-tolerability for evolocumab in patients with real statin-intolerance and opened the door to a trial aimed to explore the efficacy and tolerability of evolocumab plus ezetimibe versus evolocumab plus placebo.

g) Neurocognitive Security Trial

Robert Giugliano *et al.,* in August 17th, 2017 published the *"Evaluating PCSK9 Binding Antibody Influence on Cognitive Health in High Cardiovascular Risk Subjects"* or EBBINGHAUS trial [42]. This trial is the first published RCT designed to determine the neurocognitive safety MAbs-PCSK9, in this case AMG-145 (evolocumab) in patients with ASCVD optimally treated with statins. Justified on the non-definitive evidence between neurocognitive deterioration and MAbs-PCSK9 or the low LDL-cholesterol levels that result from their use, the study EBBINGAUSS was planned with the aim of excluding the connection between evolocumab use and neurocognitive impairment.

The EBBINGHAUS study is a multinational RCT which included adult subjects derived from the FOURIER trial [37]. The selected subjects were randomly assigned in a 1:1 ratio to receive, evolocumab 140 mg S.C/2 weeks or 420 mg S.C/4 weeks and placebo S.C/2 weeks or placebo S.C/4weeks according to the patient choice. The primary end-point was the score on the spatial working memory strategy index on executive function (principal component of the Cambridge Neuropsychological Test Automated Battery or CANTAB test; there were three secondary end points (working memory, episodic memory and psychomotor speed). The study included 1,974 (1,204 in the primary cohort and 774 in the secondary cohort); the baseline characteristics of the patients in the two groups were well matched and the median duration of follow-up was 19.4 months (19 to 21.8).

Primary Efficacy Endpoint: The trial was designed as a non-inferiority trial with a non-inferiority margin of 20% versus placebo (inferior boundary 0.80 - superior boundary 1.2). The primary efficacy endpoint evaluated by the spatial working memory strategy index was 17.8 and 17.8 in the baseline evaluation, and 17.6 and 17.5 in the post-treatment evaluation in the placebo and evolocumab groups, respectively with a mean change of -0.21 in the evolocumab group and -0.29 in the placebo groups, with a non-inferiority superior boundary of 1.06 (p value of <0.001 for non-inferiority). The mean changes with respect to the secondary end points did not differ between the evolocumab and the placebo groups. These results were homogeneous among different subgroups and independent of the nadir LDL-cholesterol achieved during the follow-up, including LDL-cholesterol levels <40 mg/dL or <25 mg/dL (661 patients). Self-assessment of everyday cognition and cognitive adverse events did not show difference between placebo and evolocumab groups.

EBBINGHAUS study confirms that among patients who received either evolocumab or placebo in addition to statin therapy, did not exist an association between adverse cognitive effects and evolocumab, as compared with placebo over a median follow up of 19 months.

h) Atherosclerosis Regression by Intracoronary Ultrasound Study

Stephen Nichols *et al.,.,* published in November 15th 2016 the *"Global Assessment of Plaque Regression with a PCSK9 Antibody as Measured by Intravascular Ultrasound"* -GLAGOV- [43]. Based on the evidence of atheroregression with the use of high-intensity statins -SATURN study- [44], the GLAGOV trial was planned with the aim of exploring at what extent the progression of coronary atherosclerosis is reduced by the use of evolocumab as assessed by intracoronary ultrasound.

The GLAGOV study included adult subjects with clinical indication of coronary angiography for suspicion of coronary atherosclerosis. Subjects included were required to have been treated with a stable statin therapy for 4 weeks and to have an LDL-cholesterol level between 60-80 mg/dL (very-high risk cohort) or >80 mg/dL (high-risk cohort). In all included subjects, a coronary ultrasound was performed at baseline and at week 78; the analysis of the segments selected for analysis was centralized, standardized and blinded. The selected subjects were randomly assigned in a 1:1 ratio to receive, evolocumab 420 mg S.C/4 weeks or placebo S.C/4 weeks for 76 weeks. The primary endpoint of the study was the change in percent atheroma volume [PAV = (EEM area – luminal area) / (EEM area) x100] and the secondary endpoint was the change in normalized total atheroma volume [TAV = (EEM area – luminal area) / (individual images number x cohort average images number)]. Other, exploratory, objectives included the analysis of the relationship between LDL-cholesterol reduction and atheroregression and the adjudicated incidence of cardiovascular events.

The study included 968 individuals, 484 in the evolocumab group and 484 in the placebo group; 87.2% of the individuals included had baseline and follow-up evaluations and 423 individuals in each group were included in the analysis. The mean follow-up was 17.6 months. With a baseline, LDL-cholesterol of 92.5 mg /dL in both groups, the mean LDL-cholesterol level at week 78 in the evolocumab group was 36.6 mg/dL versus 93 mg/dL in the placebo group with an absolute difference of -56.5 mg/dL (-59.7 to -53.4% with a p value of <0.001). The numbers of apolipoprotein-B, triglycerides and lipoprotein (a) had an absolute difference of -40.6 mg/dL, -19.1 mg/dL and -6.7 mg/dL, respectively; HDL-cholesterol levels had an absolute difference of +2.5 mg/dL and hsCRP did not differ between groups (1.4 mg/L in both groups).

The PAV increased +0.05% in the control group and reduced -0.95% in the evolocumab group, with an absolute difference of -1.0% (-1.8% to -0.64% with a p value of <0.001). Similarly, the TAV decreased -0.9 mm3 in the placebo group and -5.8 mm3 in the evolocumab group, with an absolute difference of -4.9 mm3 (-7.3 mm3 to -2.5 mm3 with a p value of <0.001). Regression by PAV was observed in 64.3% of the evolocumab group versus 47.3% of the placebo group (p <0.001) and by TAV in 61.5% versus 48.9%, respectively (p <0.001), with no difference or interaction between the pre-specified groups.

In 144 subjects with baseline LDL-cholesterol levels <70 mg/dL, the PAV reduced -1.97% in the evolocumab group versus -0.35% in the placebo group (absolute difference -1.62%: -2.5% to -0.74% with a p value of <0.001), with a regression by PAV of 81.2% versus 48% in the evolocumab group versus placebo, respectively. The results showed a linear association between levels of 90 to 20 mg/dL of LDL-cholesterol and the PAV; the lower the LDL-cholesterol, the greater the atherosclerosis regression.

The safety and tolerability profile of the evolocumab group did not show significant differences compared to that observed in the placebo group, and the incidence of blinded-evaluated cardiovascular events was numerically lower in the evolocumab group (12.2%) than in the placebo group (15.3%).

GLAGOV study demonstrates for the first time that the addition of a Mab-PCSK9, in this case evolocumab, to the optimal treatment with statins with or without ezetimibe is associated with atheroregression, whereas the treatment with statins/ezetimibe only favors stabilization or a non-progression status. The above with an appropriate safety and tolerability profile and a coherent with other evolocumab trials, sign of reduction of cardiovascular events by atherosclerosis.

APPROVED INDICATIONS FOR EVOLOCUMAB

As of the writing of this chapter, evolocumab (Repatha®), has been approved in the United States, the European Union and other counties [45].

Evolocumab (Repatha®) is approved in patients with HeFH and Non-FH as a complement to diet, in combination with statins or other non-statin lipid lowering therapies in subjects who do not achieve LDL-cholesterol target levels with maximum therapeutic statin doses or either alone or in combination with other non-statin lipid lowering therapies when there is intolerance and/or contraindication for statins. The evolocumab recommended doses are 140 mg S.C/2 weeks or 420 mg S.C/4 weeks; the scheme selection (both having the same effectiveness) is made by the patients [45]. Based in the TESLA pilot and TESLA-B trial results [26, 27], evolocumab 420 mg S.C/4 weeks is indicated in individuals ≥12 years of age with HoFH. Based in FOURIER trial results [38] evolocumab would be submitted to the Regulatory Agencies in order to obtain its approval for prevention of recurrent ASCVD events.

RECOMENDATIONS FOR MABS-PCSK9

ESC/EAS 2016 Recommendations

In 2016, an ESC/EAS Task Force Consensus on PCSK9: practical guidance for use in patients at very-high cardiovascular risk was published by Landmesser *et al.* [46]. This paper aims to provide support in appropriately allocating a highly effective LDL-cholesterol lowering therapy considering the high cost of PCSK9 inhibitors and financial restraints within healthcare budgets. Specifically, very-high risk patients for whom PCSK9 inhibitors may be considered are the following:

1.- Individuals with ASCVD or Diabetes Mellitus with target organ damage or other major risk factor on maximally tolerated efficacious statins (atorvastatin or rosuvastatin) plus ezetimibe and LDL-cholesterol >140 mg/dL.
2.- Individuals with rapid progression of ASCVD on maximally tolerated efficacious statins (atorvastatin or rosuvastatin) plus ezetimibe and LDL-cholesterol >100 mg/dL.
3.- Severe HeFH without ASCVD on maximally tolerated efficacious statins (atorvastatin or rosuvastatin) plus ezetimibe and LDL-cholesterol >200 mg/dL.
4.- Severe HeFH without ASCVD with ≥1 other major risk factor or very high risk on maximally tolerated efficacious statins (atorvastatin or rosuvastatin) plus ezetimibe and LDL-cholesterol >175 mg/dL.
5.- HoFH without ASCVD on maximally tolerated lipid lowering therapy with or

without apheresis, except individuals with negative/negative LDLR mutations.
6.- Statin intolerant individuals on ezetimibe and any of the above conditions.

2017 Expert Consensus Decision Pathway Recommendations

The *2017 Focused Update of the 2016 Expert Consensus Decision Pathway on the Role of Non-Statin Therapies for LDL-Cholesterol Lowering in the Management of Atherosclerotic Cardiovascular Disease* [47], follows the philosophy of the United States Institute of Medicine (IOM) *"to update and publish the recommendations when new evidence with high scientific value is available"*. Thus, following the publication of the results for the IMPROVE-IT trial with ezetimibe [48], FOURIER trial with evolocumab [38] and SPIRE-I and -2 trials with bococizumab [49, 50], the American College of Cardiology Experts Group endorsed by the National Lipid Association updated the 2016 document and published an Expert Consensus known as *"Lipid Pathway 2017"*. In resume, the expert's recommendation for using MAbs-PCSK9 are the following:

1. – Patients ≥21 years of age with stable clinical ASCVD (secondary prevention) without comorbidities on maximally tolerated statin dose plus ezetimibe with LDL-cholesterol reduction <50% (may consider LDL-cholesterol level >70 mg/dL or non-HDL-cholesterol level >100 mg/dL).
2. – Patients ≥21 years of age with clinical ASCVD (secondary prevention) with comorbidities (diabetes mellitus, recent ACS -<3 months-, recurrent ASCVD on-statins, primary LDL-cholesterol ≥190 mg/dL, other uncontrolled cardiovascular risk factors, Lp (a) ≥50 mg/dL, chronic kidney disease) on maximally tolerated statin dose plus ezetimibe with LDL-cholesterol reduction <50% (may consider LDL-cholesterol level >70 mg/dL, or non-HDL-cholesterol level >100 mg/dL.
3. – Patients ≥21 years of age with clinical ASCVD (secondary prevention) and primary LDL-cholesterol ≥190 mg/dL without other comorbidities on maximally tolerated statin dose plus ezetimibe (may consider resins) with LDL-cholesterol reduction <50% (may consider LDL-cholesterol level >70 mg/dL or non-HDL-cholesterol level >100 mg/dL).
4. – Patients ≥21 years of age without ASCVD (primary prevention) and primary LDL-cholesterol ≥190 mg/dL without other comorbidities on maximally tolerated statin dose plus ezetimibe (may consider resins) with LDL-cholesterol reduction <50% (may consider LDL-cholesterol level >100 mg/dL or non-HDL-cholesterol level >130 mg/dL). Recommendations for patients in this subgroup with comorbidities are similar than recommendation for patients with ASCVD and LDL-cholesterol level >190 mg/dL.
5. – Mabs-PCSK9 are not recommended for primary prevention in patients with diabetes mellitus or patients with ASCVD risk >7.5% without clinical ASCVD

and/or severe hypercholesterolemia.

The authors of *"Lipid Pathway"* make it clear that before starting a non-statin treatment, especially a MAbs-PCSK9, Doctors should address statin adherence, intensify a healthy lifestyle, increase the statin to a high-intensity or a maximally tolerated dose and evaluate for statin intolerance, control other cardiovascular risk factors, consider referral to a lipid specialist and, very important to inform patients and family on the benefit, the risk, and the alternatives for the proposed treatment. In the same way, the authors make it clear that the *"Lipid Pathways"* are a bridge to the new Guideline that will emerge once currently published/ongoing studies are evaluated, terminated and analyzed.

CONCLUSION

In conclusion, all evidence analyzed in this chapter allow us to conclude that in the PCSK9 inhibition era we can be sure that continued cardiovascular benefit can be accrued even when LDL-cholesterol levels are reduced to 20 to 25 mg/dL, a level that is well below of the current therapeutic targets, in other words, a level that is well close to the biologic LDL-cholesterol level postulated for Myant, Reich, Goldstein and Brown in 1978.

Evolocumab beyond to confirm a consistent and excellent safety and tolerability profile without immunogenicity signals, in phase I trials demonstrates significant and proportional reduction in LDL-cholesterol and other atherogenic lipoproteins with doses of 140 mg S.C/2 weeks and 420 mg S.C/4 weeks with a direct relationship between the reduction of the level of circulating PCSK9 and LDL-cholesterol. In patients with HoFH, evolocumab 420 mg S.C/4 weeks, significantly reduces LDL-cholesterol levels by 31% compared with placebo, with a surprising LDL-cholesterol reduction of 41% in individuals with LDLR defective activity mutations. In the same direction in patients with HeFH evolocumab, provides significant additional LDL-cholesterol reduction in individuals treated with background high intensity statins with or without ezetimibe, achieving LDL-cholesterol levels <70 mg/dL in 6-7 of each 10 individuals treated with evolocumab 140 mg S.C/2 weeks or 420 mg S.C/4 weeks; this response in patients with HeFH, was not related to the underlying genetic mutations. In patients with HC without pharmacologic treatment, evolocumab as monotherapy corroborates that inhibition of PCSK9 with evolocumab versus placebo and ezetimibe, provides significant LDL-cholesterol reduction in individuals with HC drug-naïve; finding potentially relevant for patients with moderate or severe HC with high cardiovascular risk and statin intolerance or contraindication. That assumption was subsequently confirmed and evolocumab demonstrates that among individuals with real statin intolerance, LDL-cholesterol is lowered by 50%, achieving a LDL-C level <70 mg/dL in 27.4% of real statin-intolerant patients with excellent muscle-tolerability and very low rates of discontinuation. In multiple phase III studies in patients with HC and cardiovascular risk, evolocumab versus placebo reduced LDL-cholesterol from 60% to 70%, achieving and LDL-C level <70 mg/dL in >80% of individuals treated with moderate-intensity statins and >90% of individuals treated with high-intensity statins, with similar percent reductions in LDL-cholesterol regardless of statin type, dose or intensity. Finally, evolocumab demonstrates that its addition to the optimal treatment with statins with or without ezetimibe in a median period of 26 months is associated with a significant 20% reduction in the risk of cardiovascular death, myocardial infarction, or stroke, both with an excellent safety and tolerability profile; this result is concordant with the significant atheroregression confirmed by evolocumab 420 mg S.C/4 weeks through intracoronary ultrasound All this evidence, accumulated in 14 years of research - reflected in the indications and recommendations for its use -, allow us to conclude that evolocumab by a highly efficient PCSK9 inhibition has confirmed to reach safely physiologic LDL-cholesterol levels, to reduce the coronary atherosclerotic burden and especially to reduce significantly the incidence of new ASCVD events, without doubt a full therapeutic landscape.

CONFLICT OF INTEREST

The author (editor) declares no conflict of interest, financial or otherwise.

ACKNOWLEDGEMENTS

The author acknowledges the editorial support of Glanser Services.

ABBREVIATIONS

LDLR	LDL Receptor
PCSK9	Proprotein Convertase Subtilisin Kexin type 9
MAbs-PCSK9	Monoclonal antibodies vs PCSK9
LDL	Low Density Lipoprotein
NARC-1	Neural Apoptosis-Regulated Convertase 1
SKI-1/S1P	Subtilisin Kexin Isozyme 1/Site-1 Protease
SREBP	Sterol Regulatory Element-Binding Proteins
BDNF	Brain-Derived Neurotrophic Factor
ApoB100	Apolipoprotein B100 (LDLR ligand)
HMGCoAR	Hydroxy-methyl-glutaryl-coenzyme A Reductase
FH3	Familial Hypercholesterolemia type 3

HeFH	Heterozygous Familial Hypercholesterolemia
Non-FH	No-Familial Hypercholesterolemia
ARIC	Atherosclerosis Risk in Communities Study
ASCVD	Atherosclerotic Cardiovascular Disease
EMA	European Medicines Agency
FDA	U.S. Food and Drug Administration
TEAE	Treatment-Emergent Adverse Events
RCT	Randomized and Controlled Trials
CPK	Creatine phosphokinase
ACS	Acute Coronary Syndrome
ABI	Ankle-Brachial Index

REFERENCES

[1]   Seidah NG, Benjannet S, Wickham L, *et al.* The secretory proprotein convertase neural apoptosis-regulated convertase 1 (NARC-1): liver regeneration and neuronal differentiation. Proc Natl Acad Sci USA 2003; 100(3): 928-33.
[http://dx.doi.org/10.1073/pnas.0335507100] [PMID: 12552133]

[2]   Seidah NG, Prat A. The proprotein convertases are potential targets in the treatment of dyslipidemia. J Mol Med (Berl) 2007; 85(7): 685-96.
[http://dx.doi.org/10.1007/s00109-007-0172-7] [PMID: 17351764]

[3]   Lopez D. PCSK9: An enigmatic protease. Biochimica and Biophysica Acta 2008; 1781: 184-91.

[4]   Seidah NG, Prat A. The biology and therapeutic targeting of the proprotein convertases. Nat Rev Drug Discov 2012; 11(5): 367-83.
[http://dx.doi.org/10.1038/nrd3699] [PMID: 22679642]

[5]   Seidah NG, Sadr MS, Chrétien M, Mbikay M. The multifaceted proprotein convertases: their unique, redundant, complementary, and opposite functions. J Biol Chem 2013; 288(30): 21473-81.
[http://dx.doi.org/10.1074/jbc.R113.481549] [PMID: 23775089]

[6]   Seidah NG, Awan Z, Chétien M, Mbikay M. 2014.http//circres.ahajournals.org

[7]   Mayne J, Raymond A, Chaplin A, *et al.* Plasma PCSK9 levels correlate with cholesterol in men but not in women. Biochem Biophys Res Commun 2007; 361(2): 451-6.
[http://dx.doi.org/10.1016/j.bbrc.2007.07.029] [PMID: 17645871]

[8]   Benjannet S, Rhainds D, Essalmani R, *et al.* NARC-1/PCSK9 and its natural mutants: zymogen cleavage and effects on the low density lipoprotein (LDL) receptor and LDL cholesterol. J Biol Chem 2004; 279(47): 48865-75.
[http://dx.doi.org/10.1074/jbc.M409699200] [PMID: 15358785]

[9]   Brown MS, Goldstein JL. A receptor-mediated pathway for cholesterol homeostasis 1985.

[10]   Zhang DW, Lagace TA, Garuti R, *et al.* Binding of proprotein convertase subtilisin/kexin type 9 to epidermal growth factor-like repeat A of low density lipoprotein receptor decreases receptor recycling and increases degradation. J Biol Chem 2007; 282(25): 18602-12.
[http://dx.doi.org/10.1074/jbc.M702027200] [PMID: 17452316]

[11]   Tavori H, Fan D, Blakemore JL, *et al.* Serum PCSK9 and cell surface LDL-R: Evidence for a reciprocal regulation. Circulation 2013; 127: 2403-13.
[http://dx.doi.org/10.1161/CIRCULATIONAHA.113.001592] [PMID: 23690465]

[12]   Jeong HJ, Lee HS, Kim KS, Kim YK, Yoon D, Park SW. Sterol-dependent regulation of proprotein convertase subtilisin/kexin type 9 expression by sterol-regulatory element binding protein-2. J Lipid Res 2008; 49(2): 399-409.
[http://dx.doi.org/10.1194/jlr.M700443-JLR200] [PMID: 17921436]

[13]   Stein EA, Raal FJ. Insights into PCSK9, LDLR, and LDL-C metabolism: Of mice and man. Circulation 2013; 127: 2372-4.
[http://dx.doi.org/10.1161/CIRCULATIONAHA.113.003360] [PMID: 23690464]

[14]   Morales-Villegas E. PCSK9 and LDLR. The yin-yang in the cellular uptake of cholesterol. Curr Hypertens Rev 2014; 9: 310-23.
[http://dx.doi.org/10.2174/1573402110666140702092415] [PMID: 24993279]

[15]   Nassoury N, Blasiole DA, Tebon Oler A, *et al.* The cellular trafficking of the secretory proprotein convertase PCSK9 and its dependence on the LDLR. Traffic 2007; 8(6): 718-32.
[http://dx.doi.org/10.1111/j.1600-0854.2007.00562.x] [PMID: 17461796]

[16]   Maxwell KN, Breslow JL. Adenoviral-mediated expression of Pcsk9 in mice results in a low-density lipoprotein receptor knockout phenotype. Proc Natl Acad Sci USA 2004; 101(18): 7100-5.
[http://dx.doi.org/10.1073/pnas.0402133101] [PMID: 15118091]

[17]   Al-Mashhadi RH, Sorensen CB, Kragh PM, *et al.* Familial hypercholesterolemia and atherosclerosis in cloned minipigs created by DNA transposition of a human PCSK9 gain-of-function mutant 2013.

[18]   Denis M, Marcinkiewics J, Zaid A, *et al.* Gene inactivation of PCSK9 reduces atherosclerosis in mice. Circulation 2012; 125: 894-901.
[http://dx.doi.org/10.1161/CIRCULATIONAHA.111.057406] [PMID: 22261195]

[19]   Abifadel M, Varret M, Rabès JP, *et al.* Mutations in *PCSK9* cause autosomal dominant hypercholesterolemia. Nat Genet 2003; 34(2): 154-6.
[http://dx.doi.org/10.1038/ng1161] [PMID: 12730697]

[20]   Cohen J, Pertsemlidis A, Kotowski IK, Graham R, Garcia CK, Hobbs HH. Low LDL cholesterol in individuals of African descent resulting from frequent nonsense mutations in PCSK9. Nat Genet 2005; 37(2): 161-5.
[http://dx.doi.org/10.1038/ng1509] [PMID: 15654334]

[21]   Cohen JC, Boerwinkle E, Mosley TH Jr, Hobbs HH. Sequence variations in PCSK9, low LDL, and protection against coronary heart disease. N Engl J Med 2006; 354(12): 1264-72.
[http://dx.doi.org/10.1056/NEJMoa054013] [PMID: 16554528]

[22]   Kotowski IK, Pertsemlidis A. Luke A y cols. A spectrum of PCSK9 alleles contributes to plasma levels of LDL-C. Am Hum Genet 2006; 78: 410-22.
[http://dx.doi.org/10.1086/500615]

[23]   Chan JC, Piper DE, Cao Q, *et al.* A PCSK9 neutralizing antibody reduces serum colesterol in mice and nonhuman primates. Proc Natl Acad Sci USA 2009; 106: 9820-5.
[http://dx.doi.org/10.1073/pnas.0903849106] [PMID: 19443683]

[24]   Foltz IN, Karow M, Wasserman SM. Evolution and emergence of therapeutic monoclonal antibodies: what cardiologists need to know. Circulation 2013; 127(22): 2222-30.
[http://dx.doi.org/10.1161/CIRCULATIONAHA.113.002033] [PMID: 23733968]

[25]   Dias CS, Shaywitz AJ, Wasserman SM, *et al.* Effects of AMG-145 on LDL-C levels. Results from two randomized, double-blind, placebo-controlled, ascending-dose phase 1 study in healthy volunteers and hypercholesterolemic subjects on statins. J Am Coll Cardiol 2012; 60: 1888-98.
[http://dx.doi.org/10.1016/j.jacc.2012.08.986] [PMID: 23083772]

[26]   Stein EA, Honarpour N, Wasserman SM, Xu F, Scott R, Raal FJ. Effect of the proprotein convertase subtilisin/kexin 9 monoclonal antibody, AMG 145, in homozygous familial hypercholesterolemia. Circulation 2013; 128(19): 2113-20.
[http://dx.doi.org/10.1161/CIRCULATIONAHA.113.004678] [PMID: 24014831]

[27]   Rall FJ, Honarpour N, Blom DJ, *et al.* www.thelancet.com

[28]   Raal F, Scott R, Somaratne R, *et al.* Low-density lipoprotein cholesterol-lowering effects of AMG 145, a monoclonal antibody to proprotein convertase subtilisin/kexin type 9 serine protease in patients with heterozygous familial hypercholesterolemia: the Reduction of LDL-C with PCSK9 Inhibition in Heterozygous Familial Hypercholesterolemia Disorder (RUTHERFORD) randomized trial. Circulation 2012; 126(20): 2408-17.
[http://dx.doi.org/10.1161/CIRCULATIONAHA.112.144055] [PMID: 23129602]

[29]   Raal FJ, Stein EA, Dufour R, *et al.* PCSK9 inhibition with evolocumab (AMG 145) in heterozygous familial hypercholesterolaemia (RUTHERFORD-2): a randomised, double-blind, placebo-controlled trial. Lancet 2015; 385(9965): 331-40.
[http://dx.doi.org/10.1016/S0140-6736(14)61399-4] [PMID: 25282519]

[30]   Giugliano RP, Desai NR, Kohli P, *et al.* www.thelancet.com

[31]   Koren MJ, Scott R, Kim JB, *et al.* www.thelancet.com

[32]   Koren MJ, Giugliano RP, Raal FJ, *et al.* Efficacy and safety of longer-term administration of evolocumab (AMG 145) in patients with hypercholesterolemia: 52-week results from the Open-Label Study of Long-Term Evaluation Against LDL-C (OSLER) randomized trial. Circulation 2014; 129(2): 234-43.
[http://dx.doi.org/10.1161/CIRCULATIONAHA.113.007012] [PMID: 24255061]

[33]   Blom DJ, Hala T, Bolognese M, *et al.* A 52-week placebo-controlled trial of evolocumab in hyperlipidemia. N Engl J Med 2014.
[http://dx.doi.org/10.1056/NEJMoa1316222]

[34]   Robinson JG, Nedergaard BS, Rogers WJ, *et al.* Effect of evolocumab or ezetimibe added to moderate- or high-intensity statin therapy on LDL-C lowering in patients with hypercholesterolemia: the LAPLACE-2 randomized clinical trial. JAMA 2014; 311(18): 1870-82.
[http://dx.doi.org/10.1001/jama.2014.4030] [PMID: 24825642]

[35]   Koren MJ, Lundqvist P, Bolognese M, *et al.* Anti-PCSK9 monotherapy for hypercholesterolemia: the MENDEL-2 randomized, controlled phase III clinical trial of evolocumab. J Am Coll Cardiol 2014; 63(23): 2531-40.
[http://dx.doi.org/10.1016/j.jacc.2014.03.018] [PMID: 24691094]

[36]   Sabatine MS, Giugliano RP, Wiviott SD, *et al.* Efficacy and safety of evolocumab in reducing lipids and cardiovascular events. N Engl J Med 2014.
[http://dx.doi.org/10.1056/NEJMoa1500858]

[37]   Koren MJ, Sabatine MS, Giugliano RP, *et al.* Long-term low-density lipoprotein cholesterol-lowering efficacy, persistence, and safety of evolocumab in treatment of hypercholesterolemia. Results up to 4 years from the open-label OSLER-1 extension study. JAMA Cardiol 2017; 2(6): 598-607.
[http://dx.doi.org/10.1001/jamacardio.2017.0747] [PMID: 28291870]

[38]   Sabatine MS, Giugliano RP, Keech AC, *et al.* Evolocumab and clinical outcomes in patients with cardiovascular disease. N Engl J Med 2017; 376(18): 1713-22.
[http://dx.doi.org/10.1056/NEJMoa1615664] [PMID: 28304224]

[39]   Sullivan D, Olsson AG, Scott R, *et al.* Effect of a monoclonal antibody to PCSK9 on low-density lipoprotein cholesterol levels in statin-intolerant patients: the GAUSS randomized trial. JAMA 2012; 308(23): 2497-506.
[http://dx.doi.org/10.1001/jama.2012.25790] [PMID: 23128163]

[40]   Stroes E, Colquhoun D, Sullivan D, *et al.* Anti-PCSK9 antibody effectively lowers cholesterol in patients with statin intolerance: the GAUSS-2 randomized, placebo-controlled phase 3 clinical trial of evolocumab. J Am Coll Cardiol 2014; 63(23): 2541-8.
[http://dx.doi.org/10.1016/j.jacc.2014.03.019] [PMID: 24694531]

[41]   Nissen S. Efficacy and tolerability of evolocumab vs ezetimibe in patients with muscle-related statin

intolerance. The GAUSS-3 randomized, clinical trial. JAMA
[http://dx.doi.org/10.1001/jama.2016.3608]

[42]   Giugliano RP, Mach F, Zavitz K, *et al.* Cognitive function in a randomized trial of evolocumab. N Engl J Med 2017; 377(7): 633-43.
[http://dx.doi.org/10.1056/NEJMoa1701131] [PMID: 28813214]

[43]   Nicholls SJ, Puri R, Anderson T, *et al.* Effect of Evolocumab on progression of coronary disease in statin-treated patients 2016.
[http://dx.doi.org/10.1001/jama.2016.16951]

[44]   Nicholls SJ, Ballantyne CM, Barter PJ, *et al.* Effect of two intensive statin regimens on progression of coronary disease. N Engl J Med 2011; 365(22): 2078-87.
[http://dx.doi.org/10.1056/NEJMoa1110874] [PMID: 22085316]

[45]   Markham A. Evolocumab: First Global Approval. Drugs 2015; 75(13): 1567-73.
[http://dx.doi.org/10.1007/s40265-015-0460-4] [PMID: 26323342]

[46]   Landmesser U, Chapman MJ, Farnier M, *et al.* European Society of Cardiology/European Atherosclerosis Society Task Force consensus statement on proprotein convertase subtilisin/kexin type 9 inhibitors: practical guidance for use in patients at very high cardiovascular risk. Eur Heart J 2016; 0: 1-11.
[http://dx.doi.org/10.1093/eurheartj/ehw480] [PMID: 27789571]

[47]   Lloyd-Jones DM, Morris PB, Ballantyne CM, *et al.* Focused Update of the 2016 ACC Expert Consensus Decision Pathway on the Rose of Non-Statin Therapies for LDL-Cholesterol Lowering in the Management of Atherosclerotic Disease Risk. J Am Coll Cardiol 2017; 2017
[http://dx.doi.org/10.1016/j.jacc.2017.07.745]

[48]   Cannon CP, Blazing MA, Giugliano RP, *et al.* Ezetimibe added to statin therapy after acute coronary syndromes. N Engl J Med 2015; 372: 2387-97.

[49]   Ridker PM, Tardiff JC, Amarenco P, *et al.* Lipid-reduction variability and anti-drug antibody formation with bococizumab. N Engl J Med 2017.
[http://dx.doi.org/10.1016/NEJMoa1614082]

[50]   Ridker PM, Revkin J, Amarenco P, *et al.* Cardiovascular efficacy and safety of bococizumab in high-risk patients. N Engl J Med 2017.
[http://dx.doi.org/10.1056/NEJMoa1701488]

SUBJECT INDEX

A

Accelerated platelet turnover 1, 2, 3, 6, 7
Activity 40, 41, 96, 103, 104
  antiplatelet 40, 41
  phosphatase 96, 103, 104
Acute 5, 7, 65, 67, 68, 77, 78, 83, 84, 87, 94, 102, 113, 114
  coronary syndrome 5, 7, 65, 67, 68, 77, 78
  rejection 83, 84, 87, 94, 102, 113, 114
Adenosine 16, 17, 18, 19, 20, 21, 22, 23, 24, 25, 26, 27, 35, 39, 41, 44, 45, 46, 47, 48, 69, 73
  agonists 26
  deaminase 18, 19
  diphosphate 69, 73
  effects of 20, 24, 47
  extracellular production 18, 19
  extracellular concentrations of 17, 18
  generation 17, 18
  kinase 18, 19
  levels 24
  production 18, 43
  receptor drug targets 35
  receptor family 35
Adenosine receptors 16, 17, 19, 20, 21, 22, 23, 24, 25, 26, 28, 29, 34, 35, 36, 37, 39, 41, 45, 46, 47
  agonists structures 25
  and Signaling Pathways 19
  antagonists 29
  cyclic structures classes 28
  blocks 24
  crystal structure 35
  dimerization 34, 35, 36
  ligands 16, 26
  ligands, selective 25
  nonselective activation of 39
  subtypes 20, 21, 25
Adenosinergic system 16, 17, 26, 39, 45, 46, 47, 48
Adverse events 83, 85, 87, 94, 102, 161, 166, 167, 168, 169, 174
  of therapy 83, 85
  muscle-related 174

Agents 94, 106, 127, 131, 132
  antiproliferative 94, 106, 132
  antiretroviral 127, 131
  lowering 124
Aggregation 66, 69, 73, 74
Agonists 19, 25, 26, 27, 32, 33, 36, 39, 40, 41, 45, 65, 69, 71, 72, 74, 78
  low-affinity 40
  non-adenosine 26
  platelet 69, 71, 74, 78
Alemtuzumab 86
Alirocumab 149
Alleles 156, 157
Allopurinol 97, 122, 133
Allosteric 16, 31, 32, 33, 34
  modulators 16, 31, 32, 33, 34
  site 31
Alopecia 96, 97, 106, 107
Amiloride 33, 34
  analogs 33
Amino acids 36, 37, 38, 149, 150
Amiodarone 96, 97, 129
AMP, dephosphorylation of 17, 25
Anemia 68, 89, 96, 97, 103, 106, 107, 110
Angiotensin receptor blockers 118, 120
Antagonists 25, 26, 29, 30, 31, 32, 33, 35, 36, 42, 43, 45, 46, 47, 86
  dual 42, 45
Antibodies 19, 86, 87, 89, 91, 154, 167, 171, 174
  circulating 91
  new anti-evolocumab binding 171
  polyclonal 86, 87, 89
Antibody induction 87, 88, 90, 91
  -mediated rejection (AMR) 88, 90, 91
  polyclonal 87
Antidepressants 128
Anti-evolocumab antibodies 157, 161, 163, 165, 166, 168, 171, 172, 173, 174
  developed 174
  developed binding 174
  transient binding 161, 163
Anti-thymocyte globulin (ATG) 86, 89, 91, 92, 93, 113
Antihistamines 88, 89

www.ingramcontent.com/pod-product-compliance
Lightning Source LLC
Chambersburg PA
CBHW080020240326
41598CB00075B/466